Paediatrics for the FRCS (Tr and Orth) Examination

T0177644

Paediatrics for the FRCS (Tr and Orth) Examination

Edited by

Yael Gelfer
Consultant Paediatric Orthopaedic Surgeon
St. George's Hospitals, NHS foundation Trust
London, UK

Deborah Eastwood
Consultant Paediatric Orthopaedic Surgeon
Great Ormond Street Hospital
London, UK

Karen Daly
Consultant Paediatric Orthopaedic Surgeon
St George's Hospitals, NHS foundation Trust
London, UK

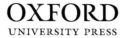
OXFORD
UNIVERSITY PRESS

OXFORD
UNIVERSITY PRESS

Great Clarendon Street, Oxford, OX2 6DP,
United Kingdom

Oxford University Press is a department of the University of Oxford.
It furthers the University's objective of excellence in research, scholarship,
and education by publishing worldwide. Oxford is a registered trade mark of
Oxford University Press in the UK and in certain other countries

© Oxford University Press 2018

The moral rights of the authors have been asserted

First Edition published in 2018

Impression: 1

All rights reserved. No part of this publication may be reproduced, stored in
a retrieval system, or transmitted, in any form or by any means, without the
prior permission in writing of Oxford University Press, or as expressly permitted
by law, by licence or under terms agreed with the appropriate reprographics
rights organization. Enquiries concerning reproduction outside the scope of the
above should be sent to the Rights Department, Oxford University Press, at the
address above

You must not circulate this work in any other form
and you must impose this same condition on any acquirer

Published in the United States of America by Oxford University Press
198 Madison Avenue, New York, NY 10016, United States of America

British Library Cataloguing in Publication Data
Data available

Library of Congress Control Number: 2017941748

ISBN 978–0–19–874930–1

Printed and bound by
CPI Group (UK) Ltd, Croydon, CR0 4YY

Oxford University Press makes no representation, express or implied, that the
drug dosages in this book are correct. Readers must therefore always check
the product information and clinical procedures with the most up-to-date
published product information and data sheets provided by the manufacturers
and the most recent codes of conduct and safety regulations. The authors and
the publishers do not accept responsibility or legal liability for any errors in the
text or for the misuse or misapplication of material in this work. Except where
otherwise stated, drug dosages and recommendations are for the non-pregnant
adult who is not breast-feeding

Links to third party websites are provided by Oxford in good faith and
for information only. Oxford disclaims any responsibility for the materials
contained in any third party website referenced in this work.

CONTENTS

A&E	Accident and Emergency
AAOS	American Academy of Orthopaedic Surgeons
AARD	atlantoaxial rotatory displacement
ACL	anterior cruciate ligament
AER	apical ectodermal ridge
AIS	abbreviated Injury Scale
AIS	adolescent idiopathic scoliosis
A-K	above knee
AP	anteroposterior
ASIS	anterior superior iliac spine
ATLS	advanced trauma life support
AVN	avascular necrosis
BAPRAS	British Association of Plastic, Reconstructive and Aesthetic Surgeons
BMI	body mass index
BMP	Bone Morphogenetic protein
BOAST	British Orthopaedic Association Standard for Traumas
BoS	base of support
CAVE	cavus, adductus varus, and equinus
CoM	centre of mass
CORA	centre of rotation angulation
CP	cerebral palsy
CRP	C-Reactive Protein
CT	computed tomography
CTEV	club foot
CVT	Congenital vertical talus
DDH	developmental dysplasia of the hip
DGH	district general hospital
ENT	ear, nose, and throat
EOS	early onset scoliosis

ESIN	elastic stable Intra medullary nailing
ESR	erythrocyte sedimentation rate
EUA	examination under anaesthesia
FBC	full blood count
FGFR3	fibroblast growth factor receptor 3
FHL	Flexor hallucis longus
GA	general anaesthetic
GABA	gamma-aminobutyric acid
GCS	Glasgow Coma Scale
GMFCS	gross motor function classification system
GRF	ground reaction force
HSMN	hereditary sensorimotor neuropathy
ISS	Injury Severity Score
IV	intravenous
JIA	juvenile inflammatory arthritis
LCNT	lateral cutaneous nerve of the thigh
LEA	lateral epiphyseal artery
LLD	Leg length difference
LSCB	Local Safeguarding Children Board
LT	ligamentum teres
MCA	medial femoral circumflex artery
MCP	metacarpophalangeal
MDT	multidisciplinary team
MISME	multiple inherited schwannomas, menigiomas, and ependymomas
MISS	Modified Injury Severity Score
MR	magnetic resonance
MSK	Musculoskeletal
MTP	Metatarsophalangeal
NAI	non-accidental injury
NF1	neurofibromatosis type 1
OCD	osteochondritis dissecans
OI	osteogenesis imperfecta
OT	occupational therapy
PA	postero anterior
PAO	postero anterior
QoL	quality of life
RF	rectus femoris

RGO	reciprocating gait orthosis
RMI	Reimer's migration index
RVAD	rib-vertebral angle difference
SCFE	Slipped capital femoral epiphysis
SCM	sternocleidomastoid muscle
SDR	Selective Dorsal Rhizotomy
SESA	Subtalar extra-articular screw arthroereisis
SHH	Sonic Hedgehog
SHOX	Short Stature Homeobox
SIJt	sacroiliac joint
SUFE	slipped upper femoral epiphysis
TAR	thrombocytopaenia-absent radius
TFL	tensor fasciae latae
TIS	thoracic insufficiency syndrome
U&E	urea and electrolytes
VACTERL	vertebral, anal atresia, cardiac, trachea, esophageal, renal, and limb defects
VDRO	varus derotational osteotomy
WCC	white cell count
WHO	World Health Organization

CONTRIBUTORS

Anna Allan Specialty Trainee, London Deanery, London, UK

Anthony Catterall Emeritus Consultant Paediatric Orthopaedic Surgeon, London, UK

John Dabis Trauma and Orthopaedic registrar, St George's Hospitals, London, UK

Karen Daly Consultant Paediatric Orthopaedic Surgeon, St George's Hospitals, NHS Foundation Trust, London, UK

Deborah Eastwood Consultant Paediatric Orthopaedic Surgeon, Great Ormond Street Hospital, London, UK

Yael Gelfer Consultant Paediatric Orthopaedic Surgeon, St George's Hospitals, NHS Foundation Trust, London, UK

Yaser Jabbar Consultant Paediatric Orthopaedic Surgeon, Great Ormond St Hospital, London, UK

Leonora Mills Consultant Paediatric Orthopaedic Surgeon, Royal Aberdeen Children's Hospital, Aberdeen, UK

Kuldeep Stohr Consultant Paediatric Orthopaedic Surgeon, Addenbrooke's Hospital, Cambridge, UK

Roger Walton Consultant Paediatric Orthopaedic Surgeon, Alder Hey Children's Hospital, Liverpool, UK

Andrea Yeo Consultant Paediatric Orthopaedic Surgeon, St George's Hospitals, NHS Foundation Trust, London, UK

INTRODUCTION

This book aims to cover the Paediatric Orthopaedic curriculum for FRCS (Orth) including children's trauma. Please remember that the syllabus is constantly changing so we advise you to check the intercollegiate exam website as well as the JSCT website on a regular basis.

The book consists of SBAs, EMQs and although there is no particular sequence to them, there are about two SBAs and one EMQ per topic. The answers will often complement each other. The Vivas are arranged according to topics. The reference lists are suggested further reading for each topic; some references such as Tachdjian's Paediatric Orthopaedic Textbook are quoted frequently but some are more specific when we felt it was necessary for you to be familiar with a recent advance/a good review/or an important randomized controlled trial.

The SBAs have only one correct answer: so read the question carefully! There is no negative marking in the exam so it is always worth answering all the questions. The EMQs offer several statements with a list of possible answers; each answer can be used as many times as appropriate or not at all.

The Viva section aims to cover most paediatric orthopaedic topics. It is important to remember that the paediatric Viva table covers six topics and the examiners are all paediatric orthopaedic consultants. They will be well informed and experienced in the topics chosen so will find it easy to identify lack of experience and confidence in their field. Please remember that you are not expected to know how to perform a specific pelvic osteotomy, for example, but you are expected to be safe and sound in the assessment of a child particularly one who presents following trauma. You are also expected to be capable and confident in evaluating the limping child, abnormalities of gait and of function and identifying scenarios that require urgent attention either by 'yourself' as a T&O Consultant in a DGH or that may require discussion with or onward referral to a paediatric centre. If you have not worked in a paediatric 'centre of excellence' you should still be able to pass this section of the exam by ensuring you make the most of the paediatric trauma and general outpatient clinics that exist in most DGHs and supplement this with your reading, attendance at your training programme sessions and tutorials.

Each Viva starts with a prompt like a radiograph, a picture or a question and progresses from there through the marking scheme from four (fail) to eight (excellent) mark. The Viva section will not teach you all you need to know about the topic but will give you a good idea of how to answer important questions on that topic and where to continue reading if you feel you need to know more. There are obviously many styles in which you may answer the question and our answers are simply one way of doing so. Be guided by the verbal and non-verbal cues from your examiner: whilst you may wish to list 101 causes of a particular problem they may lose interest after the first few! Please remember that common things are common but that you must not miss the rare, serious situations either.

Good luck!

Yael Gelfer
Karen Daly
Deborah Eastwood
2017

1. **With respect to the pathology of a congenital vertical talus (CVT) foot deformity, which of the following statements is incorrect?**

   Select the single most appropriate answer.

   A. The forefoot is abducted
   B. The heel is in valgus
   C. The hindfoot lies in equinus
   D. The peroneal tendons are not a deforming force
   E. The talonavicular joint is subluxed/dislocated

2. **Which of the following statements regarding CVT is correct?**

   Select the single most appropriate answer.

   A. 50% of cases are associated with neuromuscular conditions or an identified syndrome
   B. Bilateral cases are unusual
   C. Girls are more commonly affected than boys
   D. Many feet only have a postural deformity
   E. The Ponseti technique is the treatment of choice

3. **What is a normal mechanical Medial Proximal Tibial Angle?**

   Select the single most appropriate answer.

   A. 81°
   B. 95°
   C. 87°
   D. 79°
   E. 93°

4. **What is the most appropriate initial management of Cozen's phenomenon?**

   Select the single most appropriate answer.

   A. Distraction osteogenesis with circular frame
   B. Observation
   C. Hemi-epiphysiodesis
   D. Epiphysiodesis with monitoring for LLD
   E. Acute corrective osteotomy and internal fixation

5. **Which of the following statements regarding genu varum secondary to Vitamin D deficiency rickets is true?**

    Select the single most appropriate answer.

    A. It can improve spontaneously by the age of 24 months
    B. It only affects the tibial physes
    C. The deformity will always improve after Vitamin D treatment
    D. The tibio-femoral angle will be at least 10°
    E. There will be an accompanying lateral thrust

6. **Which of the following statements regarding infantile Blount's disease is incorrect?**

    Select the single most appropriate answer.

    A. The tibial metaphyseal-diaphyseal angle (Drennan angle) will be greater than 16°
    B. Langenskiöld stages I and II may regress over time or with treatment
    C. The articular surface is usually normal
    D. Bracing is useful in children over 4 years old
    E. A lateral thrust is a common sign

7. **Which of the following statements regarding Osteogenesis Imperfecta (OI) is incorrect?**

    Select the single most appropriate answer.

    A. A quantitative or qualitative abnormality in type 1 collagen
    B. The disease is associated with low vitamin D levels that cause fragile teeth
    C. Can be lethal with the patient stillborn
    D. Short stature can result from growth deficiency and/or secondary bone deformity
    E. Fractures heal at a normal rate

8. **Which of the following statements about Osteogenesis Imperfecta (OI) is correct?**

    Select the single most appropriate answer.

    A. The frequency of fractures declines after adolescence
    B. Spinal deformity is rare in OI
    C. Blue sclera is the most typical manifestation of OI and is always present
    D. Radiographic findings are only present after walking age
    E. Fractures in OI heal without callus, only intramembranous ossification is present

9. **An 8-year-old girl falls off a horse whilst galloping and sustains a proximal femoral fracture. A radiograph demonstrates a displaced transcervical (type II) proximal femoral fracture. Which of the following is the best treatment option?**

Select the single most appropriate answer.

A. Spica cast with the affected leg in abduction

B. Capsulotomy, reduction and internal fixation as an emergency

C. Closed reduction and internal fixation with percutaneous screw fixation

D. Open reduction and internal fixation with dynamic hip screw

E. Open reduction and internal fixation on the next available trauma list

10. **Which is the most common complication following management of a displaced femoral neck fracture in a child?**

Select the single most appropriate answer.

A. Infection

B. Physeal arrest

C. Avascular necrosis

D. Chondrolysis

E. Coxa valga

11. **Which of the following is a clinical manifestation of Vitamin D deficiency rickets?**

Select the single most appropriate answer.

A. Osteoporosis

B. Growth on 95th centile

C. Growth on 5th centile

D. Epiphyseal cupping on X-ray

E. Metaphyseal beaking at proximal tibia

12. **Which single answer best describes hypophosphataemic rickets?**

Select the single most appropriate answer.

A. All cases are X-linked recessive

B. Patients have high serum phosphate levels

C. The urinary phosphate levels are low

D. Vitamin D treatment does not lead to clinical improvement

E. Renal calculi are not associated with this condition

13. **Which of the following statements relating to pelvic osteotomy for acetabular dysplasia is incorrect?**

Select the single most appropriate answer.

A. The bikini skin incision and anterior tensor fascia lata-sartorius interval does not provide adequate exposure for pelvic osteotomies and can only be used for open reduction

B. The Salter osteotomy redirects the acetabulum and is used in patients younger than 9-years-old

C. The Pemberton and Dega osteotomies restructure the acetabulum and decrease acetabular volume

D. The Ganz osteotomy (Periacetabular osteotomy or PAO) achieves maximal redirection of the acetabulum in patients with a fused tri-radiate cartilage

E. The triple pelvic osteotomy achieves maximal redirection of the acetabulum in patients with an open tri-radiate cartilage

14. **Which of the following statements is true about Salter osteotomies?**

Select the single most appropriate answer.

A. It is performed when open reduction of the hip cannot be achieved

B. It is indicated when acetabular anterolateral deficiency is present either after primary treatment of DDH or in an untreated child

C. It aims to change the acetabular index by 25°

D. The lower age limit for this osteotomy is 18 months: below this age, there is a higher rate of re-dislocation

E. There is no risk of subsequent posterior dislocation

15. **In fractures of the proximal third of the forearm, the proximal radius is:**

Select the single most appropriate answer.

A. Pronated and flexed

B. Supinated and flexed

C. Pronated and extended

D. Supinated and extended

E. In neutral alignment

16. **A 5-year-old boy sustains greenstick fractures of both forearm bones with minimal angulation and rotation. You decide to place him in a full above elbow plaster cast. Which of the following increase the risk of thermal injury?**

Select the single most appropriate answer.

A. Water temperature >24°C when the plaster is 'dipped'

B. Folding over the edges of casts that are too long

C. Placing the arm on a pillow during the curing process of the cast

D. Overwrapping the plaster cast with fibreglass

E. All of the above

17. Regarding leg lengths which of the following statements is true?

Select the single most appropriate answer.

A. Beckwith Wiedemann syndrome is associated with shortening of the affected side

B. An apparent leg length discrepancy (LLD) is that which is perceived by the patient

C. Growth arrest secondary to physeal injury causes a static LLD

D. Skeletal age is assessed by a postero-anterior radiograph of the non-dominant wrist and hand

E. A 15 mm LLD alters gait parameters significantly

18. An 11-year-old, pre-menarchal girl sustains an isolated subtrochanteric femoral fracture. You decide to treat it with a plate, with screws into the femoral neck. Assuming her leg lengths are currently equal, crossing the growth plate with your screws will most likely lead to the following amount of shortening at maturity?

Select the single most appropriate answer.

A. 30 mm

B. 36 mm

C. 6 mm

D. 12 mm

E. 27 mm

19. A 12-year-old child presents with a Gustilo-Anderson II open tibial fracture. According to the BOAST 4 guidelines what is the ideal next step in management of this child?

Select the single most appropriate answer.

A. Immediate debridement and closure on the emergency theatre list

B. Delayed debridement and soft tissue cover the next morning

C. Paediatric orthopaedic and plastic surgical input on the next appropriate paediatric trauma list within 50 hours

D. Combined orthopaedic and plastic surgical care on the next available specialist list within 24 hours

E. Immediate skeletal stabilization and vac pump application until next available paediatric trauma list within 36 hours

20. Guidelines for the management of open fractures in children are published by?

Select the single most appropriate answer.

A. British Trauma Society

B. British Society of Children's Orthopaedic Surgeons

C. British Orthopaedic Association Standards for Trauma (Guideline 4)

D. British Orthopaedic Association Standards for Trauma (Guideline 1)

E. British Association of Plastic, Reconstructive and Aesthetic Surgeons

21. In a triplane ankle fracture, what fracture pattern is seen on the AP radiograph?

Select the single most appropriate answer.

A. Salter-Harris I
B. Salter-Harris II
C. Salter-Harris III
D. Salter-Harris IV
E. Salter-Harris V

22. Which of the following ankle fracture patterns has the lowest rate of growth arrest?

Select the single most appropriate answer.

A. Tillaux fracture
B. 2-part triplane fracture
C. 3-part triplane fracture
D. Extra-articular triplane fracture
E. Salter-Harris II fracture

23. Achondroplasia is caused by a mutation in which gene?

Select the single most appropriate answer.

A. FGFR3 (fibroblast growth factor receptor)
B. COL1A (collagen)
C. FGF1B (fibroblast growth factor)
D. TNF-α (tumour necrosis factor)
E. FBN1 (fibrillin)

24. Which of the following is not a feature of achondroplasia?

Select the single most appropriate answer.

A. Autosomal dominant inheritance
B. Rhizomelic dwarfism
C. Kyphoscoliosis
D. Spinal canal stenosis
E. Genu valgum

25. **A 14-year-old boy is tackled during a rugby match and sustains a twisting injury to the knee, it immediately swells up and he is unable to play on. In A&E he is treated as an MCL injury and managed in a knee brace. 2 weeks later he presents to fracture clinic with ongoing symptoms and is found to have a positive anterior drawer test. Which of the following is true?**

Select the single most appropriate answer.

A. ACL injuries can be differentiated from tibial eminence injuries by clinical examination
B. An open physis is a contraindication to surgical reconstruction
C. Paediatric ACL injuries are more common in girls than boys
D. Physiological and skeletal age do not play a role in management decision making
E. ACL injuries in this age group are self-limiting

26. **The following statements relate to the management of ACL ruptures in children. Which one is incorrect?**

Select the single most appropriate answer.

A. A transphyseal reconstruction is an accepted surgical technique
B. An 'all epiphyseal' reconstruction is an accepted surgical technique
C. A physeal sparing reconstruction is an accepted surgical technique
D. An extra-articular reconstruction is an accepted surgical technique
E. Management is always operative

27. **Which of the following statements relating to cerebral palsy is true?**

Select the single most appropriate answer.

A. It is a condition caused by a non-progressive permanent injury to the immature brain which gives rise to non-progressive peripheral manifestations
B. Spasticity refers to a velocity dependent increase in tone
C. The prevalence of children living with cerebral palsy is decreasing
D. The GMFCS (Gross Motor Function Classification Scale) is based on anatomical distribution
E. A child who does not sit by 2 years of age is unlikely to walk

28. **Regarding the management of spasticity:**

Select the single most appropriate answer.

A. Selective dorsal rhizotomy is useful in some ambulant patients who exhibit weakness
B. Botulinum toxin causes presynaptic blockade of acetylcholine release at the neuromuscular junction
C. Intrathecal baclofen risks more sedation and cognitive impairment than oral baclofen
D. Surgery for children with crouch gait should include an Achilles tendon lengthening
E. Surgical interventions should be undertaken on a staged basis: one level at a time

29. What is the definitive way to diagnose CTEV?

Select the single most appropriate answer.

A. Clinical examination

B. X-ray

C. US

D. MRI

E. Genetic analysis

30. What is the position of the clubfoot before correction?

Select the single most appropriate answer.

A. forefoot supination, heel valgus, midfoot cavus and ankle equinus

B. forefoot pronation, heel varus, midfoot planus and ankle dorsiflextion

C. forefoot adduction, hindfoot varus, midfoot cavus and ankle equinus

D. forefoot abduction, hindfoot valgus, midfoot cavus and ankle equinus

E. forefoot abduction, hindfoot varus, midfoot cavus and ankle calcaneus

31. Which type of congenital spinal anomaly is associated with the highest curve progression and poorest prognosis?

Select the single most appropriate answer.

A. Hemivertebra

B. Wedge vertebra

C. Block vertebra

D. Unilateral unsegmented bar

E. Unilateral unsegmented bar with a convex-sided hemivertebra

32. Which one of the following is not a recognized cause of congenital scoliosis?

Select the single most appropriate answer.

A. Maternal diabetes mellitus

B. Maternal exposure to alcohol

C. Maternal family history

D. Maternal hyperthermia

E. Maternal exposure to valproic acid

33. Which of the following statements about the aetiology of Developmental Dysplasia of the Hip (DDH) is true?

Select the single most appropriate answer.

A. Afrocaribbean and Asian populations have a low incidence of DDH

B. Post natal positioning has no affect on DDH as the condition is present at birth

C. The most common aetiological factor for DDH is primary acetabular dysplasia

D. High collagen type I content in the newborn increases connective tissue tightness

E. Antenatal positioning has an association with DDH only in cases with oligohydramnios

34. Which of the following statements is true regarding management of a child with DDH?

Select the single most appropriate answer.

A. In the child younger than 12 months of age with a dislocated hip traction should not be attempted due to the risk of causing AVN

B. If the hip remains unstable and Ortolani positive 1 week following application of a Pavlik Harness, the harness should be discontinued and closed reduction considered

C. In closed reduction of the hip, an adductor tenotomy facilitates maximal abduction which ensures joint stability

D. A medial dye pool wider than 6 mm on the arthrogram during a closed reduction implies the hip is neither reduced nor stable

E. The position in SPICA following the Arthrogram is not significant as long as reduction of the hip was achieved

35. A 6-year-old boy falls off his bicycle onto his dominant right arm. His wrist looks swollen and is very painful. His X-rays show an isolated distal radius metaphyseal fracture that is not translated but dorsally angulated 15°. Which is the most appropriate treatment?

Select the single most appropriate answer.

A. Closed reduction of the fracture and place in a cast, review in 7–10 days

B. Open reduction and fixation with semi-tubular plate, review in 10–14 days

C. Closed reduction and fixation with K-wire(s), review in 5 days

D. Below elbow cast only with radiographic review in 5 days

E. Closed reduction and fixation with flexible nail, review in 7–10 days

36. **A 14-year-old boy sustains a Galeazzi fracture to his wrist (Fig. 1.1). Which is the best manoeuvre to reduce this fracture closed?**

Select the single most appropriate answer.

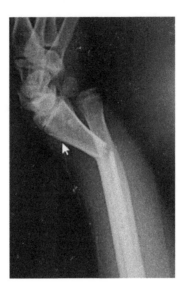

Fig. 1.1 X-ray

A. Forearm supination with volar to dorsal force on the distal radius
B. Forearm pronation with volar to dorsal force on the distal radius
C. Forearm pronation with dorsal to volar force on the distal radius
D. Forearm supination with dorsal to volar force on the distal radius
E. None of the above, this fracture pattern always requires open, direct reduction

37. **Which of the scoring systems listed can be used to suggest features compatible with a diagnosis of Ehlers-Danlos syndrome in a child?**

Select the single most appropriate answer.

A. Brighton score
B. DASH score
C. Beighton score
D. Marfan score
E. Carter and Wilkinson score

38. Which of the following is not a feature of Benign Joint Hypermobility Syndrome?

Select the single most appropriate answer.

A. Joint pain in small and large joints > 3 months

B. Blue sclerae

C. Entheseopathies

D. Aortic arch dilatation

E. Carpal tunnel syndrome

39. In a 3-year-old child with a radio-ulnar synostosis which of the following statements is incorrect?

Select the single most appropriate answer.

A. The site of the synostosis is usually distal

B. Pronation-supination movement is absent

C. Elbow flexion-extension may be restricted

D. Bilateral involvement is rare

E. There is often an associated dislocation of the radial head

40. The preferred management of a 6-year-old child with a radioulnar synostosis and a non-dominant hand position in 10° of supination is:

Select the single most appropriate answer.

A. Physiotherapy to improve range of pronation

B. Excision of the associated dislocated radial head

C. Corrective osteotomies of both the radius and ulna

D. Excision of the synostosis and insertion of interpositional graft

E. No treatment

41. A 10-year-old child is hit by a motor vehicle at 30 mph. He sustains a transverse mid-shaft femoral fracture. What is the recommended treatment?

Select the single most appropriate answer.

A. External fixation

B. Bridge plating

C. Flexible (elastic stable) intramedullary nailing (FIN or ESIN)

D. Rigid antegrade trochanteric intramedullary nailing

E. Spica cast

42. What is the recommended treatment for a 12-year-old boy with a comminuted femoral shaft fracture?

Select the single most appropriate answer.

A. External fixation
B. Bridge plating
C. Flexible intramedullary nailing
D. Rigid antegrade trochanteric intramedullary nailing
E. Spica cast

43. A 3-year-old child was playing on a set of monkey bars in the presence of her family. She fell from a height of about 4 feet. She sustained an isolated femoral shaft fracture. There is 15° of varus angulation, 15° of posterior angulation and 15 mm of shortening. What is the optimal treatment option for this injury?

Select the single most appropriate answer.

A. External fixation
B. Bridge plating with a locking plate
C. Elastic stable intramedullary nails
D. Gallows traction
E. Spica cast

44. When treating femoral shaft fractures in children younger than 6 months of age, both a Pavlik harness and a spica cast are effective treatment options. Which complication is more common with the spica cast?

Select the single most appropriate answer.

A. Loss of reduction
B. Shortening during treatment
C. Femoral neuropraxia
D. Superficial reactive dermatitis
E. Skin breakdown

45. Femoral shaft fractures in children aged 3 months or less are best treated with which treatment modality?

Select the single most appropriate answer.

A. Elastic Stable Intramedullary Nailing (ESIN)
B. External fixation
C. Spica cast
D. Pavlik Harness
E. Straight leg traction

46. A lytic, expansile lesion in the proximal humerus of a 5-year-old child with a ground-glass appearance is most likely to represent:

Select the single most appropriate answer.

A. Fibrous dysplasia

B. Fibrous cortical defect

C. Simple bone cyst

D. Aneurysmal bone cyst

E. Ollier's disease

47. Which one of the following might you see in a patient with tibial and mandibular fibrous dysplasia?

Select the single most appropriate answer.

A. Vestibular acoustic nerve neuroma

B. Precocious puberty

C. Smooth-edged café-au-lait spots

D. Pigmented villonodular synovitis

E. Dysplastic spondylolysis

48. In the flexible flat foot the heel swings in which direction on single stance heel raise?

Select the single most appropriate answer.

A. Equinus and Valgus

B. Equinus and Varus

C. Calcaneus and Valgus

D. Calcaneus and Varus

E. Planus

49. Arthroereisis commonly involves which joint?

Select the single most appropriate answer.

A. Chopart joint

B. Talo-navicular

C. Calcaneo-cuboid

D. Sub-talar joint

E. Tibio-talar joint

50. Which one of these statements best describes the pathology in a child with Madelung's deformity?

Select the single most appropriate answer.

A. There is an autosomal recessive inheritance pattern
B. The condition is usually unilateral
C. The Vickers ligament tethers the radial aspect of the distal ulna growth plate causing deformity
D. There is dorsal subluxation of the carpus on the distal forearm
E. Deformity is due to abnormal growth of the ulnar and volar aspects of the distal radial physis

51. An infant is referred to your clinic with a radial club hand. Which of the following statements is incorrect?

Select the single most appropriate answer.

A. In the Holt Oram syndrome, there is associated renal agenesis
B. It represents a longitudinal deficiency of the forearm.
C. In TAR (Thrombocytopaenia-absent radius) syndrome, there is a platelet deficiency and a good quality thumb.
D. The condition affects both limbs in >50% cases
E. The genetic defect is associated with the Homeobox gene

52. Which of the following is not a pre-requisite for a normal gait?

Select the single most appropriate answer.

A. Stability in stance phase
B. Centre of mass that remains within the base of support
C. Foot clearance in swing phase
D. Foot pre-positioning in terminal swing
E. Adequate step length

53. Which of the following statements about the ankle rockers is incorrect?

A. The 1st rocker is controlled by the eccentrically acting gastrocnemius
B. Progressive ankle dorsiflexion in the 2nd rocker allows the centre of gravity to progress over the foot
C. Concentric gastrocnemius contraction provides pushoff in the 3rd rocker.
D. In patients with heel pain the first rocker is absent
E. In patients with a painful forefoot, the 3rd rocker is lost.

54. Which of the following statements is correct?

Select the single most appropriate answer.

A. Fibroblast growth factor 2 is implicated in achondroplasia
B. Bone morphogenetic proteins are types of transforming growth factor
C. Bone morphogenetic proteins are osteoconductive
D. Each molecule of cartilage oligomeric matrix protein binds 4 type II collagen molecules
E. Type X collagen is mainly found in the proliferative zone of the growth plate

55. The following statement is true of a typically developing child:

Select the single most appropriate answer.

A. 90% of children will walk independently, before 12 months of age
B. Children should develop hand preference before the age of 18 months
C. All primitive reflexes have usually disappeared by the age of 12 months
D. Most children will sit unsupported by 4 months of age
E. A child who bottom-shuffles will walk early.

56. In an 11-year-old girl with a prominent hallux valgus which of the following statements is true?

A. There is unlikely to be a family history of 'bunions'
B. A basal osteotomy of the first metatarsal is a popular surgical option
C. The intermetatarsal angle is within normal limits
D. Surgery is best delayed until late adolescence
E. Surgical treatment is associated with a low risk of recurrence

57. In a 12-year-old girl with symptomatic hallux valgus, surgical treatment options do not include:

Select the single most appropriate answer.

A. Concomitant osteotomy of the proximal phalanx
B. A soft tissue release of the MTP joint
C. Osteotomy of the medial cuneiform
D. A Scarf 1st metatarsal osteotomy
E. A basal 1st metatarasal osteotomy

58. When treating patients with idiopathic scoliosis, all of the following are indications for a whole spine MRI except:

Select the single most appropriate answer.

A. Right thoracic curves
B. Hyperkyphosis
C. Patients younger than 10 years
D. Abnormal neurological findings
E. Severe pain

59. Factors predictive for curve progression in idiopathic scoliosis include all the following apart from:

Select the single most appropriate answer.

A. Risser stage 0–1
B. Pre-menarchal status
C. Female gender
D. Curve severity
E. Café-au-lait spots

60. What is the definition of Scheuermann's kyphosis as per the Sorenson criteria?

Select the single most appropriate answer.

A. Thoracic kyphosis caused by 4 or more consecutive vertebrae with more than 10° of anterior wedging each
B. Thoracic kyphosis caused by 3 or more consecutive vertebrae with more than 5° of anterior wedging each
C. Thoracolumbar kyphosis caused by 3 or more consecutive vertebra with more than 10° of anterior wedging each
D. Lumbar kyphosis caused by 4 consecutive vertebra with more than 5° of anterior wedging each
E. Thoracic kyphosis caused by 2 consecutive vertebra with more than 5° of anterior wedging each

61. Which of the following statements are not true regarding Scheuermann's kyphosis?

Select the single most appropriate answer.

A. Due to a developmental error in collagen aggregation resulting in disturbance of endochondral ossification of the vertebral end plates
B. Pulmonary compromise is not a concern unless curvature exceeds 100°
C. More common in the thoracic spine than in the lumbar spine
D. Curves greater than 75°, are more likely to cause thoracic pain
E. Autosomal recessive inheritance

62. In addition to the AP and lateral X-rays of the elbow, which other view is the most useful in assessing the degree of fracture displacement in paediatric lateral condyle fractures?

Select the single most appropriate answer.

A. Valgus stress view
B. Varus stress view
C. External oblique view
D. Internal oblique view
E. Lateral in full flexion

63. Which complication is most commonly associated with non-union of a lateral condyle elbow fracture?

Select the single most appropriate answer.

A. Lateral spur formation
B. Ulnar nerve palsy
C. Cubitus varus
D. Fishtail deformity
E. Radial nerve palsy

64. Which of the following is an absolute indication for operative treatment for medial epicondyle fracture?

Select the single most appropriate answer.

A. Incarcerated medial epicondyle in the elbow joint
B. Ulnar nerve injury
C. Valgus instability of the elbow
D. Fracture displacement >5 mm
E. All of the above

65. What is the order of appearance of the secondary ossification centres of the elbow?

Select the single most appropriate answer.

A. Capitellum—medial epicondyle—olecranon—radial head—trochlea—lateral epicondyle
B. Medial epicondyle—capitellum—radial head—lateral epicondyle—trochlea—olecranon
C. Olecranon—radial head—medial epicondyle—trochlea—capitellum—lateral epicondyle
D. Lateral epicondyle—olecranon—trochlea—radial head—medial epicondyle—capitellum
E. Capitellum—radial head—medial epicondyle—trochlea—olecranon—lateral epicondyle

66. Which nerve is most at risk of injury in Monteggia fractures?

Select the single most appropriate answer.

A. Median nerve
B. Anterior interosseous nerve
C. Posterior interosseous nerve
D. Ulnar nerve
E. Radial nerve

67. Which Monteggia fracture-dislocation pattern is most common?

Select the single most appropriate answer.

A. Bado type I
B. Bado type II
C. Bado type III
D. Bado type IV
E. Bado type III B

68. In the multiple-injured child which site carries the highest risk for mortality and morbidity?

Select the single most appropriate answer.

A. Pelvis
B. Femur
C. Spine
D. Abdomen
E. Head

69. Which of the following is a priority in Paediatric Trauma?

Select the single most appropriate answer.

A. GCS
B. Temperature
C. Long bone fracture
D. Fluid resuscitation
E. Airway

70. The following is true of normal development:

Select the single most appropriate answer.

A. Genu varum is physiological in a 3-year-old girl
B. 50% of the growth of the foot is complete by the age of 7 years old
C. A heel-toe gait pattern is usually present at the age of 2 years old
D. The femoral neck is retroverted at birth and becomes progressively more anteverted with growth
E. The medial arch of the foot usually develops by the age of 7 years old

71. Concerning types of ossification:

Select the single most appropriate answer.

A. Endochondral ossification is affected in cleidocranial dysostosis
B. Intramembranous ossification is affected primarily in achondroplasia
C. Intramembranous ossification results in appositional bone growth
D. Endochondral ossification occurs from the periosteum of long bones
E. Intramembranous ossification involves the replacement of a cartilage precursor with bone

72. Which of the following conditions is not associated with myelomeningocele?

Select the single most appropriate answer.

A. Rigid clubfoot
B. Hip dysplasia
C. Scoliosis and Kyphosis
D. Trisomy 21
E. Learning difficulties

73. Which of the following is not a risk factor for developing myelomeningocele?

Select the single most appropriate answer.

A. Maternal hyperthermia
B. Pre-gestational maternal diabetes
C. In utero exposure to valproic acid
D. History of a previously affected pregnancy
E. B12 deficiency

74. Which of the following injuries has the highest specificity for non-accidental injury (NAI)?

Select the single most appropriate answer.

A. Femoral fracture
B. Rib fracture
C. Humeral fracture
D. Skull fracture
E. Vertebral fracture

75. Which of the following is a risk factor for non-accidental injury?

Select the single most appropriate answer.

A. Twins
B. Child with disability
C. Single parent
D. All of the above
E. None of the above

76. Hyperpigmented spots with rounded edges are most frequently associated with:

Select the single most appropriate answer.

A. McCune Albright syndrome
B. Fibrous dysplasia
C. Charcot-Marie-Tooth syndrome
D. Neurofibromatosis Type 1
E. Neurofibromatosis Type 2

77. Which of the following is not one of the criteria for the diagnosis of neurofibromatosis Type 1?

Select the single most appropriate answer.

A. Axillary freckling
B. More than 6 café-au-lait spots
C. Dystrophic kyphoscoliosis
D. Optic glioma
E. First degree relative with NF1

78. Regarding osteochondritis dissecans (OCD) in children:

Select the single most appropriate answer.

A. OCD usually occurs secondary to a traumatic event
B. It is more common in girls than boys
C. Anatomically it is commonly found in the medial aspect of the lateral femoral condyle
D. OCD is generally associated with meniscal pathology
E. None of the above

79. A 14-year-old boy presents to clinic with a several week history of knee pain, swelling and feeling of giving way when he is playing football. He denies any specific traumatic event or injury to the knee. Radiographs are suggestive of an osteochondral defect in keeping with osteochondritis dissecans. Which of the following is true?

Select the single most appropriate answer.

A. This occurs only in the knee
B. Notch views are unhelpful
C. The same system is used to grade both MRI and arthroscopic findings
D. Retrieval of loose bodies is the main surgical indication
E. Lesions are broadly defined in terms of their stability

80. Which of the following statements about Ollier's disease is correct?

Select the single most appropriate answer.

A. It is also called hereditary multiple exostoses
B. The inheritance pattern is X-linked recessive
C. There are abnormal intra-osseous deposits of fibrous tissue
D. There are abnormal intra-osseous deposits of cartilaginous tissue
E. Malignant change is very rare

81. Which of the following statements is incorrect in relation to Ollier's disease?

Select the single most appropriate answer.

A. Maffuci's syndrome is Ollier's disease and soft tissue haemangiomas
B. Bisphosphonates may be useful in improving bone pain
C. McCune-Albright syndrome is Ollier's disease with precocious puberty
D. Chondrosarcoma complicates upto 20–25% of cases
E. Bone healing post osteotomy/fracture is not delayed

82. **A 7-year-old is referred with a short history of left knee pain, no history of trauma, raised inflammatory markers and a negative ultrasound scan of the left hip and left knee. MRI subsequently confirms osteomyelitis of the proximal tibia. Which of the following is true?**

Select the single most appropriate answer.

A. Only a short course of antibiotics (approximately 7 days) is required
B. The first line treatment is surgical
C. Kingella Kingae is the most likely pathogen
D. Osteomyelitis can result in physeal growth arrest
E. In uncomplicated cases typical management is 6–8 weeks of IV antibiotics

83. **In the diagnosis and management of osteomyelitis which of the following is true?**

Select the single most appropriate answer.

A. Radiographic changes are usually seen within the first week of symptoms
B. Radiographic changes are distinguishable from those of sarcoma
C. Osteomyelitis typically occurs in the diaphyseal region
D. The most common causative organism is Staph aureus
E. Subperiosteal collections can only be detected on MRI

84. **In a Salter Harris type I, the fracture line runs through which zone of the physis?**

Select the single most appropriate answer.

A. Resting
B. Hypertrophic
C. Primary Spongiosa
D. Proliferative
E. Groove of Ranvier

85. **Which of these is an example of a Salter Harris type III fracture?**

Select the single most appropriate answer.

A. Monteggia fracture
B. Triplane fracture
C. Lateral condyle fracture
D. Slip of the capital femoral epiphysis
E. Tillaux fracture

86. Which is the most common proximal humeral fracture pattern in neonates?

Select the single most appropriate answer.

A. Salter-Harris type I
B. Salter-Harris type II
C. Salter-Harris type III
D. Salter-Harris type IV
E. Salter-Harris type V

87. In fractures of the proximal humerus, what position does the proximal fragment (epiphysis) lie in?

Select the single most appropriate answer.

A. Adducted and externally rotated
B. Adducted and internally rotated
C. Abducted and internally rotated
D. Abducted and externally rotated
E. Neutral position

88. An 11-year-old girl presents with a 2-week history of right thigh pain and a limp. She is generally well and radiographs confirm a unilateral SCFE with a lateral epiphyseal shaft (Southwick) angle of 30° on the right and 10° on the left. Which of the following is true?

Select the single most appropriate answer.

A. SCFE generally present at a younger age in boys than girls
B. SCFE occur through the proliferation zone of the physis
C. Patients with a SCFE are described as having obligatory internal rotation in flexing up of the hip
D. SCFE can be associated with renal osteodystrophy
E. Small/ mild slips are more easily seen on AP than lateral radiographs

89. A 14-year-old boy with autistic spectrum disorder presents to A&E with a 24 hour history of severe groin pain. He had presented to his GP 4 months earlier with thigh pain which was treated with reassurance alone. Radiographs confirm a severe SCFE with signs of a chronic process present. Which of the following is true?

Select the single most appropriate answer.

A. Loder's Classification is based on the chronicity of the slip
B. Patients with unstable slips should all have prophylactic pinning of the contralateral hip
C. Acute slips should undergo closed reduction prior to percutaneous cannulated screw fixation
D. Chondrolysis is secondary to avascular necrosis
E. Stable slips have a lower rate of osteonecrosis

90. A 16-year-old boy presents with a 12 month history of groin pain. He weighs 100 kg, plays rugby and has been treated so far for recurrent groin strains. His physiotherapist referred him in as he gives a 2-day history of further thigh pain but he is still able to weightbear and straight leg raise. Radiographs confirm a SCFE with some remodelling. Which of the following statements is true?

Select the single most appropriate answer.

A. The SCFE is unstable and has an increased risk of avascular necrosis

B. Impingement from CAM deformities are only associated with acute slips

C. The entry point for pinning in situ should be below the level of the lesser trochanter

D. Intertrochanteric osteotomies have a lower risk of AVN than osteotomies closer to the deformity

E. The preceding 12 months of symptoms gives him a higher risk of developing AVN after pinning in situ

91. A 12-year-old boy is referred to your clinic with unilateral out-toeing on the right. On further questioning the family describe a vague history of thigh pain for the past 9 months since a heavy rugby tackle. On examination there is a minor leg length discrepancy and the right hip flexes up in to obligatory external rotation. Radiographs confirm a SCFE. Which of the following statements is correct?

Select the single most appropriate answer.

A. The direction of the neck relative to the head is posterior and superior

B. The SCFE is stable and therefore no operative intervention is required

C. A stable SCFE is not associated with secondary osteoarthritis

D. The entry point for pinning in situ should be slightly anterior and not below the level of the lesser trochanter

E. The guide wire for the cannulated screw fixation should be centred up the femoral neck on both the AP and lateral radiographs

92. Which of the statements is true regarding septic arthritis?

Select the single most appropriate answer.

A. The Kocher criteria include a raised CRP, temperature and white cell count

B. The Kocher criteria include a temperature greater than 38.5°

C. Septic arthritis of the shoulder is more common than the knee

D. Septic arthritis commonly occurs around the age of physeal closure

E. Children with sickle cell disease commonly grow salmonella species

93. A 2-year-old child is brought to A&E by his parents with a 2-day history of a sore lower thigh and knee and an inability to walk, he is otherwise systemically well but there is a history of a recent ear infection. The child gets upset whenever you try to examine his leg. The WCC is 17, CRP 27 and he is apyrexial. An ultrasound scan of the knee has been requested. Which of the following is true?

Select the single most appropriate answer.

A. A normal ultrasound (no effusion) of the knee rules out septic arthritis

B. An effusion on ultrasound would confirm the diagnosis of septic arthritis

C. Antibiotics should be commenced

D. The possibility of osteomyelitis cannot be excluded

E. 4 weeks of IV antibiotics is indicated

94. Regarding shoulder dislocation in the adolescent, which of the following statements is true?

Select the single most appropriate answer.

A. Gender is a risk factor

B. Recurrent dislocation within the first 2 years is rare

C. Voluntary dislocation is more frequent than traumatic

D. Posterior instability is more common than anterior instability

E. Surgical stabilization is recommended after the first dislocation

95. Regarding shoulder instability in pre-teenage children, which of the following statements is true?

Select the single most appropriate answer.

A. Multidirectional instability is more common than in adolescence

B. Immobilization for 2 weeks is recommended following each episode

C. An open physis increases the risk of recurrence

D. An open physis is a contraindication to surgical stabilization

E. Physiotherapy is usually unnecessary

96. Which of the following statements relating to congenital/dysplastic spondylolisthesis (compared to other types of spondylolisthesis) is incorrect?

Select the single most appropriate answer.

A. More likely to have significant neurological symptoms

B. The posterior neural arch will be intact

C. Bilateral pars defects are present

D. Anatomical abnormalities are present at the lumbosacral articulation

E. The pars interarticularis is poorly developed, elongated or lysed

97. Which of the following are not considered to be risk factors for isthmic spondylolisthesis?

Select the single most appropriate answer.

A. Repetitive flexion/extension activities

B. Female gender

C. Inuit race

D. A known relative with the defect

E. Participation in competitive sports

98. Which is the most common fracture that occurs in conjunction with a supracondylar elbow fracture?

Select the single most appropriate answer.

A. Ipsilateral proximal humerus fracture

B. Contralateral supracondylar elbow fracture

C. Contralateral elbow dislocation

D. Ipsilateral forearm fracture

E. Ipsilateral distal radius fracture

99. Which of the following concurrent injuries increases the risk of compartment syndrome in a supracondylar elbow fracture?

Select the single most appropriate answer.

A. Distal radius fracture

B. Forearm fracture

C. Radial head fracture

D. Proximal humeral fracture

E. Humeral shaft fracture

100. With respect to tarsal coalitions, which of the following statements is true?

Select the single most appropriate answer.

A. The 45° oblique radiograph identifies the talocalcaneal coalition

B. This congenital abnormality is due to failure of mesenchymal segmentation

C. The child usually presents in early childhood with a flat foot

D. Calcaneonavicular coalitions demonstrate a 'C' sign on the lateral radiograph

E. Fibrous coalitions are treated by surgical excision

101. Which of the following is not a clinical symptom/sign of a tarsal coalition?

Select the single most appropriate answer.

A. A history of recurrent ankle sprains

B. A painful flat foot with swelling in the sinus tarsi

C. A painful flat foot with swelling medially

D. A rigid, painfree flatfoot

E. Dynamic contracture of peroneus longus/brevis

102. An 8-year-old girl presented to A&E after sustaining a grade 2 tibial eminence fracture of her left knee whilst playing touch rugby, which of the following statements is true?

Select the single most appropriate answer.

A. It is a fracture that is most commonly sustained with the knee in an extended position
B. It is associated with a traction apophysitis
C. Occurs predominantly in children over the age of 8 years
D. The fracture fragment is best reduced by flexing the knee
E. Should be managed conservatively unless associated with a locked knee

103. Which of the following statements is true regarding fractures of the tibial eminence?

Select the single most appropriate answer.

A. They are defined by the Ogden classification
B. They are associated with a 10% risk of meniscal injury
C. They occur around the time of physeal closure
D. The fracture involves the proximal tibial physis
E. They are defined by the Meyers–McKeever classification

104. With regards to tip-toe walking, which of the following statements is incorrect?

Select the single most appropriate answer.

A. It can be associated with cerebral palsy
B. Idiopathic toe walking is a diagnosis of exclusion
C. Children with autism frequently toe walk
D. Surgery is often advisable as soon as the diagnosis is established
E. Idiopathic cases are always bilateral

105. Which of the following statements is incorrect concerning children who tip toe walk?

Select the single most appropriate answer.

A. Autosomal dominant inheritance has been suggested for idiopathic toe walking
B. The Silfverskiold test may be positive
C. Children who continue to toe walk into adolescence will have poor functional outcomes
D. Pathology in the triceps surae muscle-tendon complex can be encountered
E. Persistent toe walking secondary to a heel contracture can potentiate forefoot splay and a wide forefoot

106. Which of the following is not associated with a torticollis in infancy?

Select the single most appropriate answer.

A. Developmental dysplasia of the hip
B. Metatarsus adductus
C. Basilar invagination
D. Traumatic delivery
E. Congenital atlanto-axial abnormalities

107. The following broad categories are recognized causes of atlantoaxial rotatory displacement or instability (AARD or AARI) in children, except:

Select the single most appropriate answer.

A. Trauma
B. Inflammation
C. Autoimmune
D. Congenital abnormalities
E. Degenerative

108. Considering a child with a fixed flexion deformity of the IPjt (interphalangeal joint) of the thumb (trigger thumb), which of the following statements is correct?

Select the single most appropriate answer.

A. Males are most commonly affected
B. Frequently associated with triggering of other digits
C. Invariably resolves by the age of 4 yrs
D. Surgical release of the A1 pulley after 12 m of age is the treatment of choice
E. An inflammatory aetiology must be excluded

SINGLE BEST ANSWERS

1. D

Congenital Vertical Talus (CVT) deformity is similar but different to that in a club foot Congenital Talipes Equino Varus (CTEV). In both conditions the heel is in equinus but in CVT the heel is in valgus and hence the talar head is plantarmedial (rather than dorsolateral) and there is dorsal subluxation/dislocation of the talonavicular joint. The forefoot is abducted (rather than adducted in CTEV). In CVT, tibialis anterior is short/tight as are the peroneal tendons and the toe extensors: all contribute to the deformity.

A true vertical talus is not a flexible or postural deformity: by definition, the talonavicular dislocation/subluxation does not reduce with plantarflexion of the forefoot.

The 'reverse-Ponseti' method is the first line treatment of choice.

Miller M, Dobbs MB. Congenital Vertical Talus: Etiology and Management. *Journal of the American Academy of Orthopaedic Surgeons*, 201; Oct; 23(10): 604–11.

Brand RA, Siegler S, Pirani S, Morrison WB, Udupa JK. Cartilage anlagen adapt in response to static deformation. *Medical Hypothese*, 2006; 66(3): 653–9.

2. A

The child with a CVT has a three-dimensional foot deformity with an incidence of 1–2 per 10,000 live births. There is no gender difference, 50% of cases are bilateral and the same number are isolated deformities. The deformity is similar but different to that in a club foot (CTEV). In both conditions the heel is in equinus but in CVT the heel is in valgus and hence the talar head is plantarmedial (rather than dorsolateral) and there is dorsal subluxation/dislocation of the talonavicular joint. The forefoot is abducted (rather than adducted in CTEV). In CVT, tibialis anterior is short/tight as are the peroneal tendons and the toe extensors: all contribute to the deformity.

A true vertical talus is not a flexible or postural deformity: by definition, the talonavicular dislocation/subluxation does not reduce with plantarflexion of the forefoot.

The 'reverse-Ponseti' method is the first line treatment of choice but the results are not as good as with the use of the true Ponseti method in an idiopathic CTEV. The first few stages of the reverse-Ponseti method are similar but opposite to those in the club foot: a limited open approach to the talonavicular joint is often used to reduce this joint which is then stabilized with a K-wire before the Achilles tenotomy is performed. In this way, all components of the deformity can be treated.

Miller M, Dobbs MB. 'Congenital Vertical Talus: Etiology and Management'. *Journal of the American Academy of Orthopaedic Surgeons*, 2015 Oct; 23(10): 604–11.

Brand RA, Siegler S, Pirani S, Morrison WB, Udupa JK. 'Cartilage anlagen adapt in response to static deformatio'. *Medical Hypotheses*, 2006; 66(3): 653–9.

Pirani S, Zeznik L, Hodges D. 'Magnetic resonance imaging study of the congenital clubfoot treated with the Ponseti method', *Journal of Pediatric Orthopaedics*, 2001 Nov-Dec; 21(6): 719–26.

3. C

Genu valgum is classically defined as an inter-malleolar distance greater than 8–10 cm up to the age of 7. Genu valgum can be physiologically normal, and if patients are followed through their lower limb development along the Salenius curve, they reach a maximum genu valgum of approximately 20° at around the age of three and a half. This then settles into physiological genu valgum of approximately 12° by age 7.

On focused radiological examination of the tibia, a normal (mechanical and anatomical) medial proximal tibial angle is quoted as 87°, with a range from 85–90°. The normal mechanical lateral distal femoral angle is quoted as 88°, with a range from 85–90° and the anatomical lateral distal femoral angle is 81°, with a range from 79–83°.

Paley D, Herzenberg J. *Principles of Deformity Correction.* Springer. 2005.

Miller MD. *Review of Orthopaedics* (5th Ed). 2008. Elsevier, P. 646t.

4. B

In Cozen's phenomenon, a post-traumatic valgus deformity develops following a low-energy proximal tibial metaphyseal fracture: it is an acquired form of genu valgum. It is most common in children 3–6 years of age. Most cases resolve spontaneously and observation and reassurance is all that is required. If the deformity fails to resolve within 18–24 months guided growth should be considered.

Cozen L. 'Knock-knee deformity in children. Congenital and acquired'. *Clinical Orthopaedics and Related Research,* 1990, Sep; 258: 191–203.

5. D

Associated features of rickets in childhood are short stature, chest wall deformities including a rachitic rosary and a pigeon chest. The ribs may become deformed and a Harrison's sulcus can be seen. The head may be enlarged. The long bones may be bowed in both the coronal and sagittal plane leading to genu varum or genu valgum with anterior bowing. The deformities are usually reversible following treatment but this depends on their severity. All bones are affected, not just the tibia.

Herring JA, *Tachdijian's Pediatric Orthopaedics* 5th edition. 2013. Elsevier.

6. D

There are 2 subtypes of Blount's disease—infantile (1–3 years) and late (> 4 years). Historically late Blount's was further subdivided into juvenile (4–10 years) and adolescent (> 10 years).

Infantile Blount's may be a physiological phenomenon and more likely to be bilateral while late is more likely to be unilateral. Milder forms of infantile Blount's may respond to conservative management, which includes bracing in some cases. Late or more severe Blount's will usually require surgical intervention: guided growth, a high tibial osteotomy to correct deformity and held with internal or external fixation and plans to deal with the risk of recurrent deformity and asymmetrical leg lengths.

The early stages / milder forms of Blount's may resolve during early childhood. The tibial metaphyseal-diaphyseal angle of Drennan helps distinguish between physiological deformity (angle <11°) and pathological deformity (>16°). There is a 'grey' area between 11 and 16.

Sabharwal S. 'Blount disease'. *The Journal of Bone & Joint Surgery,* American edition, Jul 2009; 91(7): 1758–76.

7. B

Osteogenesis Imperfecta is a genetic disorder producing either a quantitative or qualitative abnormality in type I collagen. It is characterized by bone fragility resulting in fractures that vary with the type and severity of the condition. The fractures heal at a normal rate and short stature can result from growth deficiency and/or secondary bone deformity. Skeletal deformity of long bones and spine are common along with ligamentous laxity and a tendency to bruise easily. The vast majority of affected individuals have a genetic defect that is either autosomal dominant, recessive or a spontaneous mutation.

Harrington J, Sochett E, Howard A. 'Update on the evaluation and treatment of osteogenesis imperfecta'. *Pediatric Clinics of North America*, 2014 Dec; 61(6): 1243–57.

Herring JA. *Tachdijian's Pediatric Orthopaedics*, Elsevier, 5th edition. 2013.

8. A

Osteogenesis Imperfecta is a genetic disorder producing either a quantitative or qualitative abnormality in type I collagen. It is characterized by bone fragility resulting in fractures that vary with the type and severity of the condition. The vast majority of the affected individuals have a genetic defect that is either autosomal dominant, recessive or a spontaneous mutation. Over 280 locations and disruptions in genetic coding for type I collagen have now been identified. These complement our understanding of the classic phenotypical classification systems from 40 years ago: these systems are still used although we now know their limitations.

Blue sclerae are present in 2 types of the classic classification and with some spontaneous mutations.

Harrington J, Sochett E, Howard A. 'Update on the evaluation and treatment of osteogenesis imperfecta'. *Pediatric Clinics of North America*, 2014 Dec; 61(6): 1243–57.

Herring JA. *Tachdijian's Pediatric Orthopaedics*, 5th edition. 2013. Elsevier.

9. B

Proximal femoral fractures in children are very rare and account for 0.1% of all paediatric fractures. They are challenging injuries to manage, as there is a high complication rate. AVN followed closely by coxa vara malunion are the most common problems following this injury. The described fracture is a paediatric orthopaedic emergency and should be managed with capsulotomy, reduction, and internal fixation without delay.

Song KS. 'Displaced fracture of the femoral neck in children: open versus closed reduction'. *The Bone & Joint Journal*, 2010 Aug; 92(8): 1148–51.

SM Chung, SC Batterman, CT Brighton. 'Shear strength of the human femoral capital epiphyseal plate'. *The Journal of Bone & Joint Surgery*, American edition, 1976 Jan; 58(1): 94–103.

Rockwood and Wilkins, *Fractures in Children* (7th ed) Edited by James H. Beaty and James R. Kasser. p. 1057. Philadelphia: Lippincott, Williams & Wilkins, 2010.

10. C

Proximal femoral fractures in children have a high complication rate. AVN followed closely by coxa vara malunion are the most common complications following this injury. High-energy trauma, such as a road traffic accident, causes these fractures. There are often associated pelvic, head, facial, and intra abdominal visceral injuries. The Delbet classification is used for its simplicity and reproducibility. This classification aids the management of these fractures.

Song KS. 'Displaced fracture of the femoral neck in children: open versus closed reduction'. *The Bone & Joint Journal.* 2010 Aug; 92(8): 1148–51.

SM Chung, SC Batterman, CT Brighton. 'Shear strength of the human femoral capital epiphyseal plate'. *The Journal of Bone & Joint Surgery,* American edition, 1976 Jan; 58(1): 94–103.

Rockwood and Wilkins, *Fractures in Children* (7th ed) Edited by James H. Beaty and James R. Kasser. p. 1057. Philadelphia: Lippincott, Williams & Wilkins, 2010.

11. C

The incidence of rickets and vitamin D deficiency in the UK seems to be increasing. Certain ethnic groups in Northern Europe are particularly susceptible, namely dark-skinned groups and those not exposed to sunlight. Breast milk has virtually zero levels of vitamin D in these groups. Vitamin D supplementation in babies and toddlers of Asian and Afro-Caribbean descent is now recommended. Serum calcium levels can be normal in rickets due to secondary hyperparathyroidism. The clinical manifestation of vitamin D deficiency rickets is growth on the 5th centile.

Ford L, et al. (2006). 'Vitamin D concentrations in an UK inner-city multicultural outpatient population', *Annals of Clinical Biochemistry,* 43(6): 468–73.

Vitamins and minerals—Vitamin D. National Health Service. November 26, 2012.

12. D

Hypophosphataemic rickets is also known as X-linked rickets or as vitamin D-resistant rickets. The underlying mechanism is impaired renal tubular reabsorption of phosphate resulting in high urinary concentrations of phosphate and low serum concentrations. The genetic mutation is in the PHEX gene (phosphate regulating gene on the X chromosome). Treatment is phosphate replacement together with high 1,25-dihydroxy-vitamin D doses.

Ford L, et al. 'Vitamin D concentrations in an UK inner-city multicultural outpatient population', *Annals of Clinical Biochemistry,* 2006; 43(6): 468–73.

Vitamins and minerals—Vitamin D. National Health Service. November 26, 2012.

13. A

The traditional Smith Peterson approach resulted in excessive and unsightly scarring and has largely been abandoned for routine procedures. An anterior bikini incision and dissection through the tensor fascia lata-sartorius interval is the approach of choice and it provides good exposure for all pelvic osteotomies in the child.

Different pelvic osteotomies are used in different age groups. Some are aimed at redirecting an appropriately sized but dysplastic acetabulum (Salter, PAO or periacetabular osteotomy, Triple), or reducing the volume and version of a large dysplastic acetabulum (Dega or Pemberton) and some are considered 'salvage' osteotomies (Chiari, shelf acetabuloplasties) and simply provide non articular cartilage cover of the uncovered head.

The Pemberton and Dega volume-reducing osteotomies restructure the acetabulum: there are various (conflicting) descriptions of these; the examiner will be content if you say you choose the type of correction you want based on your assessment of where the deficiency is. The Pemberton is used for anterolateral deficiency (in DDH) and repositions the acetabulum to improve the lateral cover of the femoral head. The Dega osteotomy for posterior deficiency (typically in cerebral palsy).

The triple pelvic osteotomy corrects orientation whilst preserving growth potential from the tri-radiate cartilage.

The Ganz (PAO), being closest to the acetabulum, provides the greatest correction in all planes, with the greatest risks and cannot be done until the tri-radiate cartilage is closed (age 12–14 years).

Herring JA, *Tachdijian's Pediatric Orthopaedics*, 5th edition. 2013. Elsevier.

Pemberton A. 'Pericapsular osteotomy of the ilium for treatment of congenital subluxation and dislocation of the hip'. *The Journal of Bone & Joint Surgery,* American edition, 1965; 87: 65.

Salter RB. Innominate osteotomy in the treatment of congenital dislocation of the hip. *The Journal of Bone & Joint Surgery,* American edition 1966; 48: 1413.

14. B

The Salter innominate osteotomy addresses anterolateral deficiency of the acetabulum and corrects it by redirecting the acetabulum through a single pelvic cut. It hinges/rotates on the symphysis pubis. The acetabular index reduces by up to 10°. The lower age limit for Salter osteotomy is due to the pelvic wings not being thick enough to support the bone graft. There is a risk of posterior dislocation particularly if the procedure is combined with a proximal femoral varus derotation osteotomy (VDRO).

Herring JA, *Tachdijian's Pediatric Orthopaedics*, 5th edition. 2013. Elsevier.

Salter RB. 'Innominate osteotomy in the treatment of congenital dislocation of the hip'. *The Journal of Bone & Joint Surgery,* American edition, 1966: 48: 1413.

15. B

The proximal radial fragment is supinated and flexed by the unopposed action of biceps brachii and the supinator. The distal fragment is pronated by the action of pronator teres and pronator quadratus. An appropriate reduction manoeuvre is therefore to reverse the forces acting on the distal fragment.

DeMaio M et al. 'Plaster: our orthopaedic heritage: AAOS exhibit selection'. *The Journal of Bone & Joint Surgery,* American edition, 2012; 94(20): e152.

16. E

All the scenarios mentioned can contribute to thermal injury and should be avoided.

Halanski MA et al. 'Thermal injury with contemporary cast application technqiues and methods to circumvent morbidity'. *The Journal of Bone & Joint Surgery,* American edition, 2007; 89(11): 2369–77.

17. D

Up to 20% of the normal population have a LLD of at least 5 mm and up to 10% have 1 cm or more. Discrepancies up to 2 cm, in their own right, do not negatively influence gait parameters or hip forces but they may do if they occur in combination with fixed contractures, weakness and/or deformities. Leg length discrepancies may be true (an absolute difference, as measured clinically from the ASIS to the medial malleolus), apparent (due to positioning, such as a hip adduction contracture; measured from the xiphisternum to the medial malleolus), or functional (that which is perceived by the patient and can be corrected with blocks). The discrepancy may be static or progressive. Patient age is also a factor, as is whether or not the discrepancy develops over time or is "acute". A physeal injury is likely to cause a progressive discrepancy, while a diaphyseal fracture that heals with shortening due to fragment overlap, for example, is more likely to cause a static problem.

Whilst many congenital anomalies can lead to shortening of the affected limb, the causes of hemihypertrophy are worth remembering and include 'idiopathic' hemihypertrophy and Beckwith-Wiedemann syndrome. In other overgrowth syndromes, such as Klippel-Trenaunay syndrome (and other vascular malformations) and Proteus syndrome; the incidence of LLD is variable and surprisingly the affected leg can be the short one.

Kaufman KR, Miller LS, Sutherland DH. 'Gait asymmetry in patients with limb-length inequality'. *Journal of Pediatric Orthopaedics*, 1996; 16: 144.

Gurney B, Mermier C, Robergs R, Gibson A, Rivero D. 'Effects of limb-length discrepancy on gait economy and lower-extremity muscle activity in older adults'. *The Journal of Bone & Joint Surgery*, American edition, 2001 Jun; 83-A(6): 907–15.

Song KM, Halliday SE, Little DG. 'The effect of limb-length discrepancy on gait'. *The Journal of Bone & Joint Surgery*, American edition, 1997 Nov; 79(11): 1690–8.

18. D

The proximal femoral growth plate contributes a relatively small amount to leg length (15% of leg length and 30% of femoral length). Assume that girls reach skeletal maturity at age 14 and that the proximal femur contributes 3-4 mm annually. It should be unnecessary to cross the physis in this type of injury.

Menelaus MB. 'Correction of leg length discrepancy by epiphyseal arrest'. *The Bone & Joint Journal*, 1966; 48-B: 336–9.

Westh RN, Menelaus MB. 'A simple calculation for the timing of epiphyseal arrest: a further report'. *The Bone & Joint Journal*, 1981; 63-B: 117–9.

19. D

Open fractures in children are managed according to the same principles as open fractures in adults. In the UK, the BOAST 4 guidelines from the British Orthopaedic Association and the British Association of Plastic, Reconstructive & Aesthetic Surgeons are the gold standard.

British Orthopaedic Association and British Association of Plastic, Reconstructive and aesthetic surgeons standard for trauma, 2009 https://www.boa.ac.uk/wp-content/uploads/2014/12/BOAST-4.pdf

Gustilo RB, Anderson JT. 'Prevention of infection in the treatment of one thousand and twenty-five open fractures of long bones: retrospective and prospective analyses'. *Journal of Bone & Joint Surgery*, American edition, 1976 Jun; 58(4) :453–8.

Pace JL, Kocher MS, Skaggs DL. 'Evidence-based review: management of open pediatric fractures'. *Journal of Pediatric Orthopaedics*, 2012 Sep; 32 Suppl 2: S123–7.

20. C

Standards for the management of open fractures are set by British Orthopaedic Association Standards for Trauma Guideline 4. There is no separate guideline for children.

British Orthopaedic Association and British Association of Plastic, Reconstructive and aesthetic surgeons standard for trauma, 2009, https://www.boa.ac.uk/wp-content/uploads/2014/12/BOAST-4.pdf

21. C

In triplane fractures the AP view will show a Salter-Harris III fracture and the lateral view shows a Salter–Harris II or IV depending on the number of parts (3 vs 2 respectively).

Ertl JP, Barrack RL, Alexander AH, VanBuecken K. 'Triplane fracture of the distal tibial epiphysis. Long-term follow-up'. *Journal of Bone & Joint Surgery*, American edition,. 1988; 70(7): 967–76.

Wuerz TH, Gurd DP. 'Pediatric physeal ankle fracture'. *Journal of the American Academy of Orthopaedic Surgeons*, 2013; 21: 234–44 [Review].

22. A

Tillaux fractures have the lowest rate of growth arrest as they occur in an older age group than the triplane or Salter–Harris fracture types. Tillaux fractures occur as the distal tibial physis is closing. The risk of premature growth arrest following triplane fracture ranges from 0–21%.

Horn BD et al. 'Radiologic evaluation of juvenile Tillaux fractures of the distal tibia'. *Journal of Pediatric Orthopaedics*, 2001; 21(2): 162–4.

23. A

Achondroplasia is an autosomal dominant condition caused by a gain-in-function mutation in the FGFR3 gene. The FGFR3 protein regulates the formation of bone from cartilage.

Wright MJ et al. 'Clinical management of achondroplasia'. *Archives of Disease in Childhood*, 2012; 97: 129–34.

24. E

In Achondroplasia the limbs demonstrate rhizomelic shortening: proximal limb segments more affected than the distal segments. The pedicles of the vertebrae are shortened and thickened resulting in nerve root compression and spinal stenosis. Kyphosis and lumbar lordosis are common but scoliosis occurs predominantly in the adult patient. Achondroplasia is associated with genu varum.

Wright MJ et al. 'Clinical management of achondroplasia'. *Archives of Disease in Childhood*, 2012; 97: 129–34.

25. C

The incidence of paediatric ACL ruptures is increasing; and in girls more than boys. Treatment can be conservative, particularly in those who are young, not keen on sport and not particularly symptomatic. There is a potential risk of physeal damage but only a few cases of growth arrest have been reported. Reconstruction is certainly not contraindicated in an open physis and the gold standard treatment would be anatomical reconstruction analogous to that in an adult.

Renstrom P, Ljungqvist A, Arendt E, Beynnon B, Fukubayashi T, Garrett W, et al. 'Non-contact ACL injuries in female athletes: an International Olympic Committee current concepts statement'. *British Journal of Sports Medicine*, 2008; 42(6): 394–412.

Al-Hadithy N, Dodds AL, Akhtar KS, Gupte CM. 'Current concepts of the management of anterior cruciate ligament injuries in children.' *The Bone & Joint Journal*, 2013; 95-B(11): 1562–9.

Dodwell ER, Lamont LE, Green DW, Pan TJ, Marx RG, Lyman S. '20 years of pediatric anterior cruciate ligament reconstruction in New York State'. *American Journal of Sports Medicine*, 2014; 42(3): 675–80.

26. E

Treatment for ACL rupture can be conservative, particularly in those who are young, not keen on sport and not particularly symptomatic. The gold standard repair would be anatomical reconstruction analogous to that of an adult however, there is a potential risk of physeal damage and partial or total growth arrest. This is only a potential risk and very few cases of growth arrest have been reported.

Renstrom P, Ljungqvist A, Arendt E, Beynnon B, Fukubayashi T, Garrett W, et al. 'Non-contact ACL injuries in female athletes: an International Olympic Committee current concepts statement'. *British Journal of Sports Medicine*, 2008; 42(6): 394–412.

Al-Hadithy N, Dodds AL, Akhtar KS, Gupte CM. 'Current concepts of the management of anterior cruciate ligament injuries in children'. *The Bone & Joint Journal*, 2013; 95-B(11): 1562–9.

Dodwell ER, Lamont LE, Green DW, Pan TJ, Marx RG, Lyman S. '20 years of pediatric anterior cruciate ligament reconstruction in New York State'. *The American Journal of Sports Medicine*, 2014; 42(3): 675–80.

27. B

Cerebral palsy is the term used for a group of non-progressive disorders of movement and posture related to abnormal development or perinatal damage to the motor control centres of the brain. The peripheral MSK manifestations of this condition usually do progress with time and growth. The more severe the insult to the developing motor centres, the more likely it is that other central centres will be affected leading to a range of other neurological abnormalities e.g. epilepsy, visual problems, and learning difficulties.

The prevalence of children living with CP is actually increasing. This may be attributable to advances in neonatal care for very low birth-weight infants. CP can be classified according to type of muscle tone, anatomic distribution of the effects and functional abilities (GMFCS). Children with CP who manage to walk usually do so by the age of 7. Those who have not walked by the age of 7 are unlikely to walk. Other negative predictors include:

- Primitive reflexes still present beyond 1 year of age
- No head control by 20 months
- Not sitting by 2 years

Herring JA. *Tachdijian's Pediatric Orthopaedics*, 5th edition. 2013. Elsevier.

PL Rosenbaum, RJ Palisano, DJ Bartlett, BE Galuppi, DJ Russell. 'Development of the Gross Motor Function Classification System for cerebral palsy'. *Developmental Medicine & Child Neurology*, 2008 Apr; 50(4): 249–53.

V Bhushan, N Paneth, JL Kiely. 'Impact of improved survival of very low birth weight infants on recent secular trends in the prevalence of cerebral palsy'. *Pediatrics*, 1993; 91: 1094.

EE Bleck. 'Locomotor prognosis in cerebral palsy'. *Developmental Medicine & Child Neurology*, 1975; 17: 18.

AC da Paz Junior, SM Burnett, LW Braga. 'Walking prognosis in cerebral palsy: a 22-year retrospective analysis'. *Developmental Medicine & Child Neurology*, 199; 36: 130.

Sewell MD, Eastwood DM, Wimalasundera N. 'Managing common symptoms of cerebral palsy in children'. *BMJ*, 2014; 349: 5474.

28. B

There are several management options for spasticity, including physiotherapy and orthotics, medical and surgical treatment. Baclofen is a GABA agonist of unknown mechanism which has traditionally been administered orally, although this can be associated with sedation and cognitive impairment. The placement of an intrathecal catheter with a reservoir (lying within the abdominal cavity) allows a lower dose to be administered with less side effects. Other risks, such as infection are higher and the reservoir needs to be re-filled periodically.

Botulinum toxin injections work by causing a presynaptic blockade of acetylcholine release at the neuromuscular junction. The medical effect lasts 3–4 months (until new nerve terminals sprout and become active) but the benefits may last 6–12 months or more. A classic use would be to try and improve the flexed knee and tip toe posture by injecting the 'strong' hamstrings and gastrocnemius muscles to reduce spasticity whilst working on strengthening the antagonists, such as the quadriceps muscle.

Lower limb orthopaedic surgery is concerned with improving gait efficiency. A detailed surgical plan is made, often with information gained from a 3D gait analysis and will often involve procedures to several levels of the lower limbs at the same time: SEMLS – single event multilevel surgery.

Selective Dorsal Rhizotomy (SDR) involves lumbar laminectomy or laminotomy and division of a select number of dorsal nerve rootlets. 2010 NICE guidelines state that it should be carried out in an MDT setting in a specialized paediatric centre with access to the full range of treatments for spasticity. The division of sensory lumbar nerves clearly carries the risks of sphincter dysfunction and weakness and therefore children who exhibit weakness (more than spasticity) are not candidates.

National Institute for Health and Clinical Excellence (NICE) 2012. Spasticity in children and young people with non-progressive brain disorders: Management of spasticity and co-existing motor disorders and their early musculoskeletal complications. Online, available at https://www.nice.org.uk/guidance/cg145 http://www.england.nhs.uk/wp-content/uploads/2014/03/ce-sdr-guide2.pdf

JF Mooney 3rd, LA Koman, BP Smith. 'Pharmacologic management of spasticity in cerebral palsy'. *Journal of Pediatric Orthopaedics*, 2003; 23: 679.

29. A

CTEV or clubfoot is a three-dimensional foot deformity with an incidence of 1–2 per 1000 live births. Several etiological theories have been suggested from genetic factors, embryological arrest in development, a fibrotic response to injury and neuromuscular pathologies. Idiopathic clubfoot is considered to have a multifactorial aetiology. The diagnosis can be made on antenatal ultrasound but is still most commonly made at or soon after birth: no imaging is required to confirm the diagnosis but may occasionally be required to exclude a congenital anomaly causing a similar appearance. In addition to identifying the deformity it is important to search for associated abnormalities, both neuromuscular and syndromic that will define the deformity as non-idiopathic as this will imply a different prognosis and management. Antenatal diagnosis is accurate in terms of identifying the problem but less good at defining its severity.

Herring JA, *Tachdijian's Pediatric Orthopaedics*, 5th edition. 2013. Elsevier.

Ponseti IV. *Congenital Clubfoot: Fundamentals of Treatment.* Oxford: Oxford Medical Publications 1996.

30. C

The classic appearance of a clubfoot (both idiopathic and syndromic) is CAVE: midfoot cavus, forefoot adduction, hindfoot varus, and ankle equinus.

Herring JA. *Tachdijian's Pediatric Orthopaedics*, 5th edition. 2013. Elsevier.

Ponseti IV. *Congenital Clubfoot: Fundamentals of Treatment,* Oxford: Oxford Medical Publications 1996.

31. E

Curve progression in congenital scoliosis is determined by the exact morphology of the congenital abnormality and the growth potential of the vertebrae. Curve progression is certain with a unilateral unsegmented bar and a contralateral (convex–sided) hemivertebra. Deformities, in order of severity, are also caused by unilateral unsegmented bars, fully segmented hemivertebrae, unsegmented hemivertebrae, and lastly block vertebrae. The worst potential outcome is the development of thoracic insufficiency syndrome, which is the result of significant growth retardation of the thorax and results in abnormal lung development.

Hedequist D, Emans J. 'Congenital scoliosis: a review and update'. *Journal of Pediatric Orthopaedic,* 2007 Jan-Feb; 27(1): 106–16.

32. C

There is no evidence that congenital anomalies leading to scoliosis are inherited. All the listed reasons could be associated with congenital scoliosis.

Hedequist D, Emans J. 'Congenital scoliosis: a review and update'. *Journal of Pediatric Orthopaedics*, 2007 Jan-Feb; 27(1): 106–16.

Hedequist DJ. 'Instrumentation and fusion for congenital spine deformities'. *Spine*, 2009 1; 34(17): 1783–90.

33. A

There is no one single cause of DDH but several predisposing factors have been identified. Racial predilection plays a role in DDH; certain ethnic groups have a higher incidence of DDH such as Native Americans (15 per 1000) where others such as Afrocaribbeans and Asians have a much lower incidence (0.1–5 per 1000). Ligamentous laxity and a higher collagen III to I ratio suggest a connective tissue abnormality. A breech position at any time in the last trimester or at delivery (particularly when the knees are extended) is strongly associated with DDH. Swaddling in the post natal period, is a significant aetiological factor influencing the development of DDH particularly if babies are positioned with the hips extended. Primary acetabular dysplasia is an unlikely cause of DDH: the foetal acetabulum covers most of the femoral head, coverage decreases towards/around birth and then deepens again with growth and weightbearing.

Herring JA, *Tachdijian's Pediatric Orthopaedics*, 5th edition. 2013. Elsevier.

Artz TD, Lim WN, et al. 'Neonatal diagnosis, treatment and related factors of congenital dislocation of the hip'. *Clinical Orthopaedics and Related Research*, 1975 Aug; 110: 112–36.

Dunn PM. 'Perinatal observations on the etiology of congenital dislocation of the hip'. *Clinical Orthopaedics and Related Research*, 1976: 119: 11.

34. D

The primary aim of treating a dislocated hip is to obtain and maintain a stable reduction, as soon as possible. The methods of treatment depend on the age and associated findings. A Pavlik harness is the first line of treatment of both an unstable (Barlow positive) and a dislocated but reducible hip (Ortolani positive) for the child under 6 months of age. The harness encourages reduction over time so the hip is placed in the flexed and abducted position to encourage reduction and examined with ultrasound to monitor improvement in femoral head/acetabular relationships and improved joint stability. The harness will be discontinued if stable reduction is not achieved within 6–8 weeks: if the hip is Ortolani negative at the first assessment, some surgeons would feel this to be a contra-indication to the use of the Pavlik harness and others would suggest a trial of harness use for 1–2 weeks only.

An examination under anaesthetic (EUA, arthrogram and closed reduction is attempted in cases where treatment with the Pavlik harness has failed or when the baby presents after the age of 4–6 months. An adductor tenotomy is performed to increase the safe zone of stability (between maximal abduction and the position of re-subluxation). Extreme and/or forced abduction should be avoided due to the risk of AVN. The position of the maximal diameter of the femoral head relative to the labrum and the width of medial dye pool are both important factors in judging whether the hip is reduced or not. If the maximal diameter is not under the abnormal labrum and/or the dye pool is > 5 mm; the reduction is considered unacceptable. Even if the position is judged acceptable, if there is only a small cone of stability around the reduced position, the reduction is likely to fail.

An acceptable closed reduction should be held in a spica cast with the hip flexed and abducted (in the 'human frog' position).

Herring JA. *Tachdijian's Pediatric Orthopaedics*, 5th edition. 2013, Elsevier.

35. D

In a child under 8, angulation of up to 30° is acceptable due to the excellent remodeling potential. There is evidence, including randomized prospective studies, that shows no difference in the outcome of children treated with short-arm versus long-arm casts.

Paneru SR et al. 'Randomized controlled trial comparing above- and below-elbow plaster casts for distal forearm fractures in children'. *Journal of Children's Orthopaedics*, 2010; 4(3): 233–7.

Bohm ER, Bubbar V, Yong Hing K, Dzus A. 'Above and below-the-elbow plaster casts for distal forearm fractures in children. A randomized controlled trial'. *The Journal of Bone & Joint Surgery*, 2006; 88(1): 1–8.

36. C

Dorsal to volar force with pronation to maintain the DRUJ reduction is recommended. A timely clinic review is important especially when a reduction has been performed.

Herring JA. *Tachdijian's Pediatric Orthopaedics*, 5th edition. 2013. Elsevier.

37. C

The Beighton score is a score for hypermobility (maximal points 9); features include passive dorsiflexion of little finger beyond 90° with the forearm flat on a table, passive movement of the thumb to the volar aspect of the forearm, hyperextension of elbow, hyperextension of knee, and touching palms to floor with legs straight. A score greater than 4 is considered by some to be of increased joint laxity (such as Benign Joint Hypermobility Syndrome or possibly Ehlers-Danlos) but in children, unofficially, the threshold is higher (> 5–6). The Brighton Criteria describes both joint laxity (Beighton Score) and other clinical signs as major/minor criteria: the system has not been validated in children.*

Beighton P, et al. 'Ehlers-Danlos syndromes: revised nosology'. *American Journal of Medical Genetics*, 1998; 77(1): 31–7.

38 D

Aortic arch dilatation is more specifically a feature of Marfan Syndrome (though milder dilatation can also be seen in Type IV Ehler Danlos syndrome—the so-called vascular type). In young infants, blue sclerae can be seen in some ethnic groups: they are not pathognomonic for osteogenesis imperfecta and can be seen in other collagen disorders. Carpal tunnel syndrome and entheseopathies can be found in any of the conditions that result in hypermobility.

Bravo JF et al. 'Clinical study of hereditary disorders of connective tissues in an Chilean population: Joint hypermobility syndrome and vascular Ehlers-Danlos syndrome'. *Arthritis & Rheumatology*, 2006; 54(2): 515–23.

39. A

Congenital radioulnar synostosis is a rare condition affecting boys a little more commonly than girls, the majority are bilateral. It results due to a failure of separation of the radius and ulna early during embryonic development: the synostosis is usually proximal and occurs at a time when the foetal arm is in pronation. Hence, most cases have the arm in fixed pronation with slight restriction of elbow flexion/extension. The radial head may be rudimentary and dislocated posterolaterally.

Herring JA, *Tachdijian's Pediatric Orthopaedics*, 5th edition. 2013. Elsevier.

Simcock X, Shah AS, Waters PM, Bae DS. 'Safety and Efficacy of Derotational Osteotomy for Congenital Radioulnar Synostosis'. *Journal of Pediatric Orthopaedics*, 2015 Dec; 35(8): 838–43.

* Data from *American Journal of Medical Genetics*, 77, 1998, Beighton P, et al. 'Ehlers-Danlos syndromes: revised nosology', pp. 31–7.

40. E

Congenital radioulnar synostosis occurs due to a failure of separation of the radius and ulna early during embryonic development: the synostosis is usually proximal and occurs at a time when the foetal arm is in pronation. Hence, most cases have the arm in fixed pronation with slight restriction of elbow flexion/extension. Physiotherapy will not improve motion. In children, there is rarely any indication for excision of the radial head and excision of the synostosis with/without an interposition graft as it is not usually successful. Osteotomy of the radius and ulna can be performed to exchange one fixed position for another fixed position with the aim of improving bimanual function.

Herring JA, *Tachdijian's Pediatric Orthopaedics*, 5th edition. 2013. Elsevier.

Simcock X, Shah AS, Waters PM, Bae DS. 'Safety and Efficacy of Derotational Osteotomy for Congenital Radioulnar Synostosis'. *Journal of Pediatric Orthopaedics*, 2015 Dec; 35(8); 838–43.

41. C

The factors that dictate the management in children aged between 6 and 11 years of age are the weight of the child and the fracture pattern. Length-stable fractures, such as transverse or oblique fractures, are generally managed with elastic stable intramedullary nails (ESIN) or flexible intramedullary nailing (FIN). Length-unstable fractures, such as comminuted or spiral fractures, are managed using a plating technique. The weight must be taken into consideration regardless of fracture pattern and age, as there is evidence to suggest that poor outcomes from ESIN/FIN correlate with children weighing more than 49 kg.

Garner MR, Bhat SB, Khujanazarov I, Flynn JM, Spiegel D. 'Fixation of length-stable femoral shaft fractures in heavier children: flexible nails vs rigid locked nails'. *Journal of Pediatric Orthopaedics*, 2011 Jan-Feb; 31(1): 11–6.

Kosuge D, Barry M. 'Changing trends in the management of children's fractures'. *The Bone & Joint Journal*, 2015 Apr; 97-B(4): 442–8.

Moroz LA, Launay F, Kocher MS, Newton PO, Frick SL, Sponseller PD, Flynn JM. 'Titanium elastic nailing of fractures of the femur in children. Predictors of complications and poor outcome'. *The Bone & Joint Journal*, 2006 Oct; 88(10): 1361–6.

42. B

The factors that influence management in children aged between 6 and 11 years of age are the weight of the child and the fracture pattern. Length stable fractures, such as transverse or oblique fractures, are generally managed with flexible intramedullary nails. Length unstable fractures, such as comminuted or spiral fractures, are managed using a plating technique. The weight must be taken into consideration regardless of fracture pattern and age, as there is evidence to suggest that poor outcomes correlate with children weighing more than 49 kg. There is evidence to suggest that ESIN is not a stable option in the child weighing 50 kg or more and plating using a bridging technique is safer and more predictable. External fixation can also be used effectively as time to healing is less in the skeletally immature than the adult.

Garner MR, Bhat SB, Khujanazarov I, Flynn JM, Spiegel D. 'Fixation of length-stable femoral shaft fractures in heavier children: flexible nails vs rigid locked nails'. *Journal of Pediatric Orthopaedics*, 2011 Jan-Feb; 31(1): 11–6.

Kosuge D, Barry M. 'Changing trends in the management of children's fractures'. *The Bone & Joint Journal*. 2015 Apr; 97-B(4): 442–8.

Moroz LA, Launay F, Kocher MS, Newton PO, Frick SL, Sponseller PD, Flynn JM. 'Titanium elastic nailing of fractures of the femur in children. Predictors of complications and poor outcomes. *The Bone & Joint Journal*, 2006 Oct; 88(10): 1361–6.

43. E

Children with femoral shaft fractures aged 6 months to 5 years are managed according to the presence or absence of femoral shortening. If there is less than 2 cm of femoral shortening and no other contraindications early spica casting or skin traction with delayed spica casting is suggested. However if there is more than 2 cm of shortening, spica casting should be avoided. All other modalities can be used in this scenario including FIN or ESIN, plating, or initial traction followed by spica casting. There is insufficient evidence to advocate one preferred method.

'Treatment of Paediatric Diaphyseal Femur Fracture Guideline and Evidence Report', adopted by the AAOS Board of Directors. June 19, 2009.

Brousil J, Hunter JB: 'Femoral fractures in children'. *Current Opinion in Pediatrics*, 2013 Feb; 25(1): 52–7.

44. E

The 2009 AAOS guideline is to treat infants with either a Pavlik harness or a spica cast. Both treatment modalities were reported to result in equally excellent outcome with minimal complications, although skin complications have been reported with spica treatment.

Podeszwa DA, Mooney JF 3rd, Cramer KE, Mendelow MJ. 'Comparison of Pavlik harness application and immediate spica casting for femur fractures in infants'. *Journal of Pediatric Orthopaedics*, 2004 Sep-Oct; 24(5): 460–2.

45. D

For infants aged 6 months and younger, the recommendation from the 2009 AAOS guidelines is to treat the infant with either a Pavlik harness or a spica cast. Both treatment modalities were reported to result in equally excellent outcome with minimal complications. In the UK Gallows traction is still used when the fracture is not stable with significant shortening but a Pavlik Harness can be used for 3–4 weeks in this young age group for most fractures.

Flynn JM, Curatolo E. 'Pediatric femoral shaft fractures: a system for decision-making'. *Instructional Course Lectures*, 2015; 64: 453–60.

Rush JK, Kelly DM, Sawyer JR, Beaty JH, Warner WC Jr. 'Treatment of pediatric femur fractures with the Pavlik harness: multiyear clinical and radiographic outcomes'. *Journal of Pediatric Orthopaedics*, 2013 Sep; 33(6): 614–7.

Podeszwa DA, Mooney JF 3rd, Cramer KE, Mendelow MJ. 'Comparison of Pavlik harness application and immediate spica casting for femur fractures in infants'. *Journal of Pediatric Orthopaedics*, 2004 Sep-Oct; 24(5) :460–2.

46. A

This is a classic radiographic description of Fibrous Dysplasia.

Herring JA. *Tachdijian's Pediatric Orthopaedics*, 5th edition. 2013. Elsevier.

47. B

The focus of initial investigations in fibrous dysplasia is to establish whether the condition is polyostotic or monostotic and whether there are symptoms suggestive of McCune Albright syndrome.

A thorough clinical examination, looking specifically for signs of precocious puberty and irregular café-au-lait spots is the starting point. These features would be consistent with McCune Albright syndrome. The clinical examination may also reveal other bony deformities, for example in the contralateral femur, tibiae, humeri and the jaw.

Herring JA. *Tachdijian's Pediatric Orthopaedics*, 5th edition. 2013. Elsevier.

48. B

The flexible flat foot is a common cause of concern for parents and hence they frequently present to paediatric clinics. Most feet are asymptomatic. The risk of long term pain and secondary joint damage is low. Under the age of 5, no focused intervention has been shown to alter the long term outcome: flat feet either resolve over time or they do not.

Treatment is aimed at alleviating symptoms. Physiotherapy exercises to maintain Achilles' tendon length, tibialis posterior strength and single stance stability can be helpful. Orthotics can modify symptoms and may be useful in the case of a severe flexible flat foot or in the slightly older child. Surgery is rarely required. A few centres advocate subtalar arthroereisis or, in the UK, calcaneal lengthening with appropriate medial soft tissue rebalancing for the child with significant symptoms.

Herring JA. *Tachdijian's Pediatric Orthopaedics*, 5th edition. 2013. Elsevier, pp. 775–83.

Mosca VS. 'Flexible flatfoot in children and adolescents'. *Journal of Children's Orthopaedics*, 2010 Apr; 4(2): 107–21.

De Pellegrin MI, Moharamzadeh D, Strobl WM, Biedermann R, Tschauner C, 'Wirth T Subtalar extra-articular screw arthroereisis (SESA) for the treatment of flexible flatfoot in children'. *Journal of Children's Orthopaedics*, 2014 Dec; 8(6): 479–87.

49. D

Surgery is rarely required for flexible flat foot. A few European centres advocate subtalar arthroereisis (temporary joint fusion) to reduce the valgus and prevent relative external rotation of the hindfoot driven by the talocalcaneal relationship. This is more common in the hypermobile child with painful, flexible flat feet, as long as there is no fixed medial forefoot deformity. In the UK and the USA, a calcaneal lengthening procedure with appropriate medial soft tissue rebalancing work is more popular for the child with significant symptoms.

Herring JA. *Tachdjian's Pediatric Orthopaedics* (5th edition) 2013. Elsevier, pp. 775–83.

Mosca VS. 'Flexible flatfoot in children and adolescents'. *Journal of Children's Orthopaedics*, 2010 Apr; 4(2): 107–21.

De Pellegrin MI, Moharamzadeh D, Strobl WM, Biedermann R, Tschauner C. 'Wirth T Subtalar extra-articular screw arthroereisis (SESA) for the treatment of flexible flatfoot in children'. *Journal of Children's Orthopaedics*, 2014 Dec; 8(6): 479–87.

50. E

Madelung's deformity is frequently bilateral and more common in girls, with an autosomal dominant inheritance pattern. Some cases have an abnormality in the SHOX gene and the deformity is often part of a more generalized skeletal dysplasia e.g. Leri–Weill syndrome. Vicker's ligament runs from the ulnar side of the distal radius to the lunate on the volar aspect of the wrist, tethering growth and leading to an increased radial inclination, volar angulation with shortening (and hence relative overgrowth of the distal ulna which is prominent on the dorsal aspect of the wrist). There is volar subluxation of the carpus.

Symptoms usually develop in adolescence. Treatment may be conservative if symptoms are mild with relative rest and analgesics but the pathology is progressive whilst growth remains.

Surgical treatment can involve the following:

1. Prevention of further deformity/improvement of existing deformity
   a. Release of the tether imposed by Vicker's ligament
   b. Physiolysis of the pathological portion of the distal radial physis

2. Correction of existing deformity
   a. Biplanar radial osteotomy with acute/gradual correction
   b. Concomitant distal ulnar shortening

Farr S, Kalish LA, Bae DS, Waters PM. 'Radiographic Criteria for Undergoing an Ulnar Shortening Osteotomy in Madelung Deformity: A Long-term Experience From a Single Institution'. *Journal of Pediatric Orthopaedics*, 2016 Apr-May; 36(3): 310–5.

Kozin SH, Zlotolow DA. Madelung Deformity. *Journal of Hand Surgery*, 2015 Oct; 40(10): 2090–8.

51. A

Longitudinal deficiencies of the upper limb are frequently associated with other abnormalities: in Holt–Oram syndrome there are significant cardiac anomalies and the forearm deficiency may be part of the VACTERL association. The quality of the thumb often dictates treatment and overall functional prognosis which is therefore often better in TAR (thrombocytopaenia-absent radius) syndrome than in cases with less radial deficiency but a poor quality thumb. Whilst often bilateral, the severity of symptoms can be asymmetrical.

Herring JA. *Tachdijian's Pediatric Orthopaedics*, 5th edition. 2013. Elsevier.

52. B

A,C,D and E are considered the basic elements for a normal gait and they combine to give you energy conservation. The CoM (centre of mass) should remain within the person's BoS (base of support) during stance but not during gait itself.

Herring JA. *Tachdijian's Pediatric Orthopaedics*, 5th edition. 2013. Elsevier.

53. A

The 3 ankle rockers are controlled as follows:

- 1st rocker (heel strike) by the eccentrically acting tibialis anterior
- 2nd rocker (stance phase) by the eccentrically acting gastrocnemius
- 3rd rocker (toe off) by concentric contraction of gastrocnemius (and flexor hallucis longus)

Patients with heel pain are reluctant to make a heel strike for initial contact (IC) and thus the first rocker is lost. Similarly, if the forefoot is painful, pushing off on your forefoot at the end of stance is painful and this movement is diminished.

Herring JA. *Tachdijian's Pediatric Orthopaedics*, 5th edition. 2013. Elsevier.

54. E

A mutation in the FGFR3 gene (Fibroblast growth factor receptor 3) results in achondroplasia: the mutation is inherited in an autosomal dominant pattern, although 80% cases are sporadic mutations. The effect of the mutation is to change a glycine base for an arginine base in the FGFR3 protein, the receptor becomes more active (a gain-in-in-function mutation) and growth is disturbed.

BMPs are *osteoinductive.*

Cartilage oligomeric matrix protein (COMP) is a molecule important in linking type II collagen within cartilage. Each COMP molecule binds 5 type II collagen molecules.

Type X collagen is associated with calcification. It is therefore most prevalent in the hypertrophic zone and more specifically, the zone of provisional calcification of the physis.

Herring JA. *Tachdijian's Pediatric Orthopaedics*, 5th edition. 2013. Elsevier.

TM Merritt, JL Alcorn, R Haynes, JT Hecht. 'Expression of mutant cartilage oligomeric matrix protein in human chondrocytes induces the pseudoachondroplasia phenotype'. *Journal of Orthopaedic Research*, 2006; 24(4); 700–7.

B Bragdon, O Moseychuk, S Saldanha, D King, J Julian, A Nohe. 'Bone morphogenetic proteins: a critical review'. *Cell Signal*, 2011 Apr; 23(4): 609–20.

55. C

The persistence of a primitive reflex beyond 12 months of age should raise alarm. Likewise, hand preference before the age of 2 should alert you to the possibility of a problem, often neurological, in the less used arm. Is this a mild hemiplegia?

Most babies do take their first steps by 12 m but walking well may take a few months longer. Sitting un-supported is a 6 month developmental milestone although, as with everything, some may achieve this earlier. A child who bottom-shuffles is within normal limits and may or may not walk early (it tends to be slightly later).

The more you watch children in clinic or socially—the more you will learn about normal development: remember to use your common sense.

Illingworth RS. *The development of the infant and young child. Normal and abnormal.* 9th edition. 1987. Edinburgh: Churchill Livingstone.

56. D

Most 'bunions' in the paediatric population occur in adolescent girls with a positive family history (although no true inheritance pattern has been identified). The problem is usually bilateral: in unilateral cases with no family history you may need to look for a cause of muscle imbalance (e.g. spina bifida) as a cause for the deformity. The inter-metatarsal angle, hallux valgus angle and the DMAA (distal metatarsal articular angle) particularly are all likely to be high. In children, there is a significant recurrence rate following surgery so it is best delayed until skeletal maturity and only if there are symptoms. A basal osteotomy of the first metatarsal can only be performed after skeletal maturity and closure of the proximally sited physis.

Herring JA. *Tachdijian's Pediatric Orthopaedics*, 5th edition. 2013. Elsevier.

57. E

Regarding the management of hallux valgus, there is a long list of possible surgical procedures that can be used in isolation or in combination depending on the precise pathology, however, a basal osteotomy of the first metatarsal can only be performed after skeletal maturity and closure of the proximally sited physis.

Herring JA. *Tachdijian's Pediatric Orthopaedics*, 5th edition. 2013. Elsevier.

58. A

Criteria for performing MRI are the ones mentioned plus any curve suspected of not being idiopathic.

Herring JA. *Tachdijian's Pediatric Orthopaedics*, 5th edition. 2013. Elsevier.

59. E

Curve progression is dependent on severity and time left until skeletal maturity; therefore age, sex, and Risser stage, are prognostic of progression. The presence of café au lait spots suggests the curve may not be idiopathic in origin.

Herring JA. *Tachdijian's Pediatric Orthopaedics*, 5th edition. 2013. Elsevier.

60. B

Scheuermann's kyphosis is a rigid hyperkyphosis of ≥45°: diagnosis is based on the radiographic findings of 3 or more consecutive vertebrae wedged anteriorly by 5° or more.

Sponseller PD, Akbarnia BA, Lenke LG, Wollowick AL. 'Pediatric spinal deformity: what every orthopaedic surgeon needs to know'. *Instructional Course Lectures*, 2012; 61: 481–97.

61. E

Scheuermann's kyphosis is a rigid hyperkyphosis of ≥45°: diagnosis is based on the radiographic findings of 3 or more consecutive vertebrae wedged anteriorly by 5° or more. No signs of juvenile osteoporosis or other metabolic problems have been documented. Patients with Scheuermann kyphosis are taller, heavier and have an increased BMI compared with age-matched controls. Irregular vertebral apophyseal lines combined with flattening and wedging and narrowing of the intervertebral disc spaces are further radiological features. Typically it affects the thoracic spine.

There is an atypical type which affects the spine more distally and is associated with anterior Schmorl nodes.

There is no genetic predisposition.

Sponseller PD, Akbarnia BA, Lenke LG, Wollowick AL. 'Pediatric spinal deformity: what every orthopaedic surgeon needs to know'. *Instructional Course Lectures*, 2012; 61: 481–97.

Herndon WA, Emans JB, Micheli LJ, Hall JE. 'Combined anterior and posterior fusion for Scheuermann's kyphosis'. *Spine* (Phila Pa 1976), 1981 Mar-Apr; 6(2): 125–30.

62. D

In undisplaced cases, consider performing further X-rays to confirm the degree of displacement (the internal oblique view is the most useful) as the images can be deceptive, particularly in terms of fragment rotation, as most of the lateral condyle is cartilaginous.

Song KS et al. 'Internal oblique radiographs for diagnosis of nondisplaced or minimally displaced lateral condylar fractures of the humerus in children'. *The Journal of Bone & Joint Surgery*, 2007; 89(1): 58–63.

63. B

The most common complications following lateral condyle fractures include delayed union and non-union with or without cubitus valgus and subsequent tardy ulnar nerve palsy. Growth arrest and fishtail deformity of the distal humerus can also occur. As the fracture heals, there may be formation of a lateral spur of new bone leading to the appearance of a (pseudo) cubitus varus. This has been reported to occur in as many as 40% of patients, however it is generally mild and asymptomatic.

Sullivan JA. 'Fractures of the lateral condyle of the humerus'. *Journal of the American Academy of Orthopaedic Surgeons*, 2006; 14(1): 58–62.

Launay F et al. 'Lateral humeral condyle fractures in children: a comparison of two approaches to treatment'. *Journal of Pediatric Orthopaedics*, 2004; 24(4): 385–91

Herring JA. *Tachdijian's Pediatric Orthopaedics*, 5th edition. 2013. Elsevier.

64. A

Absolute indications for operative treatment are incarceration of the medial epicondyle in the joint and open fractures. Relative indications include ulnar nerve dysfunction, gross elbow instability, displacement and desire to return to high-level sport or employment.

Mehlman CT, Howard AW. 'Medial epicondyle fractures in children: clinical decision making in the face of uncertainty'. *Journal of Pediatric Orthopaedics*, 2012; 32: S135–42.

Kamath AF et al. 'Operative versus non-operative management of pediatric medial epicondyle fractures; a systematic review'. *Journal of Children's Orthopaedics*, 2009; 3: 345–57.

65. E

The secondary ossification centres of the elbow appear in a defined sequence (CRMTOL or CRITOE I = internal rather than medial and E = external rather than lateral), starting with the capitellum between 6 months and 2 years, and the others approximately every 2 years thereafter (i.e. radial head age 4, medial epicondyle at 6, trochlea at 8, olecranon at 10, and lateral epicondyle at 12 years). The medial epicondyle fuses with the humeral diaphysis between 18–20 years of age.

Herring JA. *Tachdijian's Pediatric Orthopaedics*, 5th edition. 2013. Elsevier.

66. C

Careful examination and documentation of the neurological status of the limb is essential in these injuries, especially that of the posterior interosseous nerve which is the most commonly injured nerve, complicating around 20% of cases.

Benson M, Fixsen J, Macnicol M, Parsch K (eds). *Children's Orthopaedics and Fractures* (3rd edition) Springer-Verlag, London, UK. 2010. Chapter 44: 'Fractures of the elbow and forearm'.

Ring D, Jupiter JB, Waters PM. 'Monteggia fractures in children and adults'. *Journal of the American Academy of Orthopaedic Surgeons*, 1998; 6(4): 215–24.

67. A

Monteggia fractures can be classified by the Bado classification which is defined by the direction of the radial head dislocation. The radial head dislocation, in turn, is always in the direction of the apex of the ulnar deformity.

In Bado type I fractures, which are the most common (70%), the radial head is dislocated anteriorly with an apex anterior fracture of the ulna.

Herring JA. *Tachdijian's Pediatric Orthopaedics*, 5th edition. 2013. Elsevier.

Benson M, Fixsen J, Macnicol M, Parsch K (eds). *Children's Orthopaedics and Fractures* (3rd edition) 2010. Chapter 44: 'Fractures of the elbow and forearm'. Springer-Verlag, London, UK.

Ring D, Jupiter JB, Waters PM. 'Monteggia fractures in children and adults'. *Journal of the American Academy of Orthopaedic Surgeons*, 1998; 6(4): 215–24.

68. C

Management of the multiply injured child broadly follows the same guidelines as those applicable to the multiply injured adult. It is worth noting that as part of the anatomical and physiological variations between children and adults, the injury pattern per mechanism is different. The highest mortality and morbidity in children is associated with spinal injury but most deaths are due to brain injury. Abdominal injuries form a significant proportion of the injury risk. Long bone injuries, whilst still relatively common, are less likely to result in long term morbidity or mortality. Pelvic injuries are less common in children but are often associated with high energy trauma.

Kay RM, Skaggs DL. 'Paediatric polytrauma management'. *Journal of Pediatric Orthopaedics*, 2006; Mar-Apr; 26(2): 268–77.

69. E

Management of the multiply injured child broadly follows the same guidelines as those applicable to the multiply injured adult. The ABCD is similar and securing the airway is always the first priority.

Kay RM, Skaggs DL. 'Paediatric polytrauma management'. *Journal of Pediatric Orthopaedics*, 2006 Mar-Apr; 26(2):268–77.

Herring JA. *Tachdijian's Pediatric Orthopaedics*, 5th edition. 2013. Elsevier.

Rockwood and Wilkins. *Fractures in children* (7th Edition) 2010. Lippincott, Williams and Wilkins.

70. E

Candidates must be familiar with the curve of Salenius and Vankka and may be expected to reproduce this in the viva. Genu varum in a 3-year-old is not normal. The foot is the first musculoskeletal segment to finish growth and completes 75% of that growth by the age of 7, which is also usually the age that the medial arch has developed. Children presenting with flexible 'flat feet' before that age should not be treated. A reliable heel—toe gait pattern is usually seen by the age of three and a half. The femoral neck is anteverted at birth, with a gradual decrease towards normal adult values by age 11.

Salenius P, Vankka E. 'The development of the tibiofemoral angle in children'. *The Journal of Bone & Joint Surgery*, American edition 1975: 57(2); 259–61.

Sutherland DH, Olshen R, Cooper L. 'The development of mature gait'. *The Journal of Bone & Joint Surgery*, American edition, 1980; 62A: 336–53.

Staheli LT, Corbett M, Wyss C, King H. 'Lower-extremity rotational problems in children. Normal values to guide management'. *The Journal of Bone & Joint Surgery*, American edition, 1985; 67A: 39–47.

Staheli LT, Chew DE, Corbett M. 'The longitudinal arch'. *The Journal of Bone & Joint Surgery*, American edition, 1987; 69A: 426–8.

71. C

Both forms of ossification involve the conversion of mesenchymal tissue into bone. In intramembranous ossification, mesenchymal tissue is converted directly to bone, in comparison to endochondral ossification, where it is converted to a cartilage precursor first. Intramembranous ossification occurs in flat bones and at the periosteum of long bones, where it results in appositional bone growth. Cleidocranial dysostosis is an example of a condition affected by a defect in intramembranous ossification, resulting in problems with the skull, clavicles, and pelvis. Endochondral ossification occurs when the cartilaginous anlage of a long bone is replaced by the primary ossification centre. It then also occurs in growth plates at the sites of secondary ossification centres, resulting in longitudinal growth. Achondroplasia affects endochondral ossification.

Iannotti JP, Goldstein S, Kuhn J, Lipiello L, Kaplan FS, Zaleske DJ. 'The formation and growth of skeletal tissue'. In: Buckwalter JA, Einhorn TA, Simon SR, editors. *Orthopaedic Basic Science. Biology and Biomechanics of the Musculoskeletal System*: American Academy of Orthopaedic Surgeons; 2000.

MA Sunderland, SF Gilbert. *Developmental Biology* 6th edition. Sinauer associates 2000.

72. D

Manifestations of myelomeningocele include orthopaedic, neurosurgical and urological problems which vary with the level of the lesion. Spinal deformities such as scoliosis and kyphosis occur. Flexion contractures of the hip and hip dysplasia occur commonly when the involvement is at the mid lumbar level. Arnold–Chiari malformations are the most common congenital abnormality followed by hydrocephalus. The management of a patient with myelomeningocele requires a multidisciplinary approach. Urological and gastrointestinal manifestations such as detrusor malfunction and abnormal sphincter tone can predispose to bacterial colonization of the urinary tract. Kidney reflux and pyelonephritis can develop. Changing neurological features over time may be related to a blocked VP shunt (all limbs) or a tethered cord (lower limbs); this may lead to a progressive scoliosis.

Snow-Lisy DC, Yerkes EB, Cheng EY. 'Update on Urological Management of Spina Bifida from Prenatal Diagnosis to Adulthood'. *Journal of Urology*, 2015 Aug; 194(2): 288–96. doi: 10.1016/j.juro.2015.03.107. Epub 2015 Apr 1. Review.

Swaroop VT, Dias LS. 'Strategies of hip management in myelomeningocele: to do or not to do'. *Hip International*, 2009 Jan-Mar; 19 Suppl 6: S53–5.

Fehlings MG, Ibrahim GM. 'Spinal deformity'. *Journal of Neurosurgery: Spine*, 2010 Dec; 13(6): 663–4; discussion 664–5.

73. E

Low folic acid intake is the most common cause and is the most easily correctable with a 72–100% decrease in the overall incidence of neural tube defects with adequate folate intake during pregnancy. There is no association with B12 deficiency and spina bifida. Maternal hyperthermia and diabetes are risk factors.

Snow-Lisy DC, Yerkes EB, Cheng EY. 'Update on Urological Management of Spina Bifida from Prenatal Diagnosis to Adulthood'. *Journal of Urology* Aug; 194(2): 288–96. doi: 10.1016/j.juro.2015.03.107. Epub 2015 Apr 1. Review.

74. B

Certain radiological findings should raise suspicions for NAI including presence of multiple fractures, rib fractures (particularly posteromedial, 71% probability of NAI), fractures of different ages, X-ray evidence of occult fractures, metaphyseal corner (bucket handle) fractures of long bones, humeral fractures (1:2 chance of NAI), femoral fractures in children under 18 months old (1:3 chance), tibia/fibula fractures under 18 months old and complex skull fractures.

Maguire S, Cowley L, Mann M, Kemp A. 'What does the recent literature add to the identification and investigation of fractures in child abuse: an overview of review updates 2005–2013'. *Evidence-Based Child Health*, 2013; 8: 2044–57.

The Royal College of Radiologists/Royal College of Paediatrics and Child Health. Standards for radiological investigations of suspected non-accidental injury (March 2008). [http://www.rcr.ac.uk/docs/radiology/pdf/RCPCH_RCR_final.pdf]

75. D

Risk factors of NAI: low socioeconomic class, parents with mental health or substance-misuse issues, exposure to domestic violence, vulnerable and unsupported parents, twins, developmental delay, preterm babies, and chronic illness. All the above should alert us to the possibility of NAI and patients/families who require further investigation and support.

National Institute for Health and Clinical Excellence (2009) 'When to suspect child maltreatment'. [http://www.nice.org.uk/nicemedia/pdf/CG89FullGuideline.pdf]

Royal College of Paediatrics and Child Health (2014). 'Safeguarding children and young people: roles and competences for healthcare staff': intercollegiate document [http://www.rcpch.ac.uk/child-health/standards-care/child-protection/publications/child-protection-publications

76. D

Neurofibromatosis is the commonest single gene disorder of neural origin but the phenotype is manifested in a multisystem manner. The cutaneous features include café-au-lait spots (smooth edged 'Coast of California' lesions) and cutaneous or subcutaneous neurofibromas. Peripheral nerve neurofibromas, including plexiform neurofibromas, are found in 25% of cases. In 10% of cases there are malignant peripheral nerve sheath tumours and neurosarcomas. The orthopaedic manifestations include pseudarthrosis of the tibia (5% of cases) and scoliosis.

McCune Albright Syndrome is a genetic condition though not an inherited one. It also features café-au-lait spots; in this condition, however, they are usually unilateral and have rough, jagged edges ('Coast of Maine' lesions).

Neurofibromatosis type 2, otherwise known as multiple inherited schwannomas, meningiomas and ependymomas (MISME), is a genetic condition inherited in a autosomal dominant manner. Acoustic nerve (cranial nerve VIII) benign schwannomas are pathognomonic for NF2, other benign brain tumours such meningiomas and ependymomas are also possible.

Herring JA. *Tachdijian's Pediatric Orthopaedics*, 5th edition. 2013. Elsevier.

77. C

Neurofibromatosis is the commonest single gene disorder of neural origin but the phenotype is manifested in a multisystem manner. The cutaneous features include café-au-lait spots (smooth edged 'Coast of California' lesions) and cutaneous or subcutaneous neurofibromas. Peripheral nerve neurofibromas, including plexiform neurofibromas, are found in 25% of cases. In 10% of cases there are malignant peripheral nerve sheath tumours and neurosarcomas. The orthopaedic manifestations include pseudarthrosis of the tibia (5% of cases) and scoliosis: mild spinal deformity is common but severe scoliosis can occur when the curve starts early (< 10 years). Plexiform neurofibromas can cause growth disturbances of adjacent bones resulting in deformities and length differences.

Herring JA. *Tachdijian's Pediatric Orthopaedics*, 5th edition. 2013. Elsevier.

78. E

Juvenile OCD is fairly rare. Typically, it is more common in boys but the incidence in girls is increasing. The aetiology is unclear, there is no clear familial pattern and repetitive trauma with stress micro-fractures is postulated but unproven. Presentation is either with a history of intermittent pain, swelling and giving way or it can be an incidental finding on radiographic investigation.

AP, lateral and notch/tunnel view radiographs are usually diagnostic and MRI helps to identify the exact site and extent of the lesions: the most common site is the lateral aspect of the medial femoral condyle. MR arthrograms help assess the extent of the breach of the articular surface.

Pascual-Garrido C, Moran CJ, Green DW, Cole BJ. 'Osteochondritis dissecans of the knee in children and adolescents'. *Current Opinion in Pediatrics*, 2013; 25(1): 46–51.

Nault M KM. 'The Knee: Osteochondritis Dissecans'. *Pediatric and Adolescent Sports Traumatology*, Italy: Springer-Verlag; 2014, pp. 171–8.

79. E

There are several described classifications for Juvenile OCD; all concentrate on whether or not the lesion is considered to be stable. The Guhl (arthroscopic) and the Di Paola (MRI) systems are most widely used: both divide the pathological process in to 4 stages.

The evidence on pathology, management and long term outcome is very limited and is based on cohort studies. The AAOS report failed to recommend any clear treatment guidelines due to a lack of adequate data.

Treatment for stable lesions is initially conservative with protected load bearing, activity modification and bracing. Some studies advocate gradual increased weight bearing as symptoms allow over several months. Physiotherapy helps reduce quads wasting. MRI can be repeated at 4–6 months to assess progress. Rates of healing vary from 50–90%.

Surgical intervention is reserved for patients with loose bodies, unstable lesions and failed conservative management. Surgical options are arthroscopic debridement and drilling for stable lesions, grafting and fixation with bioabsorbable screws for unstable lesions.

There are no long term studies or RCTs to evaluate the real benefits of surgical intervention or if there is a true increased risk of secondary OA.

Kramer DE, Glotzbecker MP, Shore BJ, Zurakowski D, Yen YM, Kocher MS, et al. 'Results of Surgical Management of Osteochondritis Dissecans of the Ankle in the Pediatric and Adolescent Population'. *Journal of Pediatric Orthopedics*, 2015 Oct-Nov; 35(7): 725–33.

Pascual-Garrido C, Moran CJ, Green DW, Cole BJ. 'Osteochondritis dissecans of the knee in children and adolescents'. *Current Opinion in Pediatrics*, 2013; 25(1): 46–51.

Edmonds EW, Polousky J. 'A review of knowledge in osteochondritis dissecans: 123 years of minimal evolution from König to the ROCK study group'. *Clinical Orthopaedics and Related Research*, 2013; 471(4): 1118–26.

Dipaola JD, Nelson DW, Colville MR. 'Characterizing osteochondral lesions by magnetic resonance imaging'. *Arthroscopy*, 1991; 7(1): 101–4.

Guhl JF. 'Arthroscopic treatment of osteochondritis dissecans'. *Clinical Orthopaedics and Related Research*, 1982; (167): 65–74.

Lim HC, Bae JH, Park YE, Park YH, Park JH, Park JW, et al. 'Long-term results of arthroscopic excision of unstable osteochondral lesions of the lateral femoral condyle'. *The Bone & Joint Journal*, 2012; 94(2): 185–9.

80. D

Ollier's disease (also called multiple enchondromatosis) is a rare, sporadic condition affecting chondroblast function and leading to abnormal cartilage deposition within the medullary cavities. As it is a disorder of endochondral ossification or of the original cartilage anlage, malignant change is to a chondrosarcoma.

Krakow D and Rimoin DL. 'Review: Skeletal Dysplasias'. *Genetics in Medicine*, 2010: 12(6): 327–41.

81. C

Ollier's disease (also called multiple enchondromatosis) is a rare, sporadic condition affecting chondroblast function which leads to abnormal cartilage deposition within the medullary cavities. As it is a disorder of endochondral ossification or of the original cartilage anlage, malignant change is to a chondrosarcoma. Malignant change both in the bones, in the CNS (gliomas) and internal organs is more common in Maffuci's syndrome (enchondromatosis in assosciation with haemangiomas and occasionally, lymphangiomas). The bone pathology in McCune Albright syndrome is polyostotic fibrous dysplasia. Bone deformity is common and often painful, bisphosphonates do reduce the pain (use in children is under restricted license) but correction of malalignment is also important: bone healing/regeneration is not affected. Solitary enchondromas are rarely painful unless there is a pathological fracture.

Krakow D and Rimoin DL. 'Review: Skeletal Dysplasias'. *Genetics in Medicine,* 2010; 12(6): 327–41.

Winston MJ¹, Srivastava T, Jarka D, Alon US. 'Bisphosphonates for pain management in children with benign cartilage tumors'. *Clinical Journal of Pain*, 2012 Mar-Apr; 28(3): 268–72.

82. D

Provided that there was no collection seen on MRI, osteomyelitis can be treated with IV antibiotics, converting to oral antibiotics as soon as the patient is responding well to treatment clinically and with improvement in the inflammatory markers. If there is a subperiosteal collection drainage with or without drilling should be considered.

The duration of antibiotics has traditionally been a long course of IV administration followed by a long oral course however recent studies have advocated switching to oral antibiotics after around 3–5 days if blood markers (CRP/ WCC), temperature and weight bearing continue to improve with a total duration of 3 weeks treatment in uncomplicated cases. In complicated cases treatment is dictated by the specific case and can include sequelae of pathological fractures and physeal injury leading to growth arrest.

Dartnell J, Ramachandran M, Katchburian M. 'Haematogenous acute and subacute paediatric osteomyelitis: a systematic review of the literature'. *The Bone & Joint Journal*, 2012; 94(5): 584–95.

Peltola H, Paakkonen M. 'Acute osteomyelitis in children'. *The New England Journal of Medicine*. 2014; 370(4): 352–60.

Peltola H, Paakkonen M, Kallio P, Kallio MJ. 'Osteomyelitis-Septic Arthritis Study G. Short- versus long-term antimicrobial treatment for acute hematogenous osteomyelitis of childhood: prospective, randomized trial on 131 culture-positive cases'. *The Pediatric Infectious Disease Journal*, 2010; 29(12): 1123–8.

Jagodzinski NA, Kanwar R, Graham K, Bache CE. 'Prospective evaluation of a shortened regimen of treatment for acute osteomyelitis and septic arthritis in children'. *Journal of Pediatric Orthopedics*, 2009; 29(5): 518–25.

83. D

MRI is the gold standard test for confirmation of osteomyelitis (bone scan is an option) and changes on radiograph ie sequestrum and involucrum reflect a late/chronic presentation. Earlier changes of disordered bony architecture will take a minimum of 7-10 days to be noticeable on a plain radiograph. The femur and tibia are the most commonly affected long bones. The commonest pathogen is S. aureus but S. epidermidis, various streptococci, and Kingella kingae are on the rise. Treatment is with antibiotics. If there is any suggestion of a subperiosteal collection on ultrasound or on MRI this can be considered for aspiration if in an accessible area to aid pathogen identification. If there is a large collection or a chronic situation with a sequestrum then surgical drainage/ debridement may be required.

Dartnell J, Ramachandran M, Katchburian M. 'Haematogenous acute and subacute paediatric osteomyelitis: a systematic review of the literature'. *The Bone & Joint Journal*, 2012; 94(5): 584–95.

Peltola H, Paakkonen M. 'Acute osteomyelitis in children'. *The New England Journal of Medicine*, 2014; 370(4): 352–60.

84. B

There is a physis at the end of every long bone: it contributes primarily to longitudinal growth but also to circumferential growth. The physis is traditionally divided on a microscopic level into 4 zones: reserve zone, proliferative zone, hypertrophic zone, and spongiosa. The hypertrophic zone can be further broken down into a zone of maturation, degeneration and finally provisional calcification. The spongiosa can be divided into the primary and secondary spongiosa. Children's fractures traditionally occur through the hypertrophic zone if purely physeal, but MRI evidence suggests that, in fact, the fracture line frequently crosses the physeal zones even in type 1 fractures.

Rockwood and Wilkins. *Fractures in children*, 7th edition. 2010. Lippincott, Williams and Wilkins.

Herring JA. *Tachdjian's Pediatric Orthopaedics*, 5th edition. 2013. Elsevier.

85. E

The Salter–Harris classification is used to classify physeal injuries. The original 5-point classification describes:

> Type I: occur purely through the physis
>
> Type II: occur predominantly through the physis but with a metaphyseal extension (commonly known as the Thurston–Holland fragment)
>
> Type III: traverse the physis but then extend through the epiphysis to the joint surface
>
> Type IV: usually a linear fracture line that extends from the articular surface through all zones of the physis and exits in the metaphysis
>
> Type V: a compression injury to the physis which may only be detected once physeal failure and progressive length discrepancy or deformity occur*

A Monteggia fracture is a fracture of the ulnar shaft with an associated dislocation of the radial head. It is categorized based on the Bado classification.

A triplane fracture is a physis-traversing, partial-articular, multi-planar injury that typically demonstrates a Salter–Harris III fracture on the AP projection and a Salter–Harris II fracture on the lateral projection. The discrepancy in radiographic appearance demonstrates the fact that the fracture has coronal, sagittal and axial components. This is a Salter–Harris IV injury.

Slipped capital femoral epiphysis is essentially a type I Salter–Harris injury through the physeal plate.

Lateral condyle fractures most commonly demonstrate a Salter–Harris IV fracture pattern, and are classified according to the location of the fracture line in relation to the capitellar ossification centre using the Milch classification.

The Tillaux fracture is a transitional fracture occurring as the physis closes and is due to avulsion of the anteroinferior tibiofibular ligament. The fracture fragment represents the anterolateral portion of the distal tibial epiphysis.

Rockwood and Wilkins. *Fractures in children*, 7th edition 2010. Lippincott, Williams and Wilkins.

Herring J. *Tachdijian's Pediatric Orthopaedics*, 5th edition. 2013. Elsevier.

86. A

In comparison, adolescents tend to sustain Salter–Harris II injuries. SH III and IV physeal fractures are associated with glenohumeral joint dislocation and are rare.

Herring J. *Tachdijian's Pediatric Orthopaedics*, 5th edition. 2013. Elsevier.

87. D

In displaced fractures, the epiphysis usually remains in the glenoid fossa but is abducted and externally rotated by the pull of the attached rotator cuff. The distal fragment is displaced anteromedially by the combined action of pectoralis major, latissimus dorsi, and teres major. The periosteum tends to remain intact on the posteromedial aspect of the metaphysis. Reduction of such fractures is therefore achieved by abduction and external rotation of the arm.

Herring J. *Tachdijian's Pediatric Orthopaedics*, 5th edition. 2013. Elsevier.

88. D

Slipped capital femoral epiphysis (SCFE) is the commonest hip pathology in adolescents; it is more common in boys. It typically occurs in early adolescence, hence earlier in girls (11–13 years) than in boys (13–15 years).

---

* Reproduced from Salter R and Harris W, 'Injuries Involving the Epiphyseal Plate', *Journal of Bone & Joint Surgery*, 45, 3, pp. 587–622. Copyright (1963) with permission from Wolters Kluwer Health, Inc.

Pathogenesis is likely a combination of poor mechanical stability and a relatively weak physis. Obesity is the commonest recognized risk factor and there is racial variability. Pre-existing metabolic disorders are also a risk factor. 20–60% of cases are bilateral either at presentation or they develop contralateral symptoms later.

Clinical presentation can vary from acute, severe groin pain and inability to weight bear to a longer history of thigh/knee pain. Examination may reveal a leg that lies in external rotation and flexes up into abduction and external rotation. Flexion may be limited and a leg length discrepancy may be noticeable.

Diagnosis is based on radiographic changes, best seen on the frog lateral image.

Loder RT, Skopelja EN. 'The epidemiology and demographics of slipped capital femoral epiphysis'. *International Scholarly Research Notices: Orthopaedics*, 2011; 486512.

Novais EN, Millis MB. 'Slipped capital femoral epiphysis: prevalence, pathogenesis, and natural history'. *Clinical Orthopaedics and Related Research*, 2012; 470(12): 3432–8.

89. E

Treatment of SUFE depends mostly on the severity of the slip but also on the chronicity and patient circumstances. All slips should be treated surgically.

Stable slips: Mild slips and most moderate slips should be pinned *in situ* (PIS). Severe slips (> 60 °) are technically difficult to pin *in situ*. Dunn, Fish, and Ganz have all described osteotomies at the level of the physis to realign the capital femoral epiphysis. In moderate to severe slips, treatment can be performed acutely whilst recognizing the risk of AVN. Alternatively, if possible, the SCFE can be pinned acutely and then a realignment osteotomy can be performed at a later stage away from the CORA (centre of rotation angulation) either at the base of the neck or intertrochanteric level (Southwick, Imhauser) osteotomy, these carry a lower rate of AVN.

Unstable slips: These carry a high risk of AVN. Unstable slips are not usually mild but if the slip is mild or moderate it can be pinned in situ. Great care should be taken in positioning the patient when under GA and whilst the truly unstable slips often reduce, at least partially, under anaesthetic; forceful closed reduction should not be attempted. If pinning-*in-situ* is performed, there is a suggestion that a capsulotomy should also be performed to reduce the risk of AVN.

PIS should be done using a cannulated screw that crosses the physis by 3 threads. At no point should the subchondral bone be pierced by the guidewire, drill or screw. The screw must stay in until the physis has closed. The main complications of PIS are chondrolysis and AVN.

The risk of a contralateral slip is up to 60%, risk factors include a young age and an underlying metabolic disorder. The posterior sloping angle (PSA) is used to measure the retroversion of the contralateral hip, if it is greater than 14° the risk of a future slip is significant and prophylactic pinning should be considered.

The complications specific to SCFE are AVN and chondrolysis. Chondrolysis (2% risk) occurs within the first 12–18 months and is associated with breaching the joint space intraoperatively although it also occurs in non-operated hips.

MacLean JG, Reddy SK. 'The contralateral slip. An avoidable complication and indication for prophylactic pinning in slipped upper femoral epiphysis'. *The Bone & Joint Journal*, 2006; 88(11): 1497–501.

Sankar WN, McPartland TG, Millis MB, Kim YJ. The unstable slipped capital femoral epiphysis: risk factors for osteonecrosis. *Journal of Pediatric Orthopedics*, 2010; 30(6): 544–8.

Southwick WO. 'Osteotomy through the lesser trochanter for slipped capital femoral epiphysis'. *The Journal of Bone & Joint Surgery*, American edition, 1967; 49(5): 807–35.

Uglow MG, Clarke NM. 'The management of slipped capital femoral epiphysis. *The Bone & Joint Journal*, 2004; 86(5): 631–5.

Zenios M, Ramachandran M, Axt M, Gibbons PJ, Peat J, Little D. 'Posterior sloping angle of the capital femoral physis: interobserver and intraobserver reliability testing and predictor of bilaterality'. *Journal of Pediatric Orthopedics*, 2007; 27(7): 801–4.

90. D

This is a case of a chronic stable slip. It should be treated surgically depending on the severity of the slip. Pinning *in situ*, realignment osteotomy at a later stage away from the CORA either at the base of the neck or intertrochanteric level, carry a low rate of AVN. Pinning of the contralateral hip should be considered based on the underlying pathology and the posterior sloping angle (PSA).

Uglow MG, Clarke NM. 'The management of slipped capital femoral epiphysis'. *The Bone & Joint Journal*, 2004; 86(5): 631–5.

Zenios M, Ramachandran M, Axt M, Gibbons PJ, Peat J, Little D. 'Posterior sloping angle of the capital femoral physis: interobserver and intraobserver reliability testing and predictor of bilaterality'. *Journal of Pediatric Orthopedics*, 2007; 27(7): 801–4.

91. D

Clinical presentation of SUFE can vary from acute, severe groin pain and inability to weight bear to a mixed picture of a previous episode of bad groin pain followed by subsequent dull thigh pain to a chronic aching discomfort only. Examination may reveal a leg that lies in external rotation and flexes up into external rotation. Flexion may be limited and a leg-length discrepancy may be noticeable.

Diagnosis is based on radiographic changes, best seen on the frog lateral image, including; decreased epiphyseal height, widening of the physis, Trethowan's sign, the metaphyseal blanch sign of Steel, and if the slip is chronic, callus formation and signs of remodelling posteriorly/inferiorly.

Treatment depends mostly on the severity of the slip but also on the chronicity and patient circumstances. All slips should be treated surgically.

PIS should be with a cannulated screw that crosses the physis by 3 threads. At no point should the subchondral bone be pierced by the guidewire, drill, or screw. The screw must stay in until the physis has closed. The main complication of pinning *in situ* is chondrolysis and AVN.

The entry point for the wire is slightly anterior due to the posterior inferior position of the slipped epiphysis.

Loder RT, Skopelja EN. 'The epidemiology and demographics of slipped capital femoral epiphysis'. *International Scholarly Research Notices: Orthopaedics*, 2011;2011:486512.

Novais EN, Millis MB. 'Slipped capital femoral epiphysis: prevalence, pathogenesis, and natural history'. *Clinical Orthopaedics and Related Research*, 2012; 470(12): 3432–8.

92. B

Transient synovitis presents very similarly to septic arthritis: several parameters, including a joint effusion, occur in both. Kocher devised a set of 4 criteria to help differentiate between the two:

1. Temperature >38.5° C in the preceeding few days
2. Inability to weight bear
3. WCC >12,000/ mm^3
4. ESR > 40*

* Data from *The Journal of Bone & Joint Surgery*, American edition, 2004 Kocher MS, Mandiga R, Zurakowski D, et al, 'Validation of a clinical prediction rule for the differentiation between septic arthritis and transient synovitis of the hip in children', 86, A8, pp.1629–1635.

Initial results suggested that the probability of septic arthritis was 99% if all 4 criteria were present but less than 5% if only one factor was positive, later prospective studies reduced this to 93%. More recent publications have included or replaced ESR with CRP and found CRP > 20 and weight bearing status to be the best independent differentiating factors.

Caird MS, Flynn JM, Leung YL, Millman JE, D'Italia JG, Dormans JP. 'Factors distinguishing septic arthritis from transient synovitis of the hip in children. A prospective study'. *Journal of Bone & Joint Surgery American volume*, 2006; 88(6): 1251–7.

Singhal R, Perry DC, Khan FN, Cohen D, Stevenson HL, James LA, et al. 'The use of CRP within a clinical prediction algorithm for the differentiation of septic arthritis and transient synovitis in children'. *The Bone & Joint Journal*, 2011; 93(11): 1556–61.

93. D

Septic arthritis in children is most frequently thought of in association with the hip but it is as equally common in the knee: it also occurs in the shoulder, ankle and less frequently the elbow as well as other sites. Most cases are primary infections via a haematogenous route or by direct inoculation but secondary joint involvement can occur via direct spread of a metaphyseal osteomyelitis when pus breaks through the periosteum where the metaphysis is intracapsular (e.g. proximal femur, radius, and humerus). Septic arthritis is most frequent in the under 2 year olds and becomes less common after the age of 6 years

Mignemi ME, Menge TJ, Cole HA, Mencio GA, Martus JE, Lovejoy S, et al. 'Epidemiology, diagnosis, and treatment of pericapsular pyomyositis of the hip in children'. *Journal of Pediatric Orthopaedics*. 2014; 34(3): 316–25.

94. A

Traumatic dislocation is far more common than multidirectional or voluntary instability and most cases dislocate anteriorly. Boys are more frequently affected than girls. However, in the youngest patients (under 11 years) multidirectional a-traumatic instability is probably the most common cause and girls are more often affected than boys.

Lawton RL, Choudhury S, Mansat P, Cofield RH, Stans AA. 'Pediatric shoulder instability: presentation, findings, treatment, and outcomes'. *Journal of Pediatric Orthopedics*, 2002; 22(1): 52–61.

95. A

Unlike in the teenage years, in the youngest patients (under 11 years) multidirectional a-traumatic instability is probably the most common cause and girls are more often affected than boys. Immobilization is rarely required for the multidirectional instability and physiotherapy is essential.

Lawton RL, Choudhury S, Mansat P, Cofield RH, Stans AA. 'Pediatric shoulder instability: presentation, findings, treatment, and outcomes'. *Journal of Pediatric Orthopedics*, 2002; 22(1): 52–61.

96. C

Spondylolysis is the anatomic defect of the pars interarticularis (the bony connection between the superior and inferior processes) without displacement of the vertebral body. Spondylolisthesis describes the forward translation of one vertebra relative to the next caudal vertebral segment. The Wiltse–Newman classification is the most widely used classification of spondylolisthesis. Type I is the dysplastic type and usually occurs during the adolescent growth spurt. It is secondary to congenital abnormalities of the lumbosacral articulation, with malorientation and hypoplasia of the L5–S1 facet joint articulation. The pars is poorly developed and elongated which allows for slippage of L5 on S1.

As the posterior neural arch is intact, with a spondylolisthesis there is increasing risk of neurological symptoms due to entrapment of the nerve roots. Type II is the isthmic type. This is the most common spondylolytic disorder in adolescence. The defect develops before skeletal maturity. There are 3 subtypes; type II A occurs when there is a fatigue stress fracture which does not heal normally due to constant motion and poor mechanical environment. A resulting fibrous band of tissue develops between the fracture edges. Type II B describes an elongated intact pars interarticularis as a result of repeated micro-fractures that heal. Type II C is a result of an acute traumatic fracture. Type III is degenerative, IV is traumatic, V is neoplastic, and VI is iatrogenic. (Marchetti and Bartolozzi have proposed an alternative classification system, which is based on 2 main categories, developmental and acquired.) 25% of patients with spondylolysis have an associated spondylolisthesis. Several risk factors have been identified for isthmic spondylolisthesis including repetitive extension activities such as gymnastics, tennis players, and swimmers, male gender, and a family history.*

Hammerberg KW. New concepts on the pathogenesis and classification of spondylolisthesis. *Spine* (Phila Pa 1976), 2005 Mar 15; 30(6 Suppl): S4–11.

Cheung EV, Herman MJ, Cavalier R, Pizzutillo PD. 'Spondylolysis and spondylolisthesis in children and adolescents: II. Surgical management'. *Journal of the American Academy of Orthopaedic Surgeons*, 2006 Aug; 14(8): 488–98.

97. D

Spondylolisthesis may manifest as lower back pain produced by a 'stress fracture'. Pain may radiate to the buttocks as a result of mechanical instability and is aggravated by flexion and extension activities. Physical examination may be normal with low-grade (< 50%) slips. With an increasing slip, a step-off may be palpated at the lumbosacral junction. Hamstring tightness is common and may be associated with an abnormal gait pattern. The supine SLR (straight leg raise) is significantly reduced and there may be L5 or S1 root involvement with motor weakness and/or loss of the ankle jerk. Several risk factors have been identified for isthmic spondylolisthesis including repetitive extension activities such as gymnastics, tennis, and swimming, male gender, and a family history.

Hammerberg KW. 'New concepts on the pathogenesis and classification of spondylolisthesis'. *Spine* (Phila Pa 1976). 2005 Mar 15; 30 (6 Suppl): S4–11.

Cheung EV, Herman MJ, Cavalier R, Pizzutillo PD.' Spondylolysis and spondylolisthesis in children and adolescents: II. Surgical management'. *Journal of the American Academy of Orthopaedic Surgeons*. 2006 Aug; 14(8): 488–98.

98. E

Ipsilateral injuries occur in ~ 5% of supracondylar fractures with distal radius fractures the most common.

Abzug JM, Herman MJ. 'Management of supracondylar humeral fractures in children: current concepts'. *Journal of the American Academy of Orthopaedic Surgeons*, 2012; 20: 69–77.

99. B

Children with a displaced extension-type supracondylar fracture and ipsilateral displaced forearm fracture (i.e. floating elbow) are at significant risk of compartment syndrome (incidence 33%).

Blakemore LC et al. 'Compartment syndrome in ipsilateral humerus and forearm fractures in children'. *Clinical Orthopaedics and Related Research* 2000; 376: 32–8.

Herring JA. *Tachdijian's Pediatric Orthopaedics*, 5th edition. 2013. Elsevier.

* Data from *Clinical Orthopaedics and Related Research*, 117, 1976, Wiltse LL, Newman PH, Macnab I, 'Classification of spondylolisis and spondylolisthesis', pp. 23–29.

100. B

Oblique radiographs show a calcaneonavicular coalition and the lateral X-ray may show the 'C' sign for a talocalcaneal bar or a prominent ant-eaters sign on the distal calcaneum in cases of a calcaneonavicular bar. Many children have flat feet but coalitions do not usually present until the age of 7–8 and may present with ankle sprains and/or a painful flat foot which is semi-rigid or rigid. There may be spasm in the peroneal muscles and this may 'relax' in non-weight bearing. There may be a prominence medially at the site of the talocalcaneal bar and this can be tender or painful when the joint is stressed; similarly in the case of a calcaneonavicular bar, stressing the subtalar joint can provoke pain in the sinus tarsi (but rarely any swelling). Fibrous coalitions are not usually symptomatic (although STJt movement might be limited) and excision is not recommended.

Bouchard M and Mosca VS. 'Flatfoot deformity in children and adolescents: indications and surgical management'. Review article. *Journal of the American Academy of Orthopaedic Surgeons,* 2014 Oct; 22(10): 623–32. doi: 10.5435/JAAOS-22-10-623.

Mosca VS, et al. 'Talocalcaneal tarsal coalitions and the calcaneal lengthening osteotomy: the role of deformity correction'. *The Journal of Bone & Joint Surgery,* American edition, 2012 Sep 5; 94(17): 1584–94.

Murphy JS, Mubarak S. 'Talocalcaneal Coalitions'. *Foot And Ankle Clinics,* 2015 Dec; 20(4): 681–91. doi: 10.1016/j.fcl.2015.07.009. Epub 2015 Oct 23. Review.

101. B

Tarsal Coalition can present with ankle sprains and/or a painful flat foot around the age of 7–8 which is semi-rigid or rigid. There may be spasm in the peroneal muscles and this may 'relax' in non-weight bearing. There may be a swelling medially at the site of the talocalcaneal bar and this can be tender or painful when the joint is stressed; similarly in the case of a calcaneonavicular bar, stressing the subtalar joint can give pain in the sinus tarsi (but not swelling).

Bouchard M and Mosca VS. 'Flatfoot deformity in children and adolescents: surgical indications and management'. Review article. *Journal of the American Academy of Orthopaedic Surgeons,* 2014 Oct; **22**(10): 623–32. doi: 10.5435/JAAOS-22-10-623.

Mosca VS, et al. 'Talocalcaneal tarsal coalitions and the calcaneal lengthening osteotomy: the role of deformity correction'. *The Journal of Bone & Joint Surgery,* 2012 Sep 5; 94(17): 1584–94.

Murphy JS, Mubarak S. 'Talocalcaneal Coalitions'. *Foot And Ankle Clinics,* 2015 Dec; 20(4): 681–91. doi: 10.1016/j.fcl.2015.07.009. Epub 2015 Oct 23. Review.

102. C

Tibial eminence fractures involve avulsion of the cruciate ligament. It is considered an avulsion of the intercondylar surface rather than the spine. They tend to occur in the 8– 14 year age group whilst the physis is still fully open. The most frequent mechanism is during sport with a fall onto the flexed knee but it can occur also with knee hyperextension.

The fracture is classified according to Meyers and McKeever. Treatment for type 1 fractures is splinting the knee in extension whilst the fracture heals, type 2 fractures may be treated conservatively if reduction is achieved and maintained when the knee is extended fully but they tend to require operative fixation, type 3 fractures almost always require operative intervention to reduce and maintain reduction. 60% of patients have concomitant meniscal/ chondral/ soft tissue pathology with around a third of type 2 and 3 injuries sustaining an associated meniscal injury.*

Chotel F HJ, Bérard J. 'ACL rupture in children'. In: Bonnin, editor. *The Knee Joint.* Springer-Verlag; 2012. pp. 291–323.

* Data from *Journal of Bone and Joint Surgery,* American volume, 41, 1959, Meyers MH, McKeever RFM, 'Fracture of the intercondylar eminence of the tibia', pp. 209–222.

Leeberg V, Lekdorf J, Wong C, Sonne-Holm S. 'Tibial eminentia avulsion fracture in children—a systematic review of the current literature'. *Danish Medical Journal*, 2014; 61(3): A4792.

Merkel DL, Molony JT, Jr. 'Recognition and management of traumatic sports injuries in the skeletally immature athlete'. *International Journal of Sports Physical Therapy*, 2012; 7(6): 691–704.

Mitchell JJ, Sjostrom R, Mansour AA, Irion B, Hotchkiss M, Terhune EB, et al. 'Incidence of Meniscal Injury and Chondral Pathology in Anterior Tibial Spine Fractures of Children'. *Journal of Pediatric Orthopedics*, 2015; 35(2): 130–5.

103. E

The fracture is classified according to Meyers and McKeever as grades 1-3 , (1: undisplaced, 2: hinged fragment with half to a third displaced anteriorly, 3: total fragment separation), and a fourth subtype was added to include comminution of a type 3 injury. 60% of patients have concomitant meniscal/chondral/soft tissue pathology with around a third of type 2 and 3 injuries sustaining an associated meniscal injury.

They tend to occur prior to physeal closure and the fracture involves the proximal tibial epiphysis.

Merkel DL, Molony JT, Jr. 'Recognition and management of traumatic sports injuries in the skeletally immature athlete'. *International Journal of Sports Physical Therapy*. 2012; 7(6): 691–704.

Mitchell JJ, Sjostrom R, Mansour AA, Irion B, Hotchkiss M, Terhune EB, et al. 'Incidence of Meniscal Injury and Chondral Pathology in Anterior Tibial Spine Fractures of Children'. *Journal of Pediatric Orthopedics*. 2015; 35(2): 130–5.

104. D

The neurological examination in a child presenting with toe walking is critical as several conditions such as cerebral palsy, congenital muscular dystrophy, diastematomyelia and spina bifida, need to be excluded. Children with autism and children with global developmental delay may also toe walk. Several authors have suggested an autosomal dominant inheritance pattern for idiopathic toe walking therefore a detailed family history should be performed. Idiopathic toe walking is a diagnosis of exclusion and will present as bilateral toe walking from the time the child started to walk, unlike underlying neuromuscular conditions that can present later and could be unilateral.

Levine MS. 'Congenital short tendo calcaneus: Report of a family'. *American Journal of Diseases of Children*, 1973; 125(6): 858–9.

Katz MM, Mubarak SJ. 'Hereditary tendo Achillis contractures'. *Journal of Pediatric Orthopaedics*, 1984; 4(6): 711–4.

105. C

The neurological examination is critical as several conditions such as cerebral palsy, congenital muscular dystrophy, diastematomyelia and spina bifida, must be excluded. Children with autism and children with global developmental delay may also toe walk. Several authors have suggested an autosomal dominant inheritance pattern for idiopathic toe walking therefore a detailed family history should be performed. Idiopathic toe walking is a diagnosis of exclusion and will present as bilateral toe walking from the time the child started to walk, unlike underlying neuromuscular conditions that can present later and could be unilateral.

Levine MS. 'Congenital short tendo calcaneus: Report of a family'. *American Journal of Diseases of Children*, 1973; 125(6): 858–9.

Katz MM, Mubarak SJ: Hereditary tendo Achillis contractures. *Journal of Pediatric Orthopaedics*, 1984; 4(6):711–4.

106. C

A torticollis in infancy is caused by contracture of the sternocleidomastoid muscle and is associated with packaging deformities such as DDH and metatarsus adductus. The cause is unclear but some studies suggest there may be an intrauterine compartment syndrome of the sternocleidomastoid. In addition to congenital anomalies of the atlanto-axial joints, Klippel–Feil syndrome is characterized by failure of segmentation of the cervical spine: they present with a short, broad neck with torticollis, scoliosis, a high scapula, and jaw anomalies.

Kim HJ, Ahn HS, Yim SY. 'Effectiveness of Surgical Treatment for Neglected Congenital Muscular Torticollis: A Systematic Review and Meta-Analysis'. *Plastic and Reconstructive Surgery*, 2015 Jul; 136(1): 67e–77e.

107. E

The causes of AARD include trauma, infection, and inflammation. High-energy trauma such as cervical spine fractures can be a cause as well as low energy trauma such as a bump on the head. Many causes of inflammation and infection may cause AARD, as well as autoimmune disorders such as juvenile idiopathic arthritis. Degenerative change is not a feature of childhood torticollis.

Kim HJ, Ahn HS, Yim SY. 'Effectiveness of Surgical Treatment for Neglected Congenital Muscular Torticollis: A Systematic Review and Meta-Analysis'. *Plastic and Reconstructive Surgery*, 2015 Jul; 136(1): 67e–77e.

Neal KM, Mohamed AS. 'Atlantoaxial Rotatory Subluxation in Children'. *Journal of the American Academy of Orthopaedic Surgeons*, 2015 Jun; 23(6): 382–92.

Ishii K, Toyama Y, Nakamura M, Chiba K, Matsumoto M. 'Management of chronic atlantoaxial rotatory fixation'. *Spine* (Phila Pa 1976), 2012 Mar 1; 37(5): E278–85.

108. D

A trigger thumb usually presents within the first year of life: males and females are equally affected and there is rarely any associated generalized pathology. An inflammatory aetiology may be considered but excluded on history and examination alone. Triggering of other digits implies an associated underlying pathology (juvenile idiopathic arthritis (JIA) or mucopolysaccharidoses (MPS)).

There is some evidence to suggest thumbs that are triggering (i.e. can be actively/passively extended) may resolve on conservative treatment alone up to the age of 4 but surgical release of the A1 pulley is the treatment of choice for the fixed deformity. There is an increasing awareness of minor congenital anomalies affecting the tendon/pulley system but this has not materially affected the operative procedure.

Farr S, Grill F, Ganger R, Girsch W. 'Open surgery versus nonoperative treatments for paediatric **trigger** thumb: a systematic review'. *Journal of Hand Surgery*, European Volume, Vol. 2014. Sep; 39(7): 719–26.

Masquijo JJ, Ferreyra A, Lanfranchi L, Torres-Gomez A, Allende V. 'Percutaneous trigger thumb release in children: neither effective nor safe'. *Journal of Pediatric Orthopaedics*. 2014 Jul-Aug; 34(5): 534–6.

EXTENDED MATCHING QUESTIONS

QUESTIONS

1.

A. Genetic testing
B. Epiphysiodesis
C. Referral for limb reconstruction
D. Observation
E. Hemiepiphysiodesis
F. Vitamin D testing
G. Amputation

For each of the following scenarios select the most appropriate option from the list. Each option may be used once, more than once, or not at all.

1. Progressive valgus deformity following a distal femoral fracture in an 11-year-old girl
2. Bilateral valgus deformity in a 4-year-old child with complaints of aching knees
3. Progressive unilateral valgus with significant shortening in a 16-year-old boy

2.

A. Associated knee hyperextension is common
B. Associated with internal rotation of the tibia
C. Associated with a lateral thrust at the knee
D. Can resolve spontaneously
E. Associated with obesity

For each of the following scenarios select the most appropriate option from the list. Each option may be used once, more than once, or not at all.

1. Blount's disease
2. Physiologic genu varum
3. Focal fibrocartilaginous dysplasia

3.

A. OI type I
B. OI type II
C. OI type III
D. OI type IV

For each of the following descriptions select the most appropriate option from the list. Each option may be used once, more than once, or not at all.

1. Characterized by bony fragility
2. Characterized by blue sclerae throughout life
3. Characterized by conductive hearing loss
4. The most common type of OI with least incidence of fractures
5. Autosomal dominant inheritance
6. Characterized by bluish sclerae at birth that become less blue with age
7. Present with frequent fractures and bone deformities requiring intramedullary rodding
8. Reduction in the quantity or quality of type I collagen

4.

A. Intertrochanteric fracture
B. Transphyseal without dislocation of the epiphysis from the acetabulum
C. Open reduction and internal fixation
D. Transphyseal with dislocation of the epiphysis from the acetabulum
E. Closed reduction and spica casting
F. Threaded pins
G. Smooth pins
H. Cervicotrochanteric fracture
I. Cannulated screws
J. Open reduction
K. Transcervical fracture
L. Hip spica with affected limb in abduction
M. Hip screw and plate

For each of the following statements select the most appropriate option from the list. Each option may be used once, more than once, or not at all.

1. State the fracture type(s) associated with the classification Delbet type I fracture?
2. What is (are) the best treatment option(s) for undisplaced transphyseal and transcervical fractures?
3. Displaced transcervical fractures require anatomical reduction, what is (are) the choice(s) of implant?
4. Which fracture pattern has the lowest avascular necrosis rate?

5.

Table 2.1 Scenarios

	Serum [PTH]	Serum [Ca^{2+}]	Serum [PO$_4^{2-}$]
A	↓	↓	↑
B	↑	↓	↑
C	↑	N	↓
D	↑	↑	↓
E	↑	↓	↓

For each of the following scenarios select the most appropriate option from Table 2.1. Each option may be used once, more than once, or not at all.

1. Severe rickets which does not respond to vitamin D administration
2. A 3-year-old girl of North African descent, still breast-fed with small stature and marked bow legs
3. Patient who presents with a proximal femoral fracture: she has had a thyroidectomy in the past

6.

A. Salter innominate osteotomy
B. Pemberton osteotomy
C. Dega osteotomy
D. Ganz osteotomy
E. Triple innominate osteotomy (Steel)
F. Double innominate osteotomy (Sutherland)
G. Shelf osteotomy
H. Chiari osteotomy

For each of the following descriptions select the most appropriate osteotomy option from the list. Each option may be used once, more than once, or not at all.

1. A teenager with significant residual acetabular dysplasia and a stiff hip following multiple operations. She has significant pain
2. A 4-year-old with an AI of 27°, 3 years following a closed reduction for DDH
3. A 10-year-old with an AI of 26°, 7 years post open reduction and femoral osteotomy
4. A 12-year-old girl with significant acetabular dysplasia but no history of previous treatment

7.

    A. Closed reduction and above elbow casting

    B. Above elbow casting alone

    C. Open reduction and internal fixation with plates

    D. Closed reduction and intramedullary nailing

    E. Closed reduction and oblique cross K-wire fixation

    F. External fixation

For each of the following scenarios select the most appropriate treatment option from the list. Each option may be used once, more than once, or not at all.

1. 15-year-old girl with closed midshaft fractures of both forearm bones. The fracture is angulated (apex dorsal) 20° with significant malrotation. Her distal radial physis looks partially closed (Fig. 2.1)

2. A 7-year-old boy with plastic deformation of the ulna with bowing of 25°

3. A 5-year-old boy with greenstick fracture of both forearm bones. Both bones are angulated 10–15° and the rotation is as shown on the image

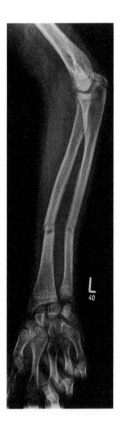

Fig. 2.1 Radiograph

8.

A. Menelaus
B. Green and Anderson
C. Shapiro
D. Paley
E. Eastwood and Cole
F. Greulich and Pyle
G. Moseley straight line graph

For each of the following descriptions select the most appropriate growth prediction from the list. Each option may be used once, more than once, or not at all.

1. An atlas used to calculate skeletal age, based on a PA radiograph of the non-dominant hand and wrist
2. A set of tables, charting chronological and skeletal age against remaining growth in the femur and tibia of boys and girls
3. A graphical method used to chart clinical leg length discrepancy over time and guide the appropriate timing and site of epiphysiodesis
4. A description of 5 ways that leg length discrepancy may develop over time, with only 1 type being linear

9.

A. Within 24 hours
B. 10 days
C. 5–6 hours
D. After initial debridement
E. Within 6 hours
F. 48 hours
G. Under 7 days

For each of the following items select the most appropriate option from the list, with respect to the management of an open fracture of the tibia in a child. Each option may be used once, more than once, or not at all.

1. Timing of antibiotics
2. Timing of initial surgery
3. Definitive skeletal stabilization and cover

10.

    A. Below knee cast with foot in external rotation

    B. Above knee cast with foot in external rotation

    C. Below knee cast with foot in internal rotation

    D. Above knee cast with foot in internal rotation

    E. Closed reduction and screw fixation

    F. Open reduction and screw fixation

    G. Open reduction and epiphysiodesis

    H. CT scan

    I. MRI scan

    J. SPECT scan

    K. Plain X-ray

For each of the following scenarios select the most appropriate option from the list. Each option may be used once, more than once, or not at all.

1. A 12-year-old boy twisted his ankle at football and sustained a 2-part triplane fracture. CT scans show the fracture to be 1.5 mm displaced. Which of the above is the next most appropriate management for this injury?

2. A 14-year-old girl falls at hockey and has a swollen ankle. A CT shows the fracture to have a 3 mm step. Which of the above is the next most appropriate management for this injury?

3. A 13-year-old girl has a 2-part triplane fracture that you decide to treat with closed reduction and K-wire fixation and she is placed in an above knee cast. Which of the above is the next appropriate management for this injury?

11.

    A. Disproportionate short stature from birth

    B. Spinal stenosis

    C. Type II collagen abnormality

    D. Genu valgum

    E. Genu varum

    F. Gross joint laxity

    G. Scoliosis

For each of the following diagnoses select the most appropriate option from the list. Each option may be used once, more than once, or not at all.

1. Achondroplasia

2. Pseudoachondroplasia

3. Spondyloepiphyseal dysplasia

12.

A. Partial transphyseal
B. Transphyseal
C. All epiphyseal
D. Physeal sparing
E. Extra-physeal intra-articular

For each of the following statements regarding ACL reconstruction select the most appropriate option from the list. Each option may be used once, more than once, or not at all.

1. An example of a non-anatomical reconstruction
2. Is very similar in technique to an adult ACL reconstruction
3. Is the technique of choice when patients are close to skeletal maturity
4. Does not require drilling across the growth plate

13.

A. Concentric contracture of tibialis anterior
B. Eccentric contracture of gastrocnemius
C. Isometric contracture of tibialis anterior
D. Concentric contracture of gastrocnemius
E. Eccentric contracture of tibialis anterior

For each of the following aspects of normal gaits select the most appropriate option from the muscle actions listed. Each option may be used once, more than once, or not at all.

1. Loading response
2. Terminal stance
3. Mid swing

14.

A. The Ponseti method
B. The severity score (Pirani, Dimeglio)
C. Complete physical examination
D. Nerve conduction studies
E. Spica cast
F. Posterior release
G. Posteromedial release

For each of the following scenarios select the most appropriate option from the list. Each option may be used once, more than once, or not at all.

1. A 1-week-old infant with bilateral Idiopathic CTEV and a strong family history of clubfeet requiring surgery
2. A 3 months old baby with severe bilateral CTEV, recently underwent a repair of her Tetralogy of Fallot. She has an amniotic band over the right ring finger
3. A 6-month-old baby with unilateral CTEV who has recently moved to your area. Treatment commenced elsewhere but apparently did not work and no medical information is available. Mum is requesting a surgical procedure

15.

    A. Observation

    B. Hemivertebra excision

    C. Bracing

    D. *In situ* posterior fusion

    E. Anterior/posterior spinal fusion +/- vertebrectomy

    F. Growing rod constructs

    G. Vertical Expanding Prosthetic Titanium Rib

For each of the following scenarios select the most appropriate option from the list. Each option may be used once, more than once, or not at all.

1. A 7-year-old boy with an unilateral unsegmented bars with significant progression
2. A 5-year-old boy with a lumbar hemivertebra and a progressive curve
3. A 4-year-old boy with a progressive scoliosis and fused ribs
4. A boy, aged 13, with a mild scoliosis and 2 hemivertebrae

16.

    A. Open Reduction—medial approach

    B. Closed Reduction

    C. Hip arthrogram

    D. Spica cast

    E. Open reduction—anterior approach

    F. Open reduction—posterior approach

    G. Pavlik Harness

    H. Repeat USS

For each of the following scenarios select the most appropriate option from the list. Each option may be used once, more than once, or not at all.

1. A 6-week-old infant with a positive family history of hip dysplasia on the maternal side but with no abnormal findings on clinical examination undergoes an USS at age 3 weeks. This shows a Graf type IIa hip with an Alpha angle of 53°
2. A 9-month-old girl recently started pulling to stand and now the family have noticed asymmetric skin creases and hip movements. AP pelvic radiograph demonstrated a dislocated right hip
3. A 10-month-old baby fails a closed reduction of his left hip

17.

A. Closed reduction and casting
B. Closed reduction and K-wiring
C. Open reduction and plate fixation
D. Open reduction and K-wiring
E. Casting alone

For each of the following scenarios select the most appropriate option from the list. Each option may be used once, more than once, or not at all.

1. A 4-year-old with a torus fracture of the distal radius
2. A 12-year-old followed up 1 week after closed manipulation and casting of a metaphyseal distal radius fracture. X-rays show re-displacement of the fracture with dorsal angulation of 25°
3. A 6-year-old followed up 1 week after closed manipulation and casting of a Salter–Harris II distal radius fracture. X-rays show re-displacement of the fracture with dorsal angulation of 25°

18.

A. Autosomal dominant inheritance
B. Widened scars
C. Type I collagen abnormality
D. Blue sclerae in childhood
E. Pain in 4 or more joints for over 3 months

For each of the following diagnoses select the most appropriate option from the list. Each option may be used once, more than once, or not at all.

1. Ehlers-Danlos Syndrome
2. Benign Joint Hypermobility Syndrome
3. Marfan syndrome

19.

A. Associated radioulnar synostosis
B. Associated cubitus valgus
C. Associated capitellar osteochondritis dissecans
D. Anterior
E. Posterior
F. Lateral
G. Posterolateral
H. Ulnar neuropathy

For each of the following questions select the most appropriate option from the list. Each option may be used once, more than once, or not at all.

1. In a traumatic dislocation of the radial head, where is the radial head most likely to be and what if any are the associated features?
2. In a congenital dislocation of not or the radial head, where is the radial head most likely to be and what if any are the associated features?
3. In a late presentation of a Monteggia fracture dislocation what are the most common features that you might see?
4. In chronic subluxation of the radial head, where is the radial head and what if any are the the associated features?

20.

    A. 45–49 kg
    B. 30–49 kg
    C. 50–60 kg
    D. Transverse fracture pattern
    E. Spiral fracture pattern
    F. Oblique fracture pattern
    G. Comminuted fracture pattern
    H. Segmental fracture pattern
    I. 30%
    J. 40%
    K. 80%

For each of the questions below, select the most appropriate option from the list above. Each option may be used once, more than once, or not at all.

1. What or which fracture pattern(s) are classified as length stable fractures?
2. What or which fracture pattern(s) are classified as length unstable fractures?
3. What is the recommended upper weight limit for the use of flexible intramedullary nailing?
4. What is the optimal individual diameter occupancy for each of the flexible nails?

21.

    A. External fixation
    B. 4
    C. Open plating
    D. 5
    E. Elastic stable intramedullary nails
    F. Spica cast
    G. 8
    H. Closed MIPO plating
    I. 2
    J. Skin traction for 2–3 weeks with subsequent spica casting
    K. 3

For each of the following scenarios select the most appropriate response from the list. Each option may be used once, more than once, or not at all.

1. Which treatment option does not have a place in the management of an open femoral fracture or in the polytrauma setting when the child is 3 years of age?
2. Which treatment option is most appropriate when a child of 5 years of age sustains a femoral shaft fracture and there is initial shortening of 10 mm?
3. What is the upper age limit for hip spica casting?
4. When using initial traction for a shortened femoral shaft fracture:
   (i) What is the weight you would apply on the traction device in a child aged 4 years? (in kg)
   (ii) How long would you apply the traction for? (in weeks)

22.

A. Elastic Stable Intramedullary Nailing (ESIN)
B. Gallows traction
C. Osteogenesis imperfecta
D. Gallows traction
E. Twisting injury
F. Metabolic bone disease
G. Pavlik harness
H. Spica cast
I. External fixation
J. Non-accidental injury
K. Gallows traction followed by spica cast
L. Road traffic accident
M. Bridge plating

For each of the following statements select the most appropriate option from the list. Each option may be used once, more than once, or not at all.

1. What is the most likely diagnosis when a non-ambulating child presents with an isolated femoral shaft deformity?
2. What is the treatment option for a child, aged 3 months weighing 7 kg, with a closed femoral shaft fracture?
3. Exclude this or these conditions after more than one fracture in a non-ambulating child?
4. What is the initial management of a femoral shaft fracture, when the child is 6 months of age, and there is initial shortening of more than 2 cm?

23.

A. Fracture will sometimes cause resolution of this lesion
B. Curettage and bone graft is an accepted treatment
C. Bisphosphonate treatment may be indicated
D. Intramedullary device is an accepted treatment
E. Radionuclide bone scan looking for other lesions is a reasonable investigation

For each of the following scenarios/conditions select the most appropriate option from the list. Each option may be used once, more than once, or not at all.

1. Aneurysmal bone cyst
2. Fibrous dysplasia
3. Simple bone cyst

24.

A. Increased Kite's angle
B. Reverse Meary's angle
C. Normal talo-navicular alignment on plantar flexion lateral view
D. Fallen leaf sign
E. Ant-eater sign
F. Additional ossification centre on oblique foot view

For each of the following items select the most appropriate option from the list. Each option may be used once, more than once, or not at all.

Match the radiological deformity to the diagnosis:

1. Congenital Vertical Talus
2. Calcaneo-navicular coalition
3. Accessory navicular

25.

A. Formation of a single bone forearm (radioulnar fusion)
B. Excision of the radial head
C. Excision of exostoses
D. Forearm lengthening
E. Correction of radial deformity
F. Excision of the distal ulna
G. Epiphysiodesis of the distal radius
H. No treatment is indicated

For each of the following scenarios select the most appropriate option from the list. Each option may be used once, more than once, or not at all.

1. A 3-year-old girl has a FH of hereditary multiple exostosis (HME) and a prominent lump over her distal ulna which is pain free
2. A 15-year-old boy presents with pain in a short, curved forearm and a known diagnosis of HME. His radiographs show marked shortening of his ulna and bowing of his radius. His radial head is located
3. A 10-year-old girl presents with marked deformity at the distal ulna and limitation of pronation/supination which has become significantly worse recently. The X-rays show a large exostosis of the distal ulna and a pressure/ modelling effect on the distal radius
4 A 16-year-old girl presents with a pain and tenderness over her radial head and significant forearm deformity. She has previously refused all treatment but is now willing to accept a surgical procedure. Her radiographs confirm a dislocated radial head

26.

    A. Thigh–foot angle

    B. Kinetics

    C. Foot progression angle

    D. Kinematics

    E. Stride

    F. Cadence

    G. Transmalleolar axis angle

    H. Step

For each of the following definitions select the most appropriate option from the list. Each option may be used once, more than once, or not at all.

1. The distance between the left-foot initial contact and the right-foot initial contact
2. The study of the relationship between movement and the forces that produce it
3. The angle the distal tibia/fibula makes with the femoral condyles
4. The study of the pattern of movement without reference to the forces that produce it
5. A measure that could help assess torsional deformity

27.

    A. 20 years

    B. 6 weeks in utero

    C. 3 years

    D. 5 years

    E. 28 weeks in utero

    F. 6 months

    G. 15 months

    H. 8 years

For each of the following scenarios select the most appropriate option from the list. Each option may be used once, more than once, or not at all.

1. Appearance of the ossific nucleus of the proximal femur
2. Appearance of the talus
3. Closure of the medial clavicular physis
4. Appearance of the trochlear secondary ossification centre at the elbow

28.

    A. Orthotic supports

    B. Chevron osteotomy

    C. First MTP joint arthrodesis

    D. Spinal MRI

    E. Night splints

    F. Mitchell osteotomy

    G. Scarf osteotomy

    H. Modified chevron osteotomy (biplanar)

For each of the following scenarios select the most appropriate intervention from the list. Each option may be used once, more than once, or not at all.

1. A 14-year-old girl who is pre-menarchal has bilateral symptomatic bunions with a IMA of 12° and a DMMA of 25° and normal arches
2. A 9-year-old boy with a unilateral flexible flat foot and a bunion that is rubbing on his football boots
3. A 18-year-old girl with spastic diplegia and a unilateral painful bunion associated with a fixed planovalgus foot deformity

29.

    A. Observation alone

    B. Bracing

    C. Posterior spinal fusion

    D. Anterior and posterior spinal fusion

    E. Dual growing rod construct

    F. Anterior spinal fusion

For each of the following scenarios select the most appropriate management option from the list. All have a diagnosis of idiopathic scoliosis. Each option may be used once, more than once, or not at all.

1. A 10-year-old girl, with a flexible 29° curve. She is 6 months post menarche and Risser grade 2
2. A 14-year-old boy, Risser grade 4 with a 20° curve
3. A 11-year-old girl, with a stiff 75° curve, Risser grade 0

30.

A. 30–60°

B. 10

C. Narrowed vertebral discs

D. 10–30°

E. Thickened ALL

F. 0

G. Thickened vertebral discs

H. 5

I. Thickened PLL

J. 20–45°

K. Collagen: proteoglycan in matrix is above normal

For each of the following questions select the most appropriate option from the list. Each option may be used once, more than once, or not at all.

1. What is the range for normal thoracic kyphosis in growing adolescents?
2. How many degrees of kyphosis are accepted as normal at the thoracolumbar junction?
3. Select 2 histological findings found in Scheuermann's kyphosis

31.

A. Above elbow cast

B. Closed reduction and above elbow cast

C. Closed reduction and K-wire fixation

D. Open reduction and K-wire fixation

E. Directly observed reduction of lateral metaphyseal fragment

F. Directly observed reduction of the articular surface

G. Directly observed reduction of the radio-capitellar joint

For each of the following scenarios select the most appropriate option from the list. Each option may be used once, more than once, or not at all.

1. A 5-year-old boy sustains a lateral condyle fracture that is clearly seen on AP, lateral and internal oblique X-rays but with less than 2 mm displacement. What is the most appropriate management?
2. A 7-year-old girl falls out of a tree and has gross swelling and obvious bruising on the lateral elbow. Her X-rays show a lateral condyle fracture that is 3mm displaced. What is the most appropriate management?
3. During open reduction of a lateral condyle elbow fracture, what is the best way to judge adequate reduction?

32.

    A. Closed reduction and long-arm casting

    B. Long-arm casting and early mobilization

    C. Open reduction and internal fixation

    D. Excision of medial epicondyle

    E. Exploration of the ulnar nerve

    F. Acute transposition of the ulnar nerve

    G. Immediate nerve conduction study

For each of the following scenarios select the most appropriate option from the list. Each option may be used once, more than once, or not at all.

1. A 10-year-old girl sustained a medial epicondyle fracture following a fall off a horse. It is displaced 5 mm. Which treatment option is the most appropriate to manage this injury?

2. An 8-year-old boy falls off a trampoline and has acute pain in the medial elbow. A&E has performed some X-rays but they tell you it is normal. You look at the AP film and notice the trochlea ossific nucleus is present but the medial epicondyle is not. Which treatment option is the most appropriate to manage this injury?

3. An 11-year-old gymnast falls off her vaulting horse onto her left-outstretched arm. She has no wounds on the elbow but has numbness in her little and ring fingers and her X-rays show a medial epicondyle fracture that is displaced 5 mm. Which treatment option is the most appropriate to manage this injury?

33.

    A. Closed reduction and long-arm casting

    B. Closed reduction and flexible intramedullary nailing of ulna

    C. Open reduction and plating of ulna

    D. Corrective osteotomy of the ulna

    E. Transcapitellar K-wire

    F. Exploration of the elbow joint

    G. Radial head excision

For each of the following scenarios select the most appropriate treatment option from the list. Each option may be used once, more than once, or not at all.

1. A 4-year-old girl sustained a greenstick fracture of the proximal ulna and anterior dislocation of the radial head.

2. An 8-year-old boy fell out of a tree and sustained a comminuted fracture of the ulna with anterior dislocation of the radial head.

3. A Bado type I injury was treated with open reduction and plating of the ulna, but the radial head remains anteriorly dislocated. You have checked the reduction of the ulna and are satisfied it is anatomically reduced. What is the next most appropriate step?

34.

    A. Physiological Response
    B. 60
    C. Anatomical
    D. 75
    E. Perineal injury
    F. 85
    G. Wound contamination

For each of the following questions select the most appropriate option from the list. Each option may be used once, more than once, or not at all.

1. An Abbreviated Injury Severity score of 6 automatically gives you what Injury Severity Score?
2. The Injury Severity Score is made up of which type of scoring?
3. Which of these is not a named part of the Injury Severity Score?

35.

    A. Wolff's law
    B. Zone of proliferating activity
    C. Sonic hedgehog gene
    D. Centrum
    E. Neural arch
    F. Apical ectodermal ridge
    G. Costal element
    H. Hueter–Volkmann law

For each of the following statements select the most appropriate option from the list. Each option may be used once, more than once, or not at all.

1. Forms the anterior part of the vertebral body
2. Governs proximal to distal growth
3. Compression across a growth plate beyond that which is physiological inhibits growth, while tension accelerates growth

36.

A. Spina bifida occulta
B. Meningocele
C. Rachischisis
D. Myelomeningocele
E. Anencephaly
F. Encephalocele
G. Lipomeningocele
H. Diastematomyelia

For each of the following diagnoses select the most appropriate option from the list. Each option may be used once, more than once, or not at all.

1. Failure of the posterior vertebral arch to close
2. Split in the spinal cord with a bony or cartilaginous septum
3. Meninges and cord protrude through a defect in the neural arch

37.

A. Allow the child to go home with follow-up in fracture clinic
B. Take a detailed history and investigate whether the child is known to social services
C. Refer immediately to the police
D. Perform forensic intimate examination
E. Perform a skeletal survey
F. Perform a bone scan
G. Perform a MRI scan
H. Perform a single film 'babygram'

For each of the following scenarios select the most appropriate option from the list. Each option may be used once, more than once, or not at all.

1. A 12-month-old baby is brought in by her crying mother with a swollen left arm. The mother is unsure what happened, she thinks her 6-year-old daughter yanked the baby's arm 3 hours ago. In your role as an orthopaedic registrar, having successfully reduced her pulled elbow, what is the next most appropriate step to take?
2. An 18-month-old toddler under joint care with orthopaedics and paediatrics with a transverse distal femoral fracture is suspected to have sustained a non-accidental injury. What is the next most appropriate step to take?
3. A 13-year-old girl has come in to A&E with a fracture of her distal radius. She has come in with her 20-year-old boyfriend only. You reduce the fracture and set it in a cast and you are preparing her discharge papers. Whilst he goes out to retrieve his car to take her home, she tells you that he has forced himself on her and in defence, she had tried to push him away but fell, fracturing her wrist. What is the next most appropriate step to take?

38.

    A. Café-au-lait spots

    B. Polyostotic fibrous dysplasia

    C. Scoliosis

    D. Pseudarthrosis of the tibia

    E. Vestibular Schwannoma

For each of the following diagnoses select the most appropriate option from the list. Each option may be used once, more than once, or not at all.

    1. Neurofibromatosis type 1

    2. McCune Albright syndrome

    3. Neurofibromatosis type 2

39.

    A. X-linked recessive inheritance

    B. Autosomal dominant inheritance

    C. Autosomal recessive inheritance

    D. X-linked dominant inheritance

    E. No genetic link

    F. Associated primarily with pathological fractures

    G. Associated primarily with deformity

    H. Associated with spinal stenosis

    I. Associated with scoliosis

For each of the following items select the most appropriate option from the list. Each option may be used once, more than once, or not at all.

    1. Achondroplasia

    2. Hypophosphataemic rickets

    3. Neurofibromatosis

    4. Osteogenesis Imperfecta

    5. Fibrous dysplasia

40.

    A. Observation

    B. Intravenous antibiotics

    C. Oral antibiotics

    D. Biopsy for pathology and microbiology

    E. Washout

For each of the following scenarios of osteomyelitis select the most appropriate management option from the list. Each option may be used once, more than once, or not at all.

1. A 3-day history of limping and lethargy in an 8-year-old boy complaining of knee pain and tenderness over the proximal tibia. Temperature 38^0 C, CRP 50, ESR 22, WCC 18.2. Radiographs and ultrasound were normal

2. A 12-year-old child with a 2-month history of thigh pain, a raised ESR and a mild pyrexia. Changes to the bone architecture are seen radiographically and there is soft tissue involvement on MRI

3. A 14-year-old boy who has had 2 inpatient admissions over the last 4 months for treatment of osteomyelitis of the humerus presents again with the same symptoms. The diagnosis had previously been confirmed on MRI and Staph epidermidis grown on blood culture

4. A 3-year-old boy with osteomyelitis in the tibia is responding well to treatment. After 3 days of IV treatment of a flucloxacillin sensitive staph aureus (blood culture results) he remains apyrexial and is now fully weight bearing

41.

    A. 3 mm

    B. 8 mm

    C. 6 mm

    D. 9 mm

    E. 13 mm

For each of the following items select the most appropriate option from the list. Each option may be used once, more than once, or not at all.

Rate of growth mm/year from the physis:

1. Distal femur

2. Proximal femur

3. Proximal tibia

42.

    A. Collar and cuff immobilization

    B. Closed reduction and fixation

    C. Open reduction and fixation

    D. Shoulder spica cast

    E. Bone scan

    F. MRI scan

    G. Ultrasound

    H. CT scan

    I. Nerve conduction study

    J. Plain X-ray

For each of the following scenarios select the most appropriate option from the list. Each option may be used once, more than once, or not at all.

1. A neonate has just been born following a long and difficult labour. Her mother is concerned she is not moving her left arm. An X-ray has excluded a fracture of the clavicle. Which further investigation would be the most useful?

2. A 6-year-old boy fell backwards off his bicycle onto his outstretched right arm. His X-rays show a Salter–Harris II proximal humeral fracture that is displaced 60° into varus and translated 50%. What is the most appropriate treatment for him?

3. A 14-year-old boy fell from a high beam at gymnastics onto his left arm. His X-rays show a Salter–Harris IV fracture of proximal humerus. What is the most appropriate treatment for him?

43.

    A. Chronic slip

    B. Acute on chronic slip

    C. Acute slip

    D. Severe slip

    E. Mild slip

    F. Prophylactic pinning of the contralateral hip should be considered

    G. Stable slip (Loder classification)

For each of the following scenarios select the most appropriate option from the list. Each option may be used once, more than once, or not at all.

1. An 11-year-old girl on thyroxine medication suddenly develops severe left-hip pain. She is is unable to weight bear or do a straight leg raise. She has had no prior symptoms. Radiographs confirm a SCFE with a slip angle of 55°

2. A 13-year-old boy with a painful left thigh for 3 days who is able to weightbear on the left. Radiographs confirm a SCFE with a PSA of 30 ° on the left and 15° on the right, Southwick grade 1

3. A 12-year-old girl, post menarche, with 4 months of right-thigh ache and 24 hour history of increasing pain and inability to weight bear. Radiographs confirm a Southwick severe SCFE

44.

    A. Osteomyelitis

    B. Transient synovitis

    C. Juvenile inflammatory arthropathy

    D. Septic arthritis

For each of the following clinical situations select the most appropriate diagnosis from the list. Each option may be used once, more than once, or not at all.

1. A child is brought to A&E with a history of a left-sided limp; further investigations find them to be apyrexial with a normal white cell count, ESR and CRP, the ultrasound confirms a small hip effusion and there is a recent past history of a URTI
2. A child is refusing to weightbear, their left ankle is painful but with no effusion on ultrasound; their WCC and CRP are elevated in association with a mild pyrexia. The ESR is normal.
3. A child presents with right-sided groin pain mild pyrexia and a CRP of 30. The ultrasound scan shows no effusion but an MRI shows acetabular changes consistent with infection
4. A 6-month-old baby is being treated by the paediatricians for cellulitis over the left shoulder. The baby has pseudoparalysis of the arm and does not like it being abducted. An ultrasound scan confirms oedema of the soft tissues and effusion of the shoulder joint.
5. A 4-year-old presents with a 10-day history of a limp and ankle swelling but is systemically well. Bloods confirm a raised ESR (50), normal CRP and mild WCC elevation. MRI confirms an effusion with synovitis

45.

    A. Immobilization for 4 weeks in a sling

    B. MR scan in addition to radiographic imaging

    C. Operative stabilization should be offered

    D. Physiotherapy focused on shoulder stability and rotator cuff strengthening

    E. Operative intervention should be delayed until skeletal maturity

For each of the following scenarios select the most appropriate option from the list. Each option may be used once, more than once, or not at all.

1. First time atraumatic shoulder dislocation in a 10-year-old girl
2. Third time shoulder dislocation in a 12-year-old boy
3. Second time shoulder dislocation in a 15-year-old boy

46.

A. Discharge

B. Follow up in 6 to 12 months

C. SPECT

D. Thoracolumbosacral orthosis

E. Rest and avoidance of inciting activities

F. Anti-inflammatories

G. Direct repair of lytic defect

H. *In-situ* fusion

I. Bone scan

J. Reduction and fusion

K. Radiographs

L. L5 vertebrectomy with L4–S1 fusion

M. MRI

For each of the following scenarios select the most appropriate management option from the list. Each option may be used once, more than once, or not at all.

1. A 13-year-old girl with a grade 2 spondylolisthesis with progression who is currently asymptomatic

2. A 14-year-old female gymnast with acute onset back pain following a training session

3. A 15-year-old boy with a progressive slip, persistent pain and L5 radiculopathy documented on MRI

4. A 12-year-old girl with chronic low back pain, a pars defect at L5 and no slip

47.

A. Above elbow cast with elbow in 90° flexion and careful monitoring of the distal neurovascular status

B. Above elbow cast with elbow in 45° flexion and careful monitoring of the distal neurovascular status

C. Urgent (out of hours) surgery with reduction and stabilization with K-wires

D. Early (first on next available trauma list) surgery with reduction and stabilization with K-wires

E. Exploration of the neurovascular structures

F. Immediate fasciotomy

G. Angiography

For each of the following scenarios select the most appropriate option from the list. Each option may be used once, more than once, or not at all.

1. It is 1 am, and a 4-year-old boy presents to A&E having jumped out of his bunk bed, sustaining a closed Gartland type III supracondylar elbow fracture. His elbow is moderately swollen, his fingers are pink with a palpable radial pulse and his nerve function is normal. Which is the most appropriate definitive treatment for him?

2. You bring a 6-year-old child to theatre urgently for a Gartland type III supracondylar elbow fracture as he has an absent radial pulse. You manage to reduce the fracture anatomically by closed means and stabilize it with K-wires. The radial pulse remains absent, the hand is pink with a capillary refill of 3 seconds. What should you do next?

3. An 8-year-old boy sustains a closed Gartland I supracondylar elbow fracture. He is neurovascularly intact. What is the most appropriate definitive treatment for him?

48.

   A. AP/Lateral weight bearing radiographs of the foot with a 45° oblique

   B. Harris axial view

   C. Excision of the coalition and insertion of fat/bone wax.

   D. CT scan of the foot/hindfoot

   E. Biplanar MRI of the foot/hindfoot

   F. Excision of the coalition and corrective osteotomy

   G. Fusion of the subtalar joint

   H. Displacement/ lengthening calcaneal osteotomy

   I. Conservative treatment

For each of the following scenarios select the most appropriate option from the list. Each option may be used once, more than once, or not at all.

1. A 14-year-old girl with a proven symptomatic talocalcaneal coalition involving solely the sustentaculum tali. Her hindfoot is in neutral. Analgesics help her pain
2. A 10-year-old boy with a 3 m history of a unilateral painful flat foot which is limiting his ability to take part in sports and a calcaneonavicular bar on an oblique radiograph
3. A 12-year-old boy with bilateral severe planovalgus feet and right-sided pain localized to the sinus tarsi, present for 12 m. His right-sided deformity is flexible. Orthotic supports have not helped
4. The same child as in 3. His left foot has a rigid deformity and some 'spasm' in the evertor muscles but no pain

49.

   A. Undisplaced fracture fragment; full knee extension on examination

   B. Complete separation of the fracture fragment from the epiphysis

   C. A Meyers–McKeever type 2 injury

   D. The anterior third to half of the fracture fragment is elevated

   E. None of the above

In relation to tibial eminence fractures, for each of the following statements select the most appropriate option from the list. Each option may be used once, more than once, or not at all.

1. For this type of fracture, conservative treatment is recommended
2. Always require an MRI scan preoperatively
3. Invariably treated by an arthroscopic rather than an open technique
4. Are often associated with meniscal pathology.

50.

A. Below knee walking cast
B. Botulinum toxin injections
C. Observation and reassurance
D. Physical stretching of posterior calf muscles
E. Shortening of triceps surae complex
F. Braces and night splints
G. Direct percutaneous or open Achilles tendon lengthening
H. Baumann/Strayer procedure (Gastrocnemius lengthening procedures)
I. Proximal gastrocnemius release

For each of the following scenarios select the most appropriate option from the list. Each option may be used once, more than once, or not at all.

1. An 18-month-old child presents to the clinic with bilateral toe walking and normal neurological examination. The parent states the child's sibling required surgery in his early teens for the same condition
2. A typically developing 4-year-old child who toe walks but has no fixed ankle contractures has been treated with physiotherapy stretches has not made any improvements
3. A 9-year-old typically developing child with persistent toe walking, has fixed equinus at both ankles with a negative Silfverskiold test and knee recurvatum in stance
4. A 6-year-old with hemiplegia presents with unilateral toe walking and has had failed non-operative measures. He has ankle equinus with the knee in extension, however is able to dorsiflex the ankle to 10° when the knee is flexed

51.

A. Refer to a paediatric neurosurgical/spinal service
B. Passive stretching /physiotherapy
C. Soft cervical collar
D. Cervical halter traction
E. Bipolar lengthening of sternocleidomastoid
F. Halo fixation
G. C1–C2 fusion

For each of the following scenarios select the most appropriate option from the list. Each option may be used once, more than once, or not at all.

1. An infant presents with a 2-month history of painless torticollis, his mother informs you that this has been present since birth. An xray has been taken but no abnormality identified
2. A patient presents with a painless torticollis, a short-webbed neck, and limited neck movements. There are several vertebral anomalies on the cervical spine radiographs
3. A child with a painful torticollis and a recent adenoid infection presents to your clinic, subsequent investigations demonstrate an abnormality of C1–C2

1. Answers: 1. E; 2. D, F; 3. C

Assessment of genu valgum centres around the age of the child, the symmetry of the deformity and the underlying cause: run through your personal list of possible aetiologies. Make a particular note of whether or not the child is of normal height and whether or not there are other associated skeletal abnormalities and symptoms.

If acquired, a unilateral genu valgum is most likely to be the result of trauma, infection or a vascular insult but it may be part of a congenital limb deformity. Benign tumours can also cause deformity.

Bilateral symmetrical genu valgum is often physiological, although skeletal dysplasias and metabolic bone disorders such as rickets must also be considered.

Cozen's phenomenon is a post-traumatic proximal tibial valgus deformity following a seemingly innocuous metaphyseal fracture. The family need to be warned about the possibility of this complication occurring and then, if it does, they should be reassured that it is usually a self-limiting process with correction over time: since the advent of guided growth techniques surgical intervention has become more common although still only indicated in a minority of cases.

Investigation and treatment for genu valgum is focused on a thorough clinical history and examination including listing the presence of pain, systemic features or progressive deformity, determination of the rotational profile and defining the cause.

Once the cause has been determined, treatment can be instituted, (a) to address the underlying cause and prevent further progressive deformity, and (b) to treat the current deformity when necessary.

Treatment for genu valgum can be divided into medical and surgical treatment. Medical treatment might range from correcting any vitamin D deficiencies to taking genetic advice if there was a major skeletal dysplasia or metabolic problem. Surgical treatment options vary considerably depending on the patient age and aetiology but could range from active observation through hemiepiphysiodesis and epiphysiodesis to deformity correction via acute or gradual means using internal or external fixation devices.

Paley D, Herzenberg J. *Principles of Deformity Correction*. Springer. 2005.

Miller MD. *Review of Orthopaedics* (5th Ed). 2008. Elsevier.

Cozen L. 'Knock-knee deformity in children. Congenital and acquired'. *Clinical Orthopaedics and Related Research*, 1990 Sep; (258): 191–203.

2. Answers: 1. B, C, D, E; 2. B, D; 3. A, C, D

Newborns are usually born with genu varum and internal tibial torsion, both of which gradually resolve. However, in many toddlers these features persist. The Salenius graph shown in Fig. 2.2 shows the 50th centile with 2SDs, it can be seen that most children should have grown straight by 2.5 y before going on to a degree of valgus and establishing an adult tibiofemoral angle at approximately 7 years.

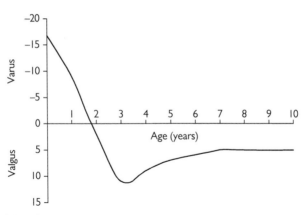

Fig. 2.2 Graph of Tibiofibular angle

Reproduced from Salenius P, Vankka E, 'The development of the tibiofemoral angle in children', *Journal of Bone & Joint Surgery, American volume*, 57, pp. 259–61. Copyright (1975) with permission from Wolters Kluwer Health, Inc.

Physiological varus is usually bilateral but in unilateral cases a diagnosis of tibia vara secondary to focal fibrocartilaginous dysplasia (or other skeletal dysplasia) should be considered. This is an uncommon condition with a distinct varus at the metaphyseal-diaphyseal junction of the tibia associated with cortical sclerosis on the medial side. Clinically it is associated with knee hyperextension and a lateral thrust (many toddlers have knee hyperextension as part of their childhood laxity). Focal fibrocartilaginous dysplasia can resolve spontaneously but in persistent cases a high tibial osteotomy may be necessary.

Blount's disease is a disorder of the posteromedial aspect of the proximal tibial physis. The most obvious deformity is tibia vara but there are elements of procurvatum and internal rotation too. When the condition is severe and long-standing there can be adaptive distal femoral changes too. There are associations of obesity, early walking and racial predisposition—with African heritage being a small risk factor. This leads to a theory that the underlying pathology is a mixture of hereditary vulnerability together with growth-restricting pressure on the medial physis compatible with the Heuter–Volkmann principles.

There are two subtypes of Blount's disease—infantile (1–3 years) and late (> 4 years). Historically late Blount's was further subdivided into juvenile (4–10 years) and adolescent (> 10 years).

Infantile Blount's is more likely to be bilateral (and is probably physiological) while late is more likely to be unilateral. Radiographically, the metaphyseal-diaphyseal angle of Drennan helps distinguish between physiological (< 11 degrees) and pathological (> 16 degrees) varus. Milder forms of infantile Blount's may respond to conservative management such as bracing. Late or severe Blount's will usually require surgical intervention which will include plans to a) correct the existing deformity via a high tibial osteotomy or hemiplateau elevation or (in mild, early cases) guided growth b) prevent recurrent deformity or accept the risk that it will occur, c) address limb length inequality.

Salenius P et al. 'The development of the tibiofemoral angle in children'. *The Journal of Bone & Joint Surgery*, American edition, 1975; 57-A: 259–61.

Sabharwal S. *Blount disease, The Journal of Bone & Joint Surgery*, American edition, Jul 2009; 91(7): 1758–76.

3. Answers: 1. A, B,C,D; 2. A; 3. A; 4. A; 5. A, D; 6. C; 7. C; 8. A,B,C,D

The original classification of Sillence and Dank (1979) divides OI into 4 types: types I and IV are autosomal dominant (AD) and types II and III are recessive (AR). More recent work has shown AR types to be extremely rare and types V–XI have now been described. These additional types are extremely rare and collectively account for less than 5% of all cases.*

Table 2.2 contains the required information about the types of OI:

Table 2.2 Table containing OI subdivision

Type	Inheritance	Bone	Growth	Hearing loss	Sclerae	Spinal deformity
IA	AD	Less severe	2–3% below mean	40%	Blue	20%
IB	AD	Less severe	2–3% below mean	40%	Blue	20%
II	AR	Extreme	Die young		Blue	
III	AR	Severe	Severe Short Stature		Bluish at birth then white	Kyphoscoliosis
IVA	AD	Moderate	Short Stature	Low frequency	Normal	Kyphoscoliosis
IVB	AD	Moderate	Short Stature	Low frequency	Normal	Kyphoscoliosis

Data from *Journal of Medical Genetics*, 16, 1979, Sillence DO, Senn A, Danks DM, 'Genetic heterogeneity in osteogenesis imperfecta', pp. 101–16.

The pattern of repeated fractures develops as a result of osteopenia, deformity, disuse, stiffness and immobilization. Bowing results from multiple microfractures fractures in long bones. Growth can be arrested as a result of micro fractures at the physis. Spinal deformities occur due to osteopenia, vertebral compression fractures, and laxity. The most common deformity is a thoracic scoliosis. The teeth are affected in type IB and IVB as a result of dentin deficiency, enamel is normal as this is ectodermal in origin.

In infancy the differential diagnosis includes hypophosphatasia, achondroplasia, and idiopathic juvenile osteoporosis. In childhood presentations, steroid use may mimic OI. When assessing any child with multiple and/or suspicious fractures, NAI must be excluded.

Herring JA. *Tachdijian's Pediatric Orthopaedics*, 5th edition. 2013. Elsevier.

4. Answers: 1. B, D; 2. F, I; 3. I, M; 4. A

The Delbet classification is used for its simplicity and reproducibility.

- Type I is a transphyseal (*through the physis*) separation, without (IA) or with (IB) dislocation of the femoral head from the acetabulum. If there is no history of trauma, non-accidental injury should be excluded. Outcomes after dislocation of the femoral head are dismal with almost 100% AVN
- Type II is a transcervical fracture. Non-displaced fractures have a lower AVN rate compared to displaced fractures regardless of the treatment received
- Type III is a cervicotrochanteric fracture. Once again displaced fractures have a higher complication rate than undisplaced fractures
- Type IV is an intertrochanteric fracture and has low AVN rates (approximately 5%)**

The Delbet classification aids the management of these fractures. Type I fractures in toddlers up to 2 years of age, which are undisplaced or truly minimally displaced, should be treated with a hip spica cast. If the fracture is unstable or displaces during treatment, small smooth kirschner wires are

* Data from *Journal of Medical Genetics*, 16, 1979, Sillence DO, Senn A, Danks DM, 'Genetic heterogeneity in osteogenesis imperfecta', pp. 101–16.
** Data from *Bulletin de la Société Chimique de France*, 35, 1907, Delbet MP, 'Fractures du col de femur', pp. 387–389.

inserted percutaneously across the physis. Children older than 2 years should normally have open reduction. If the fracture is irreducible, open reduction is mandatory.

Displaced type II and III fractures require open reduction and internal fixation. Song et al. demonstrated in his retrospective review of 27 displaced type II and type III fractures, that anatomical open reduction and internal fixation had fewer complications, including AVN, than closed reduction and internal fixation. Internal fixation is also recommended for undisplaced fractures to avoid late complications such as re-displacement. Anatomical reduction under direct vision is the key and penetration of the physis should be avoided if possible. Excellent fixation in type III fractures is possible without crossing the physis but in unstable type II fractures, fixation may have to cross the physis to achieve stability. Type IV fractures require closed reduction and internal fixation with a paediatric hip plate.

Song KS. 'Displaced fracture of the femoral neck in children: open versus closed reduction'. *The Bone & Joint Journal*, 2010 Aug; 92(8): 1148–51.

SM Chung, SC Batterman, CT Brighton. 'Shear strength of the human femoral capital epiphyseal plate'. *The Journal of Bone & Joint Surgery*, American edition, 1976 Jan; 58(1): 94–103.

Rockwood and Wilkins' *Fractures in Children* (7th ed) Edited by James H. Beaty and James R. Kasser. Philadelphia: Lippincott, Williams & Wilkins, 2010.

Delbet MP, 'Fractures du col de femur', *Bulletin de la Société Chimique de France*, 35, 1907; pp. 387–9.

5. Answers: 1. D; 2. C, E; 3. A

The blood chemistry activity in these metabolic conditions is described in Table 2.3:

Table 2.3 (refer to Table 2.1) Summary of metabolic conditions

	Serum [PTH]	Serum [Ca^{2+}]	Serum [PO$_4^{2-}$]
Hypoparathyroidism	↓	↓	↑
Pseudohypoparathyroidism	↑	↓	↑
Rickets/ Vitamin D Deficiency	↑	N	↓
X-linked or Hypophosphataemic rickets	↑	↑	↓
Rickets/ Vitamin D Deficiency	↑	↓	↓

X-linked rickets is also known as hypophosphataemic rickets or as vitamin D resistant rickets. The underlying mechanism is impaired renal tubular reabsorption of phosphate resulting in high urinary concentrations of phosphate and low serum concentrations. The genetic mutation is in the PHEX gene (phosphate regulating gene on the X chromosome). Treatment is phosphate replacement together with high 1,25-dihydroxy-vitamin D doses (note 1,25-dihydroxy-vitamin D is the hydroxylated form of vitamin D. Vitamin D is a fat-soluble steroid found in the skin).

The incidence of rickets and vitamin D deficiency in the UK seems to be increasing. Certain ethnic groups in Northern Europe are particularly susceptible, namely dark-skinned groups and those not exposed to sunlight. Breast milk has virtually zero levels of vitamin D in those groups. Vitamin D supplementation in babies and toddlers of Asian and Afro-Caribbean descent is now recommended. Serum calcium levels can be normal in rickets due to secondary hyperparathyroidism.

Hypoparathyroidism results in low parathyroid levels and subsequently low calcium and high phosphate levels. Vitamin D levels will also be low. The commonest cause is iatrogenic surgical injury after thyroidectomy.

Ford L, et al. 'Vitamin D concentrations in an UK inner-city multicultural outpatient population'. *Annals of Clinical Biochemistry*, 2006; 43(6): 468–73.

'Vitamins and minerals—Vitamin D'. National Health Service. November 26, 2012

6. Answers: 1. G, H; 2. A, B; 3. E; 4. D, E

The indication for Salter osteotomy is acetabular anteversion that persists after primary treatment for DDH or acetabular dysplasia in an untreated child. The hip must be concentrically reduced with a 'position of best fit' in flexion, abduction and IR. Children <18 months to 2 years do not have iliac wings large enough to support the osteotomy or the graft. The osteotomy is rarely indicated in children over the age of 7–9, as other osteotomies are more appropriate.

The Pemberton osteotomy repositions the acetabulum for better anterior and lateral cover: especially in the subluxated but reducible hip with a 'double diameter acetabulum'. The osteotomy hinges through the triradiate cartilage and reduces the acetabular volume: it usually requires no fixation.

The Dega osteotomy is aimed at increasing coverage, most commonly posteriorly. Although in a different direction, like the Pemberton, the osteotomy hinges through the triradiate cartilage and reduces the acetabular volume: it usually requires no fixation.

The triple osteotomy includes osteotomies through the ilium and both pubic and ischial rami. It offers greater acetabular repositioning than the Salter osteotomy, the acetabular fragment is displaced anterior and laterally with medialization offered as well. Reported results show improvement both clinically and radiographically and it is technically easier than the Ganz osteotomy.

The Ganz periacetabular osteotomy is for skeletally mature symptomatic patients with acetabular dysplasia and a hip that can be concentrically reduced. The hip should not be stiff. The osteotomy allows greater displacement and medialization whilst maintaining an intact posterior column. It is a technically challenging procedure with serious potential complications. It may be reserved for specialized hip centres.

The shelf acetabuloplasty and Chiari osteotomies are indicated when the hip is irreducible. These procedures cover the capsule of the femoral head with bone thus supporting the hip and inducing fibrocartilage formation within the capsule. The Chiari osteotomy is through the ilium with medial displacement of the acetabulum under the ilium. It provides improvement in pain and function in two thirds of patients.

Several shelf procedures are reported in the literature, the Staheli being the most popular. This can be a stand alone operation or added to a Salter osteotomy for better cover. The indications are similar to Chiari osteotomy and the anterior and lateral cover is provided from one primary bone fragment and several small bone chips from the iliac wing that are placed over the femoral head, over the hip capsule and beneath the reflected head of the rectus femoris. As the shelf matures the contour remodels into the acetabulum. If the graft is not loaded it will be resorbed.

Herring JA. *Tachdjian's Pediatric Orthopaedics*, 5th edition. 2013, Chapter 23: 'Disorders of the foot'. Elsevier.

Chiari K. 'Medial displacement osteotomy of the pelvis'. *Clinical Orthopaedics and Related Research*, 1974; 98: 55.

Ganz R, Leunig M. 'Osteotomy and the dysplastic hip: the bernes experience'. *Orthopaedics*, 2002; 25: 945.

Pemberton A. 'Pericapsular osteotomy of the ilium for treatment of congenital subluxation and dislocation of the hip'. *The Journal of Bone & Joint Surgery*, American edition, 1965; 87: 65.

Salter RB. 'Innominate osteotomy in the treatment of congenital dislocation of the hip'. *The Journal of Bone & Joint Surgery*, American edition, 1966: 48: 1413.

7. Answers: 1. C, D; 2. A; 3. A

Price's guidelines for acceptable alignment is < 15° angulation, < 30° malrotation and complete displacement in a child < 8 years old. In an older child (> 8 years old with > 2 years of growth remaining), < 10° angulation, < 30° malrotation and complete displacement is acceptable.*

Price C. 'Acceptable alignment of forearm fractures in children: open reduction indications'. *Journal of Pediatric Orthopaedics*, 2010; 30: S82–4.

8. Answers: 1. F, 2. B, 3. E, 4. C

The Green and Anderson charts and Menelaus' rule of thumb (1 cm per year growth at the distal femoral physis and 0.6 cm at the proximal tibial physis) form the basis of all calculations for the timing of epiphysiodesis. In addition to the above, Menelaus' method is referred to in other questions in this section. Paley's multiplier method uses coefficients displayed in a table. The relevant number is used to multiply current limb lengths to predict final limb length and therefore discrepancy. Shapiro has shown that not all leg length discrepancies increase in a linear fashion over time. With this in mind, repeated clinical and/or radiological measurements can be plotted in graphical form (as in Eastwood and Cole's method or the Moseley straight line graph) to give a more accurate predictor of final discrepancy. This can then be used to guide the timing and site of epiphysiodesis and its effect.

Anderson M, Green WT, Messner MB. 'Growth and predictions of growth in the lower extremities'. *Journal of Bone & Joint Surgery*, American edition, 1963; 45–A: 1-14.

Eastwood D, Cole W. 'A graphic method for timing the correction of leg-length discrepancy'. *The Bone & Joint Journal*, 1995; 77-B (5): 743–7.

Shapiro F. 'Developmental patterns in lower extremity length discrepancies. *Journal of Bone & Joint Surgery*, American edition, 1982; 64-A: 639-5 1.

Paley D, Bhave A, Herzenberg JE, et al. 'Multiplier method for predicting limb-length discrepancy'. *Journal of Bone & Joint Surgery*, American edition, 2000; 82: 1432.

9. Answers: 1. E; 2. A; 3. G

Open fractures in children are managed along the same principles as open fractures in adults. In the UK, the BOAST 4 guidelines from the British Orthopaedic Association and the British Association of Plastic, Reconstructive & Aesthetic Surgeons are the gold standard. These cover aspects such as the severity of the fracture and the open injury, the mechanism of injury, the need for urgent IV antibiotics, and suggest a combined approach between expert plastic and orthopaedic surgical teams for wound management within a sensible timeframe.

Key recommendations include assessment of the mechanism of injury, location of the injury, including marine or agricultural waste and the administration of IV antibiotics within 6 hours. Vascular injury should be treated emergently and further care should take place under a combined orthopaedic and plastic surgical team. Ideally, first debridement should take place within 24 hours and definitive wound cover should be provided within 72 hours, but within a maximum of 7 days.

'The Management of Severe Open Lower Limb Fracture, British Orthopaedic Association and British Association of Plastic, Reconstructive and Aesthetic Surgeons Standard for Trauma—2009'; https://www.boa.ac.uk/wp-content/uploads/2014/12/BOAST-4.pdf

Gustilo RB, Anderson JT. 'Prevention of infection in the treatment of one thousand and twenty-five open fractures of long bones: retrospective and prospective analyses'. *The Journal of Bone & Joint Surgery*, American edition, 1976 Jun; 58(4): 453–8.

* Data from *Journal of Pediatric Orthopaedics*, 30, 2010, Price C.T, 'Acceptable Alignment of Forearm Fractures in Children: Open Reduction Indications', pp S82-S84.

Pace JL, Kocher MS, Skaggs DL. 'Evidence-based review: management of open pediatric fractures'. *Journal of Pediatric Orthopaedics*, 2012 Sep; 32(Suppl 2): S123–7.

10. Answers: 1. D; 2. E, F; 3. H, K

Plain radiographs of distal tibial growth plate injuries have been shown to have low overall accuracy for articular surface displacement (gap and step) and subluxation as compared to CT, especially for triplane and SH III/IV fractures. CT revealed significantly more fracture fragments. A cadaveric study (Horn et al.) also reported that plain radiographs and CT were accurate within 1 mm in depicting fracture displacement approximately 50% of the time. Computed tomography was more sensitive than plain radiographs in detecting fractures with > 2 mm of displacement.

Ertl et al reported that malreduction of the articular surface of > 2 mm has been correlated with poor long-term outcomes, with 7 of 15 patients having residual symptoms after 3–13 years of follow-up.

If in doubt regarding the post op displacement following the X-rays it is appropriate to consider a post op. CT.

Lemburg SP, Lilienthal E, Heyer CM. 'Growth plate fractures of the distal tibia: is CT imaging necessary'? *Archives of Orthopaedic and Trauma Surgery*, 2010; 130(11): 1411–7.

Ertl JP, Barrack RL, Alexander AH, VanBuecken K. 'Triplane fracture of the distal tibial epiphysis. Long-term follow-up;. *The Journal of Bone & Joint Surgery*, American edition, 1988; 70(7): 967–76.

Horn BD et al. 'Radiologic evaluation of juvenile Tillaux fractures of the distal tibia'. *Journal of Pediatric Orthopaedics*, 2001; 21(2): 162–4.

11. Answers: 1. A, B, E; 2. D, E, F G; 3. A, C, G

Achondroplasia, pseudoachondroplasia and spondyloepiphyseal dysplasia congenita are different types of skeletal dysplasia: all give rise to short stature but the pseudoachondroplastic infant does not show the short stature before the age of 2 years.

Achondroplasia is an autosomal dominant condition caused by a gain-in-function mutation in the FGFR3 gene. The FGFR3 protein regulates the formation of bone from cartilage by limiting ossification and therefore increased protein function leads to decreased endochondral bone formation. Appositional growth is normal so bone width is normal; intramembranous ossification is normal so skull, clavicle and iliac crest growth is normal. It is the commonest form of disproportionate short stature affecting the legs predominantly so that the sitting height may be normal. The limbs demonstrate rhizomelic shortening: proximal limb segments more affected than the distal segments. The pedicles of the vertebrae are shortened and thickened which may result in spinal stenosis and nerve root compression in later life. Kyphosis and lumbar lordosis are common. Achondroplasia is associated with genu varum.

Pseudoachondroplasia arises from a disorder of the COMP gene (cartilage oligomeric matrix protein) which is responsible for proteins that form part of the cartilaginous extracellular matrix. Abnormalities in this protein impair natural apoptosis in chondrocytes including in growing bone. Clinical presentation is usually after the second year of life with restricted limb growth and severe joint laxity. Scoliosis does occur and limbs can be in either varus or valgus.

Spondyloepiphyseal dysplasia is a disorder of type II collagen, often caused by a mutation in the COL2A1 gene. Epiphyseal development and therefore secondary ossification centres are affected predominantly so long bones are affected more than the axial skeleton. Coxa vara and platyspondyly are characteristic features of SED and many children develop an early, severe kyphoscoliosis.

Wright MJ et al., 'Clinical management of achondroplasia', *Archives of Disease in Childhood*, 2012; 97: 129–34.

12. Answers: 1. D, E; 2. B; 3. A, B; 4. C, D, E

Several surgical techniques have been described for paediatric ACL reconstruction; some sparing the physis more than others. Animal studies suggest that providing the tunnel cross sectional area is less than 7% of that of the physis then arrest is unlikely, human studies have shown that most tunnels represent 3–5% of the physeal cross section. Physeal injury may either cause total arrest and a leg length discrepancy or a partial arrest and varus/ valgus deformity. High risk cases are prepubescent, Tanner stage 1 (bone age 12 yrs or less) with over 7 cm of lower limb growth remaining, Tanner stage 2–3 are medium risk (bone age 13–15 years) and stage 4 with a bone age of 15 years are low risk of growth complications.

Methods that spare the physis include:

1. Extra-articular techniques: 'over the top techniques' spare the epiphyseal area, however these are non-anatomical and are associated with early failure, they are usually only offered in symptomatic younger children as a temporary solution
2. All epiphyseal technique: this is a challenging method due to the limited space for fixation and II is essential. Recently new techniques have been developed with improved fixation for epiphyseal tunnels however medium and long term results are not available as yet

Most ACL surgeons will perform a transphyseal reconstruction in girls with a bone age greater than 13 years and boys over 14 years, however the tunnels will be steep and will aim to prevent fixation devices crossing (and potentially tethering) the physis. In younger patients (8–12 years) some would perform a physeal sparing procedure, others would opt for an epiphyseal sparing procedure and some would advocate delaying surgery until the child is older (particularly those under the age of 8 years) to pursue a conservative line with physio alone.

Renstrom P, Ljungqvist A, Arendt E, Beynnon B, Fukubayashi T, Garrett W, et al. 'Non-contact ACL injuries in female athletes: an International Olympic Committee current concepts statement'. *British Journal of Sports Medicine*, 2008; 42(6): 394–412.

Al-Hadithy N, Dodds AL, Akhtar KS, Gupte CM. 'Current concepts of the management of anterior cruciate ligament injuries in children'. *The Bone & Joint Journal*, 2013; 95-B(11): 1562–9.

Dodwell ER, Lamont LE, Green DW, Pan TJ, Marx RG, Lyman S. '20 years of pediatric anterior cruciate ligament reconstruction in New York State'. *The American Journal of Sports Medicine*, 2014; 42(3): 675–80.

Ramski DE, Kanj WW, Franklin CC, Baldwin KD, Ganley TJ. 'Anterior cruciate ligament tears in children and adolescents: a meta-analysis of nonoperative versus operative treatment'. *The American Journal of Sports Medicine*, 2014; 42(11): 2769–76.

Fabricant PD, Jones KJ, Delos D, Cordasco FA, Marx RG, Pearle AD, et al. 'Reconstruction of the anterior cruciate ligament in the skeletally immature athlete: a review of current concepts: AAOS exhibit selection'. *The Journal of Bone & Joint Surgery*, American edition, 2013; 95(5): e28.

13. Answers: 1. E; 2. D; 3. A

An understanding of the normal gait cycle and the muscles which function during it is essential. The gait cycle commences with 'initial contact' and can be broken down into stance and swing phases (with 7 subphases: loading response, midstance, terminal stance, preswing, initial swing, midswing, and terminal swing). Muscle contraction may be either concentric (shortens during contraction), eccentric (lengthens during contraction), or isometric (length unchanged during contraction).

Eccentric contraction is the most energy efficient. One of the key prerequisites of normal gait is energy conservation and to achieve this we use eccentric muscle contraction whenever possible.

After initial contact (which is an instantaneous moment, rather than a phase of gait), we enter the loading response phase. The natural tendency is for the ankle to rapidly plantarflex; tibialis anterior contracts eccentrically to slow this down and prevent the foot from slapping. As the centre of mass passes anteriorly, the ankle dorsiflexes during midstance, with gastrocnemius contracting eccentrically to keep this under control. In terminal stance, the ankle rapidly plantarflexes to propel the body forwards, caused by concentric contraction of gastrocnemius. During the entire swing phase, it is vital that the foot achieves clearance (avoiding a foot drop). The ankle dorsiflexes under the control of concentric contraction in tibialis anterior.

J R Gage, M H Schwartz, S E Koop, T F Novacheck. *The Identification and Treatment of Gait Problems in Cerebral Palsy,* 2nd edition. 2009, Mac Keith Press.

14. Answers: 1. A, B, C; 2. A, B, C; 3. A, B, C.

The first line treatment for the idiopathic clubfoot is the Ponseti method of serial manipulations and above knee casting followed by a tenotomy of the Achilles tendon if indicated. The Ponseti method corrects the 4 elements of the deformity in a standard order starting with midfoot cavus, forefoot adductus, heel varus, and then the equinus with a heel cord tenotomy if necessary. The management of the newly diagnosed clubfoot always entails a complete physical and neurological examination to identify associated syndromes, neuromuscular components and any other co morbidities. Evaluation of the severity of the deformity is done by using one of the established severity scores such as Pirani or Dimeglio. Both scores have high repeatability but do not offer a long term prognosis.

The treatment of non-idiopathic clubfoot is more of a challenge and the results less predictable but initial management with serial casting according to Ponseti is still the treatment of choice, although recurrence and surgery rates are higher than in the idiopathic feet.

If a patient presents to you late or is transferred in from another unit, you must always go back to the beginning with the history and examination. Unless you have documented evidence of a unit failing to achieve correction with effective use of the Ponseti Method you should always try this method first, in an idiopathic foot, before considering surgery even if this tests your communication skills with parents: they will be won over when they see an improved foot position within 2–3 weeks.

Herring JA. *Tachdjian's Pediatric Orthopaedics,* 5th edition. 2013, Chapter 23: 'Disorders of the foot'. Elsevier.

Ponseti IV. 'Clubfoot management'. *Journal of Pediatric Orthopaedics,* 2000; 20: 699–700.

Dunkley M, Gelfer Y, Jackson D, Armstrong J, Rafter C and Eastwood D. 'Mid-term results of a physiotherapist-led Ponseti service for the management of non-idiopathic and idiopathic clubfoot'. *Journal of Child Orthopaedics,* 2015; 9(3): 183–9.

15. Answers: 1. E, 2. B, 3. G, 4. A

Congenital scoliosis has been classified into 3 main categories: failure of formation, failure of segmentation or a mixture of both of these. Hemivertebrae occur as a result of a unilateral failure of formation and there are essentially 3 types:

1. The fully segmented hemivertebra has a normal disc space above and below
2. The semisegmented hemivertebra is fused to the adjacent vertebra on one side and has a normal disc present on the other side
3. In nonsegmented deformities the hemivertebra is fused to the vertebra on each side

The second major category is failure of segmentation which results in not of bony bars between vertebral bodies. There are 3 subtypes. The block vertebra is a result of bilateral failure of segmentation and has bilateral bony bars. This carries the best prognosis. Unilateral bars develop as a result of unilateral failure of segmentation. The bars are present on the concave side of the scoliotic curve. Unilateral unsegmented bars associated with a contralateral (convex side) hemivertebra have the highest risk of curve progression and ultimately the poorest prognosis.

There may be associated systemic abnormalities such as congenital heart defects or urogenital defects. Approximately half of patients with vertebral anomalies present with the VACTERL syndrome.

Thoracic insufficiency syndrome (TIS) is a result of inability of the thorax to support normal respiration and lung growth. It is associated with substantial scoliosis, a shortened thorax and rib fusions. Jarco–Levin syndrome and Jeune's syndrome are both associated with major congenital anomalies that restrict not only spinal growth but also affect lung and alveolar development.

All patients with a congenital scoliosis should have a spine MRI to exclude any neural axis abnormalities such as a Chiari malformation, tethered cord, syringomyelia, diastematomyelia, and intradural lipomas. Renal ultrasound/MRI and cardiac echocardiogram should be obtained for associated abnormalities.

Cunin V. 'Early-onset scoliosis—current treatment'. *Orthopaedics & Traumatology: Surgery & Research*, 2015 Feb; 101(1 Suppl): S109–18.

Phillips JH, Knapp DR Jr, Herrera-Soto J. 'Mortality and morbidity in early-onset scoliosis surgery'. *Spine* (Phila Pa 1976), 2013 Feb 15; 38(4): 324–7.

16. Answers: 1. H; 2. C, B, D; 3. A, D, E

The largely cartilaginous neonatal hip is best imaged using ultrasound. Graf pioneered a lateral scanning technique as the baseline for his anatomical assessment of the hip. As the sonographic findings of the newborn hip improve with age, decisions regarding treatment should be based on ultrasound examination findings that are related to age: in some centres no treatment takes place for any hip until age 6 weeks; in others the decision to start treatment is influenced by the degree of subluxation/dislocation.

The Graf Type IIa hip is described as an immature hip if the age is < 12 weeks and the alpha angle between 50–59 degrees: such hips do not require any treatment other than a repeat USS to confirm maturation by 3 m. Treatment with a Pavlik Harness is reserved for the pathological Types IIb, III and IV.

A dislocated hip in a child of 9 months requires an EUA, arthrogram and a closed reduction. If the hip reduces with a good safe zone (with or without adductor and psoas tenotomies to address the extra-articular blocks to reduction), a spica is applied.

If this fails as in scenario 3, an open reduction via either a medial or anterior approach is used to address the extra-articular, capsular and intra-articular soft tissue blocks to reduction. The choice of approach is influenced by surgeon preference: currently there is no strong evidence to guide the decision. The reduced hip position is maintained in spica cast: the duration of treatment will vary from 6 weeks to 18 weeks depending primarily on whether or not a capsulorrhaphy was performed and also on surgeon preference.

Herring JA. *Tachdijian's Pediatric Orthopaedics*, 5th edition. 2013. Elsevier.

Graf R. 'Fundamentals of sonographic diagnosis of infant hip dysplasia'. *Journal of Paediatric Orthopedics*, 1984; 4: 735.

Gardner ROE, Bradley CS, Howard A, Narayanan UG,Wedge JH, Kelley SP. 'The incidence of avascular necrosis and the radiographic outcome following medial open reduction in children with developmental dysplasia of the hip'. *The Journal of Bone & Joint Surgery*, American edition, 2014: 96-B: 279–86.

Tarassoli P, Gargan MF, Atherton WG, Thomas SR. 'The medial approach for the treatment of children with developmental dysplasia of the hip'. *The Bone & Joint Journal*, 2014 Mar; 96-B(3): 406–13

17. Answers: 1. E; 2. B; 3. E

Fractures involving the physis should not to be manipulated after 5–7 days for fear of further injury to the physis. Metaphyseal fractures may be remanipulated up to 2–3 weeks if position is lost but closed reduction will become increasingly difficult due to rapid union in young children.

Roth KC et al. 'Think twice before re-manipulating distal metaphyseal forearm fractures in children'. *Archives of Orthopaedic and Trauma Surgery*, 2014; 134(12): 1699–707.

18. Answers: 1. A, B, C, D; 2. A, C; 3. A

All the conditions have an autosomal dominant inheritance pattern although some subtypes of Ehlers-Danlos and Benign Joint Hypermobility Syndrome have variable penetrance. Widened scars are more typically associated with Ehlers-Danlos syndrome.

'Pain in four or more joints for more than 3 months' and a Beighton score ≥ 4 (probably $\geq 5/6$ in children) are diagnostic features for Benign Joint Hypermobility Syndrome.

Marfan syndrome is a disorder of fibrillin-1.

Ehlers-Danlos syndrome has some recognized subtypes, see Table 2.4:

Table 2.4 Table including Types of Ehlers-Danlos

Type	Genetic/ Phenotype	Description
Type I	Type V collagen COL5A1 gene on Chr 9	Hyperextensible skin, widened scars and joint hypermobility
Type II	Type V collagen COL1A gene on Chr 17	Hyperextensible skin, widened scars and joint hypermobility
Type III	Type I &VI collagen TNX-B gene on Chr 6	Hypermobility type. Incidence approx., 1:5000–20000. Mildly hyperextensible skin with bruising, joint and spine hypermobility, and musculoskeletal pain
Type IV	Type III collagen COL3A2 gene on Chr 2	Vascular type. Vascular rupture is possible. Thin, translucent skin with visible veins, prominent eyes, thin face, and lobeless ears. Joint laxity predominantly in hand and carpus
Type VI, VII (A, B, & C)	Type I collagen	Rare, neonatal. Kyphoscoliosis and hypotonia are common

Wolf JM, et al. 'Impact of Joint Laxity and Hypermobility on the Musculoskeletal System', *The Journal of the American Academy of Orthopaedic Surgeons*, 2011; 19: 463–71

Christophersen C, et al. 'Ehlers-Danlos Syndrome', *Journal of Hand Surgery*, American volumes, 2014 Oct; 39(10): 207104.

19. Answers: 1. D; 2. G, A; 3. D, B, H; 4. A, C,E,F, G

A congenital dislocation of the radial head is most likely to be posterolateral or posterior. The traumatic dislocation is anterior (Bado type I). In the acute situation, there is unlikely to be detectable cubitus valgus or a neuropathy but there could be a traumatic acute injury to the nerve. By the time it is a late presentation of an acute injury, the valgus is more obvious and a true ulnar nerve neuropathy may have developed. With a chronic subluxation rather than dislocation of the radial head, there is a significant incidence of troublesome capitellar osteochondritis dissecans.

Jarrett DY, Walters MM, Kleinman PK. 'Prevalence of Capitellar Osteochondritis Dissecans in Children With Chronic Radial Head Subluxation and Dislocation'. *American Journal of Roentgenology*, 2016; (6): 1329–34. doi: 10.2214/AJR.15.15513. Epub 2016 Mar 24.

20. Answers: 1. D, F; 2. E,G, H; 3. A; 4. J

When inserted correctly with a balanced construct, flexible nails resist angular, compressive and rotational forces. Pre-tensioning of the nails is an important aspect of the construct as is the material used. The titanium alloy has a Young's modulus of elasticity similar to that of a child's diaphysis. The elasticity of the construct provides the ideal micro-motion environment for rapid fracture union.

The technique involves minimal soft tissue and periosteal stripping and the fracture site remains closed. The biologically active thick periosteum (compared to an adult) is an important source of cortical blood supply and important for the growing bone. Both advantages have led to wide adoption of the FIN/ESIN technique in children.

Flynn et al. compared the use of traction and spica casts with flexible intramedullary nails in the treatment of femoral shaft fractures and found significant advantages in the nailing group. There was a significantly shorter period of hospitalization and the time taken to walk with support and independently and the return to school were all quicker in the nailing group.

The AAOS have released guidance on the weight of the patient in relation to the use of ESINs for femoral shaft fractures. One level I study and 14 level II–IV studies evaluated this recommendation. 45–9 kg is the upper weight limit in the age 5–11 years old age group.

A length stable fracture has a transverse or oblique fracture pattern. An oblique fracture is defined as a fracture whose length is less than two times the femoral diameter at the level of the fracture. These fractures should be managed with flexible intramedullary nailing.

A length unstable fracture such as a comminuted or spiral fracture may require other surgical techniques. A spiral fracture is defined as a fracture whose length is more than 2 times the femoral diameter at the level of the fracture.

Flynn JM, Schwend RM. 'Management of pediatric femoral shaft fractures'. *Journal of the American Academy of Orthopaedic Surgery*, 2004 Sep-Oct; 12(5): 347–59.

Treatment of pediatric diaphyseal femur fractures guidelines and evidence report: Adopted by the AAOS Board of Directors. June 19, 2009.

Flynn JM, Hresko T, Reynolds RA, Blasier RD, Davidson R, Kasser J. 'Titanium elastic nails for pediatric femur fractures: a multicenter study of early results with analysis of complications'. *Journal of Pediatric Orthopaedics*, 2001 Jan-Feb; 21(1): 4–8.

21. Answers: 1. F, J, 2. F, 3. D, 4. (i)—I, 4. (ii)—B

The group of paediatric femoral diaphyseal fractures aged 6 months to 5 years are generally managed with conservative methods. A spica cast is the most common method of treatment in this age group. All deformities can be addressed and the optimal position of the spica cast is with the hips and knees flexed to facilitate sitting. This position also allows control of rotation. There are specific requirements when considering use of a Spica cast to treat femoral shaft fractures, which were introduced by Staheli. The fracture pattern should be uncomplicated, initial traction should be used if there is any doubt regarding the stability of the fracture. The upper age limit previously stated was 8 years of age, however the AAOS guidelines have brought this age down to 5. There is no upper weight limit for the use of a spica cast. The guidance also quotes a threshold of 2 cm of shortening before altering the treatment plan.

With skin traction care must be taken to avoid the leg rolling into external rotation. Pillows are used to recreate the anterior bow of the femoral shaft and maintain correct torsional malalignment.

Prolonged hospital immobilization with traction and social factors, such as nursing, home tutoring, and transportation with spica casting are factors to be considered when recommending these treatment methods. Both techniques do not promote rapid mobilization and there has, in some centres, been a push to reduce the age limit for the use of elastic nails.

Park SS, Noh H, Kam M. 'Risk factors for overgrowth after flexible intramedullary nailing for fractures of the femoral shaft in children'. *The Bone & Joint Journal,* 2013 Feb; 95-B(2): 254–8.

Treatment of pediatric Disaphyseal Femur Fractures Guideline and Evident Report Adopted by the AAOS Board of Directors. June 19, 2009.

Brousil J, Hunter JB: 'Femoral fractures in children'. *Current Opinion in Pediatric,* 2013 Feb; 25(1): 52–7.

22. Answers: 1. J; 2. D, G, H, K; 3. C, F, J; 4. B, K

In a non-ambulating child presents with a femoral diaphyseal fracture there is a high index of suspicion for non-accidental injury (NAI). Studies have suggested that spiral fractures, as a result of twisting injuries, are the most common abuse-related femoral fractures in children less than 15 months. A spiral fracture of the femur is not pathognomonic of NAI, however in those under 12 months it is highly indicative of abuse. There is no clearly demonstrable association between specific fracture patterns in the femur and NAI.

Kasser et al. established acceptable criteria for femoral angulation and shortening. Up to the age of 2 years, 30° of varus/valgus malalignment, 30° of anterior/posterior malalignment and 15–20 mm of shortening were accepted.

Gallows traction has a weight limit of 16–18 kg. Applying this traction device in children heavier than this threshold will increase the risk of vascular problems, compartment syndrome and Volkmann's ischaemic contracture.

Infants up to the age of 6 months should be managed with either Pavlik harness or Gallows traction. Spica cast is rarely used in the UK for this age group. Both treatment modalities result in good outcomes with minimal complications.

Femoral overgrowth in infants is a common complication and will compensate for a degree of shortening although 15–20 mm shortening should not be exceeded. Overgrowth is a result of hypervascularity at the physeal plate secondary to the fracture. Rapid healing of diaphyseal femur fractures and post-fracture skeletal remodelling is maximal during infancy (0-6 months), which is the most rapid time of growth.

Flynn JM, Luedtke LM, Ganley TJ, Dawson J, Davidson RS, Dormans JP, Ecker ML, Gregg JR, Horn BD, Drummond DS. 'Comparison of titanium elastic nails with traction and a spica cast to treat femoral fractures in children'. *The Journal of Bone & Joint Surgery,* American edition, 2004 Apr; 86-A(4): 770–7.

Jayakumar P, Barry M, Ramachandran M: 'Orthopaedic aspects of paediatric non-accidental injury'. *The Bone & Joint Journal.* 2010 Feb; 92(2): 189–95.

Kasser JR, Beaty JH. 'Femoral shaft fractures'. *Rockwood and Wilkins' fractures in children*. 5th edition; 2001, p. 948. Lippincott Williams and Wilkins: Philadelphia.

23. Answers: 1. B; 2. C, D, E; 3. A, B, D

Curettage and bone grafting, sometimes with interim cement, is standard treatment for an aneurysmal bone cyst. By contrast simple bone cysts, though a more benign condition, can be harder to treat. A fracture will not cause resolution of the lesion in the majority of cases (85%), curettage and bone graft is an accepted treatment but associated with significant recurrence rates. Flexible nailing with 'wriggling' in the intramedullary canal to break up the septae within the cyst is a technique that provides early stability and higher rates of resolution of the cyst.

Radionuclide bone scanning is part of the workup to determine whether the Fibrous Dysplasia is monostotic or polyostotic. It is a more systemic disorder in its polyostotic form; even in the monostotic form there is no treatment that will create normal bone. Systemic bisphosphonates can be an effective management strategy: by increasing bone mineral density and reducing microfracture they reduce pain and deformity. Intramedullary fixation of the femur into the femoral neck can reduce progression of the shepherd's crook deformity by creating stability despite ongoing microfractures.

Roposch A et al. 'Flexible intramedullary nailing for the treatment of unicameral bone cysts in long bones'. *The Journal of Bone & Joint Surgery*, American edition 2000; 82: 1447.

Kushare IV et al. 'Fibrous dysplasia of the proximal femur: surgical management options and outcomes'. *Journal of Children's Orthopaedics*, 2014 Dec; 8(6): 505–11.

Herring JA. *Tachdijian's Pediatric Orthopaedics*, 5th edition. 2013. Elsevier.

24. Answers: 1. B; 2. E; 3. F

Clinical examination of the flexible flat foot centres around assessment of foot architecture, tendon power and neurological status. It is worth bearing in mind that a foot that seems flexible now, may become less flexible over time in the case of a late ossifying tarsal coalition.

On standing there is an obvious loss of the medial arch. From the posterior aspect, a 'too many toes' sign is present and the hind foot is in valgus. Asking the child to stand on tiptoes, particularly in single stance, the heel position should move from valgus in to equinus and some varus. For some children, it can be surprisingly difficult to get in to this position due to general muscle weakness and/or poor co-ordination: targeted exercises may help symptoms.

Differential diagnoses for the painful but flexible flat foot or the foot with medial column pain should include accessory navicular, apophysitis and calcaneo-navicular coalition. The ossicle representing the accessory navicular is usually seen best on the oblique or AP films. A calcaneo-navicular coalition will commonly present with an anteater sign on X-ray, denoting a lengthened, narrow, abnormal anterior process of the calcaneum, where the cartilage anlage that joins the calcaneum to the navicular ossifies but may be best seen on an oblique view where there will be no/less 'space' between the two bones. In congenital vertical talus, on the weightbearing lateral film as well as on the plantar flexion and dorsiflexion lateral film, Meary's angle is inverted: this foot is stiff not flexible.

Herring JA. *Tachdijian's Pediatric Orthopaedics*, 5th edition. 2013. Elsevier.

Miller MD. *Review of Orthopaedics*, 5th edition. 2008. Elsevier.

25. Answers: 1. H; 2. D, E; 3. C; 4. A,B,D,E

The aim of treatment is to prevent radial head dislocation and maintain joint movement at both the elbow and wrist joints. Correction of deformity and maintenance of forearm length can also be important issues. Asymptomatic lesions can be treated conservatively. Exostoses that are interfering with the function of paired bones may require early excision. Deformity correction can be achieved acutely or gradually when it is often associated with some forearm lengthening. In selected cases, it might be appropriate to limit growth of the distal radius with an epiphyseodesis. A painful dislocated radial head can be excised and a ulna-radial fusion (one bone forearm) can provide a one-stage correction of deformity

Waters PM. 'Forearm rebalancing in osteochondromatosis by radioulnar fusion'. *Techniques in Hand & Upper Extremity Surgery*, 2007 Dec; 11(4): 236–40.

26. Answers: 1. H; 2. B; 3. G; 4. D; 5. A, C, D, G

A stride is essentially two steps and is from Right IC to the next Right IC and cadence is the number of steps per minute. The foot progression angle is defined as the position of the foot relative to the line of forward progress with a negative value representing an intoeing gait. This overall observation is often a composite of hip rotation, the thigh-foot angle and the angle of the transmalleolar axis. The latter two are both clinical measures of torsion below the knee. Kinematics helps us look at and describe movement patterns and hence may be helpful in assessment of torsion whilst kinetics studies the forces that produce the movement and the moments.

Herring JA. *Tachdijian's Pediatric Orthopaedics*, Elsevier, 5th edition. 2013.

27. Answers: 1. F; 2. E; 3. A; 4. H

Questions of this type will test knowledge, but also the ability to think laterally. For example, we know from our reading that the physis at the medial end of the clavicle is the last to fuse and therefore we choose the oldest age offered. We also know the 'CRMTOL' or 'CRITOE' mnemonic for elbow ossification centres and that we will need to choose either 7 or 8 years for the trochlea. The proximal femoral ossific nucleus appears at a variable age, but when using plain X-rays for DDH we usually wait until the age of 4–5 m when we are likely to see an ossific nucleus (before that age, an ultrasound scan shows more detail). More difficult is the appearance of the talus and calcaneus but we do know that in congenital vertical talus, lateral radiographs are taken at or around birth, to look at the relative positions of the talus and the calcaneus which means that the talar ossific nucleus must appear in utero: no bones and joints have formed by the six weeks stage, so it must be later than that!

Herring JA. *Tachdijian's Pediatric Orthopaedics*, 5th edition. 2013. Elsevier.

28. Answers: 1. H; 2. A,D, E; 3. C

If you had to operate on Case 1 who is skeletally immature, then a biplanar Chevron osteotomy or an obliquely cut Mitchells osteotomy would correct her deformity and improve the DMMA. The Scarf osteotomy has had mixed results in the adolescent population. For Case 2, the gender and the unilateral deformity raises the possibility of a neurological problem which would need investigating. His flexible flat foot might be helped by orthotic supports and the symptoms might be helped by modifying his shoewear (softer boots if possible) and perhaps by night splints (the evidence is mixed). For the young woman with spastic diplegia and a painful bunion there is likely also to be significant restriction of first MTP joint movement and this in combination with her fixed hindfoot deformity means that an arthrodesis (+/- hindfoot surgery) would give her the best chance of longstanding symptomatic relief.

Agrawal Y, Bajaj SK, Flowers MJ. 'Scarf-Akin osteotomy for hallux valgus in juvenile and adolescent patients'. *Journal of Pediatric Orthopaedics*, B. 2015 Nov; 24(6): 535–40.

Barouk LS. 'The effect of gastrocnemius tightness on the pathogenesis of juvenile hallux valgus: a preliminary study'. *Foot and Ankle Clinics*, 2014 Dec; 19(4): 807–22.

29. Answers: 1. B; 2. A; 3. C, D

The management of adolescent idiopathic scoliosis is based on the skeletal maturity of the patient, the magnitude of deformity and (the risk of) curve progression. A PA and lateral weightbearing view using a 36-inch cassette should be used for assessment. When assessing the radiographs, the stable vertebrae and stable zone need to be noted, as well as the neutral vertebrae. The Cobb angle is one of the important determining factors for management of the deformity. If the Cobb angle is less than 25°, observation alone is satisfactory. Serial radiographs and measurements of the Cobb angle from the same vertebrae are imperative to reduce intra- and inter-observer error. If the curve is more than 25°, in a skeletally immature child i.e. Risser grade 0, 1, 2, bracing is recommended for 16–23 hours per day and continued until completion of skeletal growth or progression of the curve to more than 45°. The aim of the bracing is to halt curve progression, (not to correct the deformity). Bracing will only be effective for flexible deformities and is classified as successful when there is less than 5° of curve progression/time period. Operative treatment indications include a thoracic curvature exceeding 50°, a lumbar curvature more than 45°, or marked truncal imbalance with a curve exceeding 40°. Posterior spinal fusion remains the gold standard for thoracic and double major curves. Dual anterior and posterior spinal fusions are reserved for larger curves, > 75°. Younger age groups, with Risser grade 0, may also require both anterior and posterior spinal fusions to prevent a crankshaft deformity. The crankshaft phenomenon is the progression of spinal deformity after a posterior fusion due to continued anterior growth. Posterior spinal fusion aims to fuse enough levels to maintain sagittal and coronal balance whilst also preserving motion. Large, rigid curves may require posterior column osteotomies to improve the correction and spinal balance but with higher surgical risks.

Weinstein SL, Dolan LA, Wright JG, Dobbs MB. 'Effects of bracing in adolescents with idiopathic scoliosis'. *New England Journal of Medicine*, 2013 Oct 17; 369(16): 1512–21.

Helenius I. 'Anterior surgery for adolescent idiopathic scoliosis'. *Journal of Child Orthopaedics*, 2013 Feb; 7(1): 63–8.

Herring JA. *Tachdjian's Pediatric Orthopaedics*, 5th edition. 2013. Elsevier.

30. Answers: 1. J; 2. F; 3. C, E

The definition of Scheuermann's kyphosis is based on the radiographic findings, as described by Sorensen. Adolescents usually present with cosmetic deformity whereas adults present with pain. A thoracic kyphosis can be secondary to posture, Scheuermann's disease or congenital causes. Less common causes include trauma and infection. Regarding Scheuermann's kyphosis, asymptomatic children can be monitored. Bracing can be effective when the curvature is between 50–70° and the apex of the deformity is at T7 or below. If the Risser grade is 3 or less and the kyphotic curvature is between 60–80° bracing is still the favoured option. Compliance is a common problem.

Congenital kyphosis is divided into 4 types. Type I is the failure of formation of the vertebrae (anterior hemivertebra). Type II is failure of segmentation (anterior bar). Both type I and II have a rate of progression of 7° per year. Type III is mixed and type IV is rotatory/congenital dislocation of the spine. Type III has the poorest prognosis and is associated with the greatest risk of neurological injury. The other associated conditions include hyperlordosis, spondylolysis and scoliosis. If the kyphotic curvature is more than 100°, pulmonary issues may manifest. There is a high incidence of intraspinal anomalies in patients with congenital kyphosis hence an MRI of the spine is recommended. Non-surgical management of congenital kyphosis is ineffective. Surgery is indicated for most patients with type II and type III congenital kyphosis, especially those with neurological deficit. Indications for posterior spinal fusion with dual rod instrumentation and anterior release with interbody fusion include

a. kyphosis more than 75°
b. spinal cord compression
c. severe pain unresponsive to non-operative measures and
d. neurological compromise

The aim of surgery is to achieve a solid arthrodesis throughout the length of the kyphosis and to correct the kyphotic deformity. Neurological complications are higher than with surgery for idiopathic scoliosis. The anterior approach to the thoracic spine can injure the artery of Adamkiewicz, which is the main blood supply to the spinal cord from T4–T9. Junctional kyphosis can be avoided by not overcorrecting the deformity: correction should not exceed 50% of the original curve.

Bezalel T, Carmeli E, Been E, Kalichman L. 'Scheuermann's disease: current diagnosis and treatment approach'. *Journal of Back and Musculoskeletal Rehabilitation*, 2014; 27(4): 383–90.

Lamartina C. 'Posterior surgery in Scheuermann's kyphosis'. *European Spine Journal*, 2010 Mar; 19(3): 515–6.

31. Answers: 1. A; 2. C; 3. F

Significant lateral soft tissue swelling identified radiographically or clinically, palpable crepitus and the presence of lateral ecchymosis should alert the surgeon to a potentially unstable fracture, regardless of radiographic appearance. The lateral bruising implies a tear in the aponeurosis of brachioradialis. Hence it is more appropriate to stabilize a moderately displaced fracture (2–3 mm) with closed reduction and K-wire fixation rather than closed reduction and casting alone.

Song KS et al. 'Internal oblique radiographs for diagnosis of nondisplaced or minimally displaced lateral condylar fractures of the humerus in children'. *The Journal of Bone & Joint Surgery*, American edition 2007; 89(1): 58–63.

Herring JA. *Tachdijian's Pediatric Orthopaedics*, 5th edition. 2013. Elsevier.

32. Answers: 1. B; 2. C; 3. B

The secondary ossific centres of the elbow appear in sequence. It is therefore important to correlate the age of the child and the presence of each centre. An incarcerated medial epicondyle can often be missed on X-ray being completely absent on the AP film but not noticed as there is no classic fracture line, and mistaken for the trochlear ossific centre on the lateral film. It is also important to assess the concentricity of the ulnohumeral joint.

The incidence of ulnar nerve dysfunction following an epicondyle fracture ranges from 10–16%, and if the medial epicondyle is incarcerated in the joint, it can be as high as 50%. Ulnar nerve injury is a relative indication for operative treatment. In this case, it is likely to be a neuropraxia as there is no open injury and the fragment is not significantly displaced. The ulnar nerve may be more susceptible to partial devascularization after transposition following recent trauma versus transposition in an elective non-traumatic situation.

Pathy R, Dodwell ER. 'Medial epicondyle fractures in children'. *Current Opinion in Pediatrics*, 2015; 27: 58–66.

33. Answers: 1. A; 2. C; 3. F

The use of a flexible intramedullary nail is not appropriate for a 'length unstable' comminuted fracture of the ulnar. Transcapitellar K-wiring should be avoided due to high incidence of wire breakage with difficult implant retrieval and risk of joint infection. A persistently dislocated radial head must be explored to look for soft tissue interposition.

Ramski DE et al. Pediatric Monteggia fractures: a multicenter examination of treatment strategy and early clinical and radiographic results. *Journal of Pediatric Orthopaedics*, 2015; 35: 115–120.

34. Answers: 1. D; 2. C; 3. G

Priorities in initial assessment and treatment of paediatric trauma follow the same pattern as for adults. Airway is the most significant element of the assessment, can be the most difficult to manage, and can need specialist intervention. It is worth remembering that with a lower overall circulating volume but much better response to volume loss, children can maintain blood pressure and pulse within relatively normal limits before deteriorating suddenly. The increased overall surface area can also lead to rapid heat loss and hypothermia, thereby complicating resuscitation efforts.

In terms of scoring, the Abbreviated Injury Scale (AIS) and the formal Injury Severity Score (ISS) have both been used in paediatric polytrauma. There is also the Modified Injury Severity Score (MISS) that reduces the number of body areas categorized.

The Injury Severity Score is an anatomical scoring system that allows comparison of injury severity between patients. This allows prediction of mortality rate and expected outcome. The difficulty with the Injury Severity Score is that calculating the score during the initial evaluation period is difficult and time-consuming. The score does not particularly guide treatment, and is most useful as a research tool.

Baker SP et al. 'The injury severity score: a method for describing patients with multiple injuries and evaluating emergency care'. *Journal of Trauma-Injury Infection & Critical Care*, 1974; 14: 187–96.

Mayer T, Matlak ME, Johnson DG et al. 'The modified injury severity scale in pediatric multiple trauma patients'. *Journal of Pediatric Surgery*, 1980; 15: 719–26.

Rockwood and Wilkins. *Fractures in children*, 7th edition 2010. Lippincott, Williams and Wilkins, p. 75.

35. Answers: 1. D, 2. F, 3. H

Typical vertebrae are formed from 3 ossification centres. The centrum forms the anterior body, the neural arch forms the posterior body, pedicles, and posterior elements, while the costal elements form the transverse process. The zone of proliferating activity (ZPA) is closely related to the sonic hedgehog (SHH) gene, with both being responsible for anterior-posterior and radio-ulnar growth. In contrast, the apical ectodermal ridge (AER) controls proximal to distal growth.

Statement 3 is the definition for the Hueter–Volkman law. The candidate should be aware of clinical applications of this law. It may be described in pathological situations, such as Blount's disease, whereby excessive compression across a varus knee leads to reduced medial growth and worsening of the varus deformity. It may be used to the advantage of the physician, for example, in treating idiopathic genu valgum with the use of guided growth through temporary medial hemiepiphysiodesis.

IAF Stokes. 'Mechanical effects on skeletal growth'. *Journal of Musculoskeletal & Neuronal Interactions*, 2002; 2(3): 277–80.

Pownall ME, Isaacs HV. 'FGF Signalling in Vertebrate Development'. Morgan & Claypool Life Sciences; San Rafael (CA): 2010.

36. Answers: 1. A; 2. H; 3. D.

Myelodysplasia is a group of congenital abnormalities of the foetal spinal column and spinal cord caused by failure of closure of the neural tube. There are several different forms of myelodysplasia. Spina bifida occulta is the failure of the posterior vertebral arch to fuse however the cord and its meninges are essentially normal. A meningocele is a sac of dura that protrudes through the bony defect. The neural elements remain in the canal hence neurological impairment is rare. A myelomeningocele is a protruding sac, which contains neural elements and the spinal cord is no longer contained within the unfused posterior bony spine elements. Myelomeningoceles are the most common defect with an incidence of 0.9 per 1000 live births. There is a high incidence of chromosomal abnormalities including trisomy 13 and 18.

Spinal integrity at L4 or lower is considered necessary for ambulation. Motor level, ambulation and functional status have been used to classify myelodysplasia. Thoracic or high lumbar level lesions (with no quadriceps function) result in non-ambulatory patients due to lack of functioning lower limb muscle groups. As a child they may be able to 'walk' a little with a reciprocating gait orthosis (RGO) but they will be wheelchair dependant as adults. Lower level lesions are associated with improved function: a L3 level will provide a marginal household ambulator whereas a L5 level will become a community ambulator. The key level is L4, because of its contribution to quadriceps function. Patients with sacral involvement still function as community ambulators but may require ankle-foot orthoses. 94% retain walking ability as adults.

Associated conditions can be subdivided into the following categories: orthopaedic, neurosurgical and urological manifestations. Orthopaedic manifestations include pathological fractures, spine deformities, hip dysplasia, knee deformities and foot deformities. Neurosurgical manifestations include Arnold–Chiari malformations, hydrocephalus and tethered cord. Urological manifestations include neurologic bladder, renal anomalies, bladder sphincter dysfunction, and pyelonephritis.

Fletcher JM, Brei TJ. 'Introduction: Spina bifida—a multidisciplinary perspective'. *Developmental Disabilities Research Reviews.* 2010; 16(1): 1–5.

Liptak GS, Dosa NP. 'Myelomeningocele'. *Pediatric Review,* 2010 Nov; 31(11): 443–50.

Grivell RM, Andersen C, Dodd JM. 'Prenatal versus postnatal repair procedures for spina bifida for improving infant and maternal outcomes'. *Cochrane Database System Review,* 2014 Oct 28; 10: CD008825.

37. Answers: 1. B; 2. E; 3. C

If you consider a child has been maltreated, gather collateral information from other agencies (e.g. social services—there is always someone on-call who can access the child protection register) and health disciplines and discuss your concerns with a more experienced colleague(s) (your Consultant and the named or designated professional for safeguarding children in your hospital). If there is a risk of immediate serious harm, referal to the police may be appropriate as they can arrange emergency protection for the child as well as for siblings. In cases where there is genuine concern it may be sensible to admit the child even if the injury alone does not warrant that.

In cases where the skeletal survey is negative but there is ongoing clinical concern; a recent meta-analysis supports the use of repeat skeletal survey as additional imaging will reveal fractures which were not identified initially (in 8.4–37.6% of children), and which have the potential to influence the child protection decisions. The second survey may exclude the skull but include oblique views of the ribs and should be repeated 11–14 days post injury to look for callus formation.

There has been little literature regarding the 'added value' of a bone scan conducted at the time of the original skeletal survey, although what little there is would support its use in selected cases.

Maguire S, Cowley L, Mann M, Kemp A. 'What does the recent literature add to the identification and investigation of fractures in child abuse: an overview of review updates 2005–2013'. *Evidence-Based Child Health,* 2013; 8: 2044–57.

The Royal College of Radiologists/Royal College of Paediatrics and Child Health. Standards for radiological investigations of suspected non-accidental injury (March 2008).

38. Answers: 1. A, C, D; 2. A, B; 3. E

Neurofibromatosis type 1 is the commonest single gene disorder of neural origin but the phenotype is manifest in a multisystem manner. The cutaneous features include café-au-lait spots (smooth edged 'Coast of California' lesions) and cutaneous or subcutaneous neurofibromas. Peripheral nerve neurofibromas, including plexiform neurofibromas, are found in 25% of cases.

In 10% of cases there are malignant peripheral nerve sheath tumours and neurosarcomas. The orthopaedic manifestations including pseudarthrosis of the tibia (5% of cases) and scoliosis: mild spinal deformity is common but severe scoliosis can occur when the curve starts early (< 10 years). Plexiform neurofibromas can cause growth disturbances of adjacent bones resulting in deformities and limb length differences.

McCune Albright Syndrome is a genetic condition though not an inherited one. It also features café-au-lait spots; in this condition, however, they are usually unilateral and have rough, jagged edges ('Coast of Maine' lesions). Precocious puberty and polyostotic fibrous dysplasia are the other features.

Neurofibromatosis type 2, otherwise known as MISME (multiple inherited Schwannomas, menigiomas and ependymomas), is a genetic condition inherited in a autosomal dominant manner. Acoustic nerve (cranial nerve VIII) benign Schwannomas are pathognomonic for NF2, other benign brain tumours such meningiomas and ependymomas are also possible.

Herring JA. *Tachdijian's Pediatric Orthopaedics*, 5th edition. 2013. Elsevier.

39. Answers: 1. B, G, H; 2. D, G; 3. B, F, G, I; 4. B, occasionally C, F, G, I; 5. E, F, G, I

Our genetic understanding of musculoskeletal pathology is changing all the time but at the moment the genetic basis for the first 4 conditions listed is understood in that the predominant inheritance pattern for the common forms of the disease have been defined. Most conditions have a specific subgroup where the phenotype and the genotype differ slightly. Neurofibromatosis is classically associated with a specific pathological fracture (and pseudarthrosis formation) of the tibia: other bones are not affected. Spinal stenosis is common in achondroplasia but the other conditions develop a kyphoscoliosis more than a stenotic deformity.

Krakow D and Rimoin DL. 'Review: Skeletal Dysplasias'. *Genetics in Medicine* 2010; 12(6): 327–41.

Winston MJ, Srivastava T, Jarka D, Alon US. 'Bisphosphonates for pain management in children with benign cartilage tumors'. *Clinical Journal of Pain.* 2012 Mar-Apr; 28(3): 268–72.

40. Answers: 1. B; 2. D; 3. D; 4. C

Overall osteomyelitis is more common than septic arthritis in children but the two can co-exist. The femur and tibia are the most commonly affected longbones but it can affect the pelvis and occasionally it is multifocal. Risk factors include blunt trauma and recent infection.

Osteomyelitis is generally considered as acute, sub-acute (presentation > 3 weeks) or chronic. Metaphyseal areas are susceptible due to the high number of sinuous vessels with slow blood flow.

Clinical presentation has some similarity with septic arthritis (pain, temperature, reluctance to weightbear and raised inflammatory markers), however, the pain is often not so acute, movement at the joint tends to be better and the patient is not so unwell.

Results of investigations such as radiographs and blood tests vary depending on how early the presentation is and whether antibiotics have been given but inflammatory markers (ESR/CRP) tend to be raised. MRI is the gold standard test for confirmation (bone scan is an option) and changes on radiograph ie sequestrum and involucrum reflect a late/chronic presentation.

MRI is recommended as differential diagnoses are not always easy to exclude: infective myositis with/without soft tissue collections eg psoas/ pelvic abscess, septic arthritis or malignancy (Ewings, osteosarcoma, leukaemia, medulloblastoma). Any unexpected poor response or recurrence despite antibiotics should raise the suspicion of a neoplastic pathology.

The commonest pathogen is S. aureus but S. epidermidis, various streptococci and Kingella kingae are on the rise. PCR has made detection of the Kingella species possible although due to time limitation it can not help in the early decisions re antibiotic choice.

Treatment is with antibiotics after blood cultures have been taken, if there is any suggestion of a subperiosteal collection on ultrasound or MRI this can be considered for aspiration if in an accessible area to aid pathogen identification. If there is a large collection or a chronic situation with a sequestrum then surgical drainage/ debridement may be required especially if the response to intravenous antibiotics is not satisfactory.

The duration of antibiotics has traditionally been a long course of IV administration followed by a long oral course however recent studies have advocated switching to oral antibiotics after 3–5 days if blood markers (CRP/WCC), temperature and clinical function are improving with a total duration of 3 weeks treatment in uncomplicated cases. In complicated cases treatment is case by case specific and can include sequelae of pathological fractures and physeal injury leading to growth arrest.

Dartnell J, Ramachandran M, Katchburian M. 'Haematogenous acute and subacute paediatric osteomyelitis: a systematic review of the literature'. The Bone & Joint Journal, 2012; 94(5): 584–95.

Peltola H, Paakkonen M. 'Acute osteomyelitis in children'. The New England Journal of Medicine, 2014; 370(4): 352–60.

Peltola H, Paakkonen M, Kallio P, Kallio MJ. 'Osteomyelitis-Septic Arthritis Study G. Short- versus long-term antimicrobial treatment for acute hematogenous osteomyelitis of childhood: prospective, randomized trial on 131 culture-positive cases'. The Pediatric Infectious Disease Journal, 2010; 29(12): 1123–8.

Jagodzinski NA, Kanwar R, Graham K, Bache CE. 'Prospective evaluation of a shortened regimen of treatment for acute osteomyelitis and septic arthritis in children'. Journal of Pediatric Orthopedics, 2009; 29(5): 518–25.

41. Answers: 1. D; 2. A; 3. C

Physeal injuries can occur at any age. The site and extent of physeal injury can have significant long term consequences. A partial growth arrest of the physis can lead to significant angular deformity, depending on the age of the child. A complete physeal growth arrest is less common but can give rise to significant long term morbidity in terms of limb length discrepancy (but often with no or only mild angular deformity).

In practice, lower limb physeal injuries are more likely to lead to long term functional impairment. The majority of the lower limb longitudinal growth occurs from the physes around the knee, whilst in the upper limb the majority of longitudinal growth is from the proximal humeral and distal radial physes. ('From the knee we flee, to the elbow we grow.')

Typically, the distal femur gives 9 mm of growth per year, the proximal tibia gives 6 mm, the distal tibia 3–4 mm and the proximal femur 3–5 mm per year. These are average figures throughout growth and apply up until the age of 14 in girls and 16 in boys (skeletal maturity). At this skeletal age the limbs have essentially completed their longitudinal growth whilst the spine and the clavicle may continue to grow.

It is worth noting that the highest rate of significant growth arrest after physeal injury is in the distal femur. This is due to the unique geometric characteristics of the distal femoral physis. This physis has a three-dimensional undulating surface, therefore any transecting force or fracture line will tend to traverse multiple physeal zones. This makes the physis both metabolically and biomechanically vulnerable, as contact between differing physeal zones may lead to physeal bar formation and either partial or complete growth arrest.

For any physeal injury, it is worth discussing the risk of growth arrest with the family and the child at the time of injury. It should be clear that the child will be monitored for this, and that the majority of physeal arrests, if caught early, can be managed to ensure satisfactory long term functional outcome.

Anderson M, Green WT, Messner MB. 'Growth and predicitons of growth in lower extremities'. *The Bone & Joint Journal*, 1963; 45A: pp. 1–4.

Rockwood and Wilkins. *Fractures in children*, 7th edition. 2010. Lippincott, Williams and Wilkins, pp. 94–5.

Herring JA. *Tachdijian's Pediatric Orthopaedics*, 5th edition. 2013. Elsevier.

42. Answers: 1. G; 2. A; 3. C

The proximal humeral physis develops from 3 secondary ossification centres (humeral head, greater tuberosity and lesser tuberosity). The secondary ossification centre for the humeral head usually appears between the ages of 4 and 6 months. Generally, infants and small children with proximal humeral physeal injuries have Salter-Harris type I injuries. Hence X-rays may be of little help, whereas ultrasound is useful not only to confirm fractures with displacement of the bony meta-diaphysis relative to the cartilaginous humeral head but also to rule out differential diagnoses such a glenohumeral joint dislocation and septic arthritis with a joint effusion.

It is also important to consider that both neonatal shoulder injuries (fractured clavicle or a physeal separation) might be associated with a brachial plexus injury as indeed may the higher velocity scenarios outlined in 2 and 3.

Pahlavan S et al. 'Proximal humerus fractures in the pediatric population: a systemic review'. *Journal of Children's Orthopaedics*, 2011; 5(3): 187–94.

Herring JA. *Tachdijian's Pediatric Orthopaedics*, 5th edition. 2013. Elsevier.

43. Answers: 1. C, D, F; 2. C, E, F, G; 3. B, D

Clinical presentation of SUFE can vary from acute, severe groin pain and inability to weightbear to a several week/month history of thigh/knee pain, a mixed picture of a previous episode of bad groin pain followed by subsequent dull thigh pain is also common. Examination may reveal a leg that lies in external rotation and flexes up into external rotation. Flexion may be limited and a leg length discrepancy may be noticeable.

Diagnosis is based on radiographic changes, best seen on the frog lateral image, including; decreased epiphyseal height, widening of the physis, Trethowan's sign, the metaphyseal blanch sign of Steel and, if the slip is chronic, callus formation and signs of remodelling posteriorly/inferiorly.

Further imaging is not required unless the vascularity of the femoral epiphysis needs to be defined in which case a radioisotope bone scan or perfusion MRI should be performed.

There are several classification and grading systems:

The Loder Classification:

- Stable: patient is able to weightbear through the affected leg
- Unstable: patient is unable to weightbear at all (with/without crutches)

If the patient is able to lift their leg off the bed, the slip is likely to be stable. If they can not, it may well be unstable (or they are simply anxious and in pain).*

Temporal classification:

- Acute: symptoms for < 3 weeks
- Chronic: symptoms for > 3 weeks. Longer history of groin pain (often several months) with callus and remodelling changes seen on X-ray
- Acute-on-chronic: a short history of severe pain with a preceding longer history of dull pain

* Data from *International Scholarly Research Notices Orthopedics*, 2011, Randall T. Loder RT and Skopelja EN. 'The Epidemiology and Demographics of Slipped Capital Femoral Epiphysis'.

Southwick slip angle (measures the severity of the slip by comparing the affected side with the non-affected side using the lateral head shaft angle)

Grade I—Angle difference of < 30°

Grade II—Angle difference of 30–50°

Grade III—Angle difference of > 50°*

MacLean JG, Reddy SK. 'The contralateral slip. An avoidable complication and indication for prophylactic pinning in slipped upper femoral epiphysis'. *The Bone & Joint Journal*, 2006; 88(11): 1497–501.

Novais EN, Millis MB. 'Slipped capital femoral epiphysis: prevalence, pathogenesis, and natural history'. *Clinical Orthopaedics and Related Research*. 2012; 470(12): 3432–8.

Randall T. Loder RT and Skopelja EN. 'The Epidemiology and Demographics of Slipped Capital Femoral Epiphysis'. In *International Scholarly Research Notices Orthopedics*, 2011. doi: 10.5402/2011/486512

44. Answers: 1. B; 2. A; 3. A; 4. D; 5. C

Most cases of septic arthritis are primary infections via a haematogenous route or by direct inoculation but secondary joint involvement can occur via direct spread of an intra-articular (femoral neck, proximal humerus, radial head, jaw) metaphyseal osteomyelitis.

The commonest pathogens are staph aureus and streptococcus (coagulase negative, group A and group B) and the incidence of Kingella kingae is increasing. Haemophilus influenza is now rare in children who have been immunized with the HiB vaccine. Salmonella is found in immunodeficient patients and those with Sickle Cell disease although staph. aureus still remains the commonest pathogen in this group.

Presentation is typically with either a refusal to weightbear or disuse and pain on moving the limb in association with a mild pyrexia, loss of appetite and general malaise. Septic arthritis of the hip can easily be 'missed' if the child presents with knee pain.

The differential diagnosis can be wide and includes transient synovitis, juvenile idiopathic arthritis, psoas abscess, pericapsular myositis, osteomyelitis, Perthes, malignancy (e.g. lymphoma) and trauma.

An appropriate history, examination and radiographs should be supplemented by blood tests (FBC, U&Es, CRP, ESR, cultures) and ultrasound of the joint if indicated. These investigations can usually differentiate septic arthritis from all other differentials except transient synovitis which is itself, by definition, a diagnosis of exclusion. Transient synovitis presents very similarly to septic arthritis: several parameters, including a joint effusion, occur in both.

A septic arthritis must have the joint drained and irrigated, delayed treatment may result in the enzymatic degradation of cartilage secondary to the presence of neutrophils. Some centres advocate percutaneous aspiration and irrigation and only proceed to surgical arthrotomy if there is no improvement. Any aspirate should be inspected (is it clear, turbid or purulent?) and sent for urgent microscopy and Gram stain.

Antibiotics should be commenced immediately after aspiration/washout and not before unless there is clear delay and the child shows signs of systemic sepsis. Microbiology from the aspirate can be negative in over half of cases.

* Data from *American Family Physician*, 57, 1998, Loder RT, 'Slipped Capital Femoral Epiphysis', pp. 2134–2142.

Traditionally IV antibiotics have been used for several weeks but recent studies have shown that if the child presents with a short uncomplicated case of primary joint sepsis, responds promptly to treatment (by remaining apyrexial for 48 hours with improving function and/or weightbearing) and has improving inflammatory markers then 2–4 days IV followed by 7–10 days of oral antibiotics is all that is required. More complex cases that need to be treated for longer include cases with delayed presentation, septicaemia (that could result in multifocal infections), and joint involvement secondary to osteomeyelits.

Caird MS, Flynn JM, Leung YL, Millman JE, D'Italia JG, Dormans JP. 'Factors distinguishing septic arthritis from transient synovitis of the hip in children. A prospective study'. *The Journal of Bone & Joint Surgery,* American edition, 2006; 88(6): 1251–7.

Mignemi ME, Menge TJ, Cole HA, Mencio GA, Martus JE, Lovejoy S, et al. 'Epidemiology, diagnosis, and treatment of pericapsular pyomyositis of the hip in children'. *Journal of Pediatric Orthopaedics,* 2014; 34(3): 316–25.

Peltola H, Paakkonen M, Kallio P, Kallio MJ. 'Osteomyelitis-Septic Arthritis (OM-SA) Study Group. Prospective, randomized trial of 10 days versus 30 days of antimicrobial treatment, including a short-term course of parenteral therapy, for childhood septic arthritis'. *Clinical infectious diseases:* an official publication of the *Infectious Diseases Society of America,* 2009; 48(9): 1201–10.

Lyon RM, Evanich JD. 'Culture-negative septic arthritis in children'. *Journal of Pediatric Orthopaedics,* 1999; 19(5): 655–9.

45. Answers: 1. D; 2. B, C, D; 3. B, C, D

The recurrence risk is high following traumatic dislocation of the shoulder in children and does not diminish with time (up to 2 years). Adolescents presenting with a first time dislocation are thought to have a higher risk of recurrence (around 75%) compared to younger patients (10–13 years old).

Treatment for a first time traumatic dislocation of the shoulder is physiotherapy focusing on stabilization and rotator cuff strengthening following a short (1 week) period of immobilization. Patients with recurrent instability should undergo MRI imaging and surgical stabilization should be offered irrespective of whether the physis is open or closed, particularly to those shown to have a Bankart lesion. However, recurrent dislocation despite surgical intervention has been reported to be up to 20–30% and there are only a small number of studies to justify this management.

In children under 15 years of age, there is little data regarding the natural history of shoulder instability or the outcomes of surgical intervention

Cordischi K, Li X, Busconi B. 'Intermediate outcomes after primary traumatic anterior shoulder dislocation in skeletally immature patients aged 10 to 13 years'. *Orthopedics,* 2009; 32(9).

Deitch J, Mehlman CT, Foad SL, Obbehat A, Mallory M. 'Traumatic anterior shoulder dislocation in adolescents'. *The American Journal of Sports Medicine.* 2003; 31(5): 758–63.

Khan A, Samba A, Pereira B, Canavese F. 'Anterior dislocation of the shoulder in skeletally immature patients: comparison between non-operative treatment versus open Latarjet's procedure'. *The Bone & Joint Journal,* 2014; 96-B(3): 354–9.

Li X, Ma R, Nielsen NM, Gulotta LV, Dines JS, Owens BD. 'Management of shoulder instability in the skeletally immature patient'. *The Journal of the American Academy of Orthopaedic Surgeons,* 2013; 21(9): 529–37.

Roberts SB, Beattie N, McNiven ND, Robinson CM. 'The natural history of primary anterior dislocation of the glenohumeral joint in adolescence'. *The Bone & Joint Journal,* 2015; 97-B(4): 520–6.

46. Answers: 1. B; 2. E, F, K, M; 3. H, J; 4. B, E, F.

Spondylolysis and spondylolisthesis are common causes of adolescent lower back pain.
There are hereditary factors which predispose some patients to developing spondylolysis and spondylolisthesis. Repetitive and vigorous sporting activities, which involve hyperextension and rotational loads, can contribute to this pathological process in the lumbar spine. Several terms need to be clearly described to avoid confusion. The pars interarticularis is the bony connection between the superior and inferior processes. Spondylolysis is the term used to describe the anatomic defect of the pars interarticularis without displacement of the vertebral body. Spondylolisthesis describes the forward translation of one vertebra relative to the next caudal vertebral segment. The Wiltse-Newman classification is the most widely used classification of the type of spondylolisthesis. Type I is the dysplastic type and usually occurs during the adolescent growth spurt. It is secondary to congenital abnormalities of the lumbosacral articulation, with malorientation and hypoplasia of the L5–S1 facet joint articulation. The pars is poorly developed and elongated which allows for slippage of L5 on S1. As the posterior neural arch is intact, with a spondylolisthesis there is increasing risk of neurological symptoms due to entrapment of the nerve roots. Type II is the isthmic type. This is the most common spondylolytic disorder amongst adolescence. The defect develops before skeletal maturity. There are 3 subtypes; type II A occurs when there is a fatigue stress fracture which does not heal normally due to constant motion and poor mechanical environment. A resulting fibrous band of tissue develops between the fracture edges. Type II B describes an elongated intact pars interarticularis as a result of repeated micro-fractures that heal. Type II C is a result of an acute fracture due to trauma. Type III is degenerative, IV is traumatic, V is neoplastic and VI is iatrogenic. (Marchetti and Bartolozzi have proposed an alternative classification system, which is based on two main categories, developmental and acquired.) 25% of patients with spondylolysis have an associated spondylolisthesis. Several risk factors have been identified for isthmic spondylolisthesis including repetitive extension activities such as gymnastics, tennis players and swimmers, male gender and a family history.

Lee GW, Lee SM, Ahn MW, Kim HJ, Yeom JS. 'Comparison of posterolateral lumbar fusion and posterior lumbar interbody fusion for patients younger than 60 years with isthmic spondylolisthesis'. *Spine* (Phila Pa 1976), 2014 Nov 15; 39(24): E1475–80.

Martiniani M, Lamartina C, Specchia N. '"*In situ*" fusion or reduction in high-grade high dysplastic developmental spondylolisthesis (HDSS)'. *European Spine Journal,* 2012 May; 21 Suppl 1: S134–40.

47. Answers: 1. C; 2. B; 3. A

For further information on why these answers are relevant please review the British Orthopaedic Association Standards for Trauma

British Orthopaedic Association Standards for Trauma (BOAST) 11: *Supracondylar fractures of the humerus in children.*

48. Answers: 1. C; 2. I; 3. A, H; 4. A, D, E.

A symptomatic coalition limited to the anterior/middle facets of the subtalar joint is suitable for excision especially if the hindfoot is well aligned. Once it involves a substantial amount of the posterior facet, simple excision may render the joint unstable and painful and a subtalar joint fusion may be more appropriate. If the hind foot is in significant varus/valgus this will have to be corrected simultaneously at the site of the fusion or with an additional displacement/realignment calcaneal osteotomy.

A patient with a 3 m history of symptoms from a proven calcaneonavicular coalition could still be treated conservatively. Further imaging is probably only indicated if you suspect there is more than one coalition present: multiple coalitions do occur but the exact incidence is not known.

Excised coalitions can be treated with interposition of fat grafts, bone wax or nothing. EDB muscle is rarely large enough to fill the hole left by the calcaneonavicular bar excision and if used, may have a detrimental effect on the contour of the foot and occasionally on wound healing.

Most tarsal coalitions do not present with severe planovalgus deformities and with bilateral deformities and unilateral pain and asymmetric clinical findings, other causes for the problems must be excluded. The symptomatic flexible severe flat foot might require surgical treatment but should not require investigation other than plain radiographs. A calcaneal lengthening/displacement osteotomy might need to be supplemented by medial soft tissue reefing or a cuneiform osteotomy.

Bouchard M and Mosca VS. Flatfoot deformity in children and adolescents: surgical indications and management. Review article. The Journal of the American Academy of Orthopaedic Surgeons, 2014 Oct; 22(10): 623–32. doi: 10.5435/JAAOS-22-10-623

Mosca VS, et al. 'Talocalcaneal tarsal coalitions and the calcaneal lengthening osteotomy: the role of deformity correction'. The Journal of Bone & Joint Surgery, American edition, 2012 Sept 5; 94(17): 1584–94.

Murphy JS, Mubarak S. 'Talocalcaneal Coalitions'. Foot and Ankle Clinics, 2015 Dec; 20(4): 681–91. doi: 10.1016/j.fcl.2015.07.009. Epub 2015 Oct 23.

49. Answers: 1. A; 2. E; 3. C, D; 4. B, C, D

60% of these patients have concomitant meniscal/chondral/soft tissue pathology with around a third of type 2 and 3 injuries sustaining an associated meniscal injury.

Operative fixation can be done as an open or arthroscopic procedure and various methods of fixation have been described: cannulated screws are commonly used but described techniques also use K-wires, wire sutures or absorbable screws. Ideally the physis should not be crossed but this is not always possible. Any associated meniscal tears or entrapment should be addressed. Post-operatively the knee should be immobilized in full extension. Any transphyseal fixation should be removed early to reduce the risk of partial physeal arrest. Complications of treatment include ACL laxity (which may be related to the original injury rather than the treatment), physeal growth disturbance and arthrofibrosis.

Chotel F HJ, Bérard J. 'ACL rupture in children'. In: Bonnin, editor. The Knee Joint. 2012 Springer-Verlag, pp. 291–323.

Leeberg V, Lekdorf J, Wong C, Sonne-Holm S. 'Tibial eminentia avulsion fracture in children—a systematic review of the current literature'. Danish Medical Journal, 2014; 61(3): A4792.

Merkel DL, Molony JT, Jr. 'Recognition and management of traumatic sports injuries in the skeletally immature athlete'. International Journal of Sports Physical Therapy. 2012; 7(6): 691–704.

Mitchell JJ, Sjostrom R, Mansour AA, Irion B, Hotchkiss M, Terhune EB, et al. 'Incidence of Meniscal Injury and Chondral Pathology in Anterior Tibial Spine Fractures of Children'. Journal of Pediatric Orthopedics, 2015; 35(2): 130–5.

50. Answers: 1. C; 2. A, F; 3. G, 4. B, H.

After a detailed history including an account of the birth history, developmental milestones and the family history, clinical examination will ascertain if the presentation of toewalking is unilateral or bilateral. In unilateral cases always consider a dislocated hip or congenital anomaly. Occasionally, referral to a neurologist, imaging and EMG studies are required. It is important to exclude other causes of toe walking after the age of 2, such as cerebral palsy, congenital muscular dystrophy, autism, global developmental delay, HMSN (Hereditary Motor Sensory Neuropathies) and other disorders. A detailed neurological examination is essential. It is important to establish a gait history: has the child always been a toe-walker or did a normal heel-toe pattern precede the tip-toe pattern. In a boy this latter scenario suggests a diagnosis of Duchenne Muscular Dystrophy. Idiopathic toe walking may be suggested by the absence of any true shortening of the tendoachilles but, over time, a contracture does usually occur.

The Silverskiold test is important to differentiate whether the reduced range of ankle movement, is caused by the gastrocnemius alone or the entire triceps surae muscle-tendon complex.

There is no evidence to support the theory that children who continue to toe walk into adolescence will have poor functional outcomes. Patients younger than the age of 2 generally require observation, as idiopathic toe walking is often part of maturation of the normal gait cycle. Heel cord contractures can be treated with physiotherapy stretching of the posterior calf structures. If the idiopathic toe walker has the ability to passively dorsiflex the foot beyond 15°, no treatment is required apart from further follow up. BK stretching casts have shown limited success particularly if the fixed deformity is more than 10–20°.

The surgical aim for treating toe walkers consists of lengthening the triceps surae muscle-tendon complex. Indications for surgery include fixed ankle equinus contractures, compensatory knee recurvatum or recurrence following a trial of non-surgical treatment but the underlying pathoaetiology must be borne in mind.

Botulinum toxin injections have been useful in the management of dynamic contractures in children who toe walk due to a neurological disability such as cerebral palsy and such treatment may facilitate a stretching programme. There is no evidence that botulinum toxin injections are useful in idiopathic toe walking.

Oetgen ME, Peden S. 'Idiopathic toe walking'. *The Journal of the American Academy of Orthopaedic Surgeons*, 2012 May; 20(5): 292–300.

Williams CM, Tinley P, Curtin M. 'Idiopathic toe walking and sensory processing dysfunction'. *Journal of Foot and Ankle Research*, 2010 Aug 16; 3: 16.

Westberry DE, Davids JR, Davis RB, de Morais Filho MC. 'Idiopathic toe walking: a kinematic and kinetic profile'. *Journal of Pediatric Orthopaedics*, 2008 Apr-May; 28(3): 352–8.

51. Answers: 1. B; 2. A; 3. A, D

Torticollis can be an isolated pathology or part of a syndrome. Klippel–Feil syndrome is due to failure of normal segmentation and thus there are multiple abnormal cervical spine segments. It is associated with Sprengels deformity in 33% of cases. Basilar invagination and atlantoaxial instability are commonly associated with this syndrome. Radiographic imaging, specifically the lateral radiograph, is used to diagnose basilar invagination.

Congenital muscular torticollis presents with a head tilt towards the affected side and a palpable mass is often noted in the sternocleidomastoid muscle (SCM) within the first 4 weeks of life. If needed, ultrasound can be used to differentiate this mass from more serious underlying neurological or osseous abnormalities. Congenital muscular torticollis is treated initially with passive stretching exercises but may require a distal Z-plasty of the sternal head and a fascial release of the clavicular head of SCM if a significant tilt is still present at the age of 3 or more. Left untreated, significant facial asymmetry can develop.

Patients with Klippel–Feil syndrome present with the classic triad of low posterior hair line, short webbed neck and limited cervical spine range of movement. Other findings include jaw anomalies and scoliosis.

Children with atlantoaxial rotatory displacement (AARD) usually present with a tilted head, neck pain and headaches. This presentation is usually acute and in the absence of congenital muscular torticollis or congenital abnormality. Surgical reduction is indicated if there is basilar invagination, myelopathy and associated instability. Fusion of occiput to C2 or C3 is then performed.

Nilesh K, Mukherji S. 'Congenital muscular torticollis'. *Annals of Maxillofacial Surgery*, 2013 Jul; 3(2): 198–200.

Haque S, Bilal Shafi BB, Kaleem M. 'Imaging of torticollis in children'. *Radiographics*, 2012 Mar-Apr; 32(2): 557–71.

Herman MJ. 'Torticollis in infants and children: common and unusual causes'. *Instructional Course Lectures*, 2006; 55: 647–53.

Viva 1   Questions

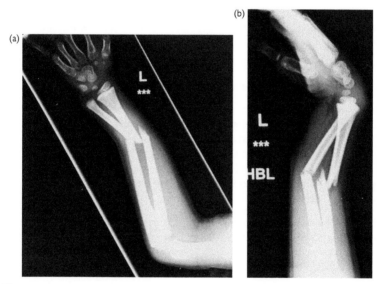

Fig. 3.1 X-rays

This seven-year-old boy fell 6 ft out of a tree onto his left arm. Describe these X-rays (Fig. 3.1).

Is the fracture malrotated? How can you tell?

What is the likely cause of the torsional deformity?

This boy has a 2 mm puncture wound on the volar aspect of his forearm. How would you manage him?

Briefly run through your surgical technique for elastic stable intramedullary nail fixation (ESIN) (or flexible intramedullary nailing FIN).

Are you aware of any complications of elastic (flexible) nailing of the forearm? Should we be plating instead?

Viva 1   Answers

This seven-year-old boy fell 6 ft out of a tree onto his left arm. Describe these X-rays (Fig. 3.1)

Anteroposterior (AP) and lateral forearm radiographs of a skeletally-immature patient showing complete midshaft fractures of both radius and ulna at the same level. The radius may be comminuted. There is significant angulation in both planes and the radius is completely translated/ 'off ended'.

Is the fracture malrotated? How can you tell?

Yes. In the X-ray on the left, the profile of the wrist is essentially AP but the elbow is a lateral view. Also, there is a discrepancy in the width and cortical thickness either side of the fracture, especially of the radius. Evans also advocated the use of the bicipital tuberosity as a landmark to ensure restoration of rotational alignment: in the AP view, the bicipital tuberosity is medial with the forearm in supination, posterior with the forearm in neutral position, and lateral with the forearm in pronation.

What is the likely cause of the torsional deformity?

In this case of a middle-third fracture of the forearm, the fracture is below the insertion of pronator teres, hence the proximal radial fragment is balanced in neutral rotation by the action of supinator and pronator teres. It is however flexed by biceps. The distal fragment is pronated and displaced in an ulnar direction by pronator quadratus.

This boy has a 2 mm puncture wound on the volar aspect of his forearm. How would you manage him?

This boy has fallen from a height, hence my priority is to ensure he has no other concurrent serious injuries. I would therefore initially assess him using ATLS protocols. Specifically, for the forearm injury, this is an open fracture (Gustilo-Anderson grade I) and I would treat it in keeping with the BOAST/BAPRAS guidelines for open fractures:

1. Commence intravenous (IV) antibiotics (Co-amoxiclav, Cefuroxime or Clindamycin) promptly (ideally within 3 h of injury)
2. Record status of tetanus immunization and prescribe immunoglobulin or booster if dictated by environment of the injury
3. Systematically and repeatedly assess the neurovascular status of the limb
4. Photograph the wound, remove any gross contaminant, cover the wound with saline-soaked gauze and impermeable film (but it is only a 2 mm puncture wound) and splint the arm in an above-elbow backslab

The child would then need his injury managed in theatre, I would do this on the first available operating list and certainly within 24 h.

The principle of management is thorough debridement followed by stabilization of the fracture.

In this case, the wound is small with no gross contamination and it is likely to be an 'inside-out' puncture. The wound should be excised. The fracture is a simple, length-stable pattern, I would proceed with elastic intramedullary nailing. (*The use of ESIN is the gold standard treatment for the stabilization of forearm fractures in children and you are required to be familiar with the indications, techniques, limitations and potential complications.)*

Briefly run through your surgical technique for ESIN

I would position the child supine with the arm on a radiolucent armboard. A tourniquet would have been used for the wound debridement but this would be deflated for the nailing procedure. An appropriately sized elastic nail is one that measures two-thirds the diameter of the medullary isthmus. I would typically nail both radius and ulna. I am aware that single bone fixation is also acceptable practice although Dietz's retrospective review highlighted the increased risk of loss of radial reduction and advocated that both bones should be nailed in open fractures and in older children.

Nails of identical diameter should be used for the radius and ulna. Typically, the ulna nail does not need to be pre-bent (as the ulna is a straight bone), but I would pre-bend the radial nail to three times the diameter of the medullary canal and ensure that the apex of the bend corresponds to the level of the fracture site. I would then insert the ulna nail antegrade from the dorsoradial surface of the proximal ulna, just distal to the physis, up to the fracture site.

I would insert the radial nail retrograde from the radial border of the distal radius under direct vision to avoid injuring the superficial radial nerve. I am also aware of the technique of inserting the nail through Lister's tubercle. Again the nail is inserted only to as far as the fracture site. The fracture is reduced and each nail is tapped gently (and alternately) into position across the fracture site.

If both nails have been pre-bent, I would ensure that the curved tip of each nail faces each other, hence splinting the interosseous membrane. The nails are then cut to an appropriate length to facilitate implant removal.

Are you aware of any complications of elastic nailing of the forearm? Should we be plating instead?

The complication rate is approximately 10%, the most serious of which is compartment syndrome with a reported incidence of 1–8%. The latter is correlated positively with increased operative time. Other complications include skin irritation by a prominent nail, infection, nerve and tendon injury (including extensor tendon rupture from poor nail placement), and re-fracture after implant removal.

Several studies have shown equivalent outcomes and complication rates for plating or elastic nailing of both bone forearm fractures.

Evans EM: 'Fracture of the radius and ulna'. *The Bone & Joint Journal*, 1952; 33: 548–61.

Colton C, Buckley R, Camuso M. 'Principles of management of open fractures. AO Surgery Reference' [https://www2.aofoundation.org]

Dietz JF et al.: 'Single bone intramedullary fixation of the ulna in pediatric both bone forearm fractures: analysis of short-term clinical and radiographic results'. *Journal of Pediatric Orthopaedics*, 2010; 30(5): 420–4.

Parikh SN et al.:' Complications of elastic stable intramedullary nailing in pediatric fracture management. AAOS exhibit selection'. *The Journal of Bone & Joint Surgery*, American edition, 2012; 94(24): me184.x.

Viva 2   Questions

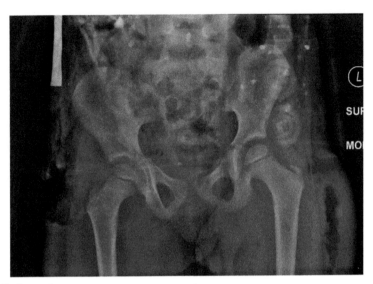

Fig. 3.2 Radiograph

Please describe this radiograph in Fig. 3.2.

Describe your approach to this patient.

Are there any special considerations in this population?

Which injuries are likely to have the greatest long-term impact in children?

Can you see any long-term potential issues for this patient?

Viva 2   Answers

Please describe this radiograph in Fig. 3.2

This AP radiograph demonstrates a pelvic fracture in an immature skeleton. There is widening of the right sacroiliac joint and what appear to be extensive soft tissue injuries with gas in the soft tissue planes. I cannot comment on the pubic symphysis in order to classify this further. Further imaging may be required after the initial resuscitation.

Describe your approach to this patient

The principles of management of this patient would follow the same principles as for adult patients. ATLS protocol should be followed, with airway and C-spine management followed by assessment of ventilation, assessment and stabilization of any circulatory deficit, and subsequent assessment of Glasgow Coma Scale (GCS) and deformity and disability.

Are there any special considerations in this population?

Special considerations centre mainly around physiological and anatomical differences, particularly in terms of airway management and cervical spine control. The physiological differences include lower circulating volume and a higher likelihood of clinical compensation for volume loss before sudden deterioration. Children often have an increased surface area, thereby leading to increased temperature loss, and hypothermia can interfere with coagulation and resuscitation.

Considerations for the medium and long term include fracture healing, remodelling potential and the risk of physeal damage.

Which injuries are likely to have the greatest long-term impact in children?

The greatest long-term impact in children is from spinal injuries and the recovery from this can be difficult to predict. However, head injuries may also have a major impact on QoL (quality of life) and independence, and physeal injuries can cause major morbidity over time.

Can you see any long-term potential issues for this patient?

Long-term potential issues for the patient include the potential for leg length discrepancy, and ongoing pain secondary to arthritis of the sacroiliac joint (SIJt), and it is possible that there may have been an associated neurological injury. Also the X-ray suggests an associated extensive soft tissue injury and I would be wary of damage to the hip joint. If, for example, there had been a momentary dislocation of the hip joint, avascular change, sciatic nerve injury, and secondary degenerative change might occur.

Kay RM and Skaggs DL: 'Paediatric polytrauma management'. *Journal of Pediatric Orthopaedics*, 2006: Mar-Apr; 26(2): 268–77.

Baker SP, et al.: 'The injury severity score: a method for describing patients with multiple injuries and evaluating emergency care'. *Journal of Trauma*, 1974: 14: 187–96.

Mayer T, Matlak ME, Johnson DG, et al.: 'The modified injury severity scale in pediatric multiple trauma patients'. *Journal of Pediatric Surgery* 1980 Dec; 15(6): 719–26.

Holden CP, Holman J, Herman MJ. 'Pediatric Pelvic Fractures'. *Journal of the American Academy of Orthopaedic Surgeons*, 2007: 15: 172–7.

Viva 3 Questions

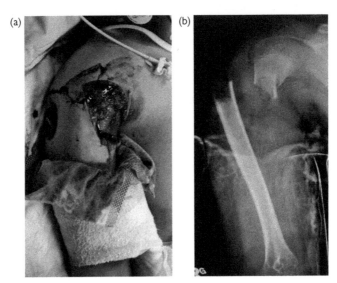

Fig. 3.3 Motorcycle accident injuries

Could you describe Fig. 3.3 of this teenager who came to A&E following a motorcycle accident, pulses are absent from the brachial artery distally.

How would you classify this injury?

Do you know any guidelines for managing this type of injury?

You are the consultant on call in a large district general hospital (DGH). What would you do next?

What are your treatment options for this limb injury?

What are your concerns for long-term outcome?

Viva 3   Answers

Could you describe Fig. 3.3 of this teenager who came to A&E following a motorcycle accident? Pulses are absent from the brachial artery distally.

The clinical photograph demonstrates a laceration to the axilla affecting what looks like the right upper limb. There is obvious deformity. It is difficult to ascertain any further information from this photograph. There is also a more posterior wound: it appears that bone may be protruding from this.

The radiographs demonstrate a completely displaced metaphyseal proximal humerus fracture. The physis is open. The soft tissue shadow is disrupted and this is in keeping with the clinical photograph.

How would you classify this injury?

This injury can be classified according to the Gustilo–Anderson classification. In the presence of a vascular injury, this becomes a Gustilo IIIC injury. This indicates a high severity limb-threatening injury.

Do you know any guidelines for managing this type of injury?

This type of injury is managed according to ATLS protocol. The airway, ventilation and circulation are addressed first, along with an assessment of the Glasgow Coma Scale. This is an open fracture, and therefore it would be managed according to BOAST 4 principles. This suggests assessment of wound severity, timely antibiotics and a combined orthopaedic and plastic surgical approach to the injury. As there is an associated vascular injury, emergency operative intervention is likely to be the next recommendation.

You are the consultant on call in a large DGH. What would you do next?

In the DGH setting, patients in this scenario need to be discussed with the local trauma unit. The ability to look after and anaesthetize significantly injured children, as well as provide orthopaedic and plastic surgical intervention, including for the vascular injury, are the priorities. If that cannot be provided on-site, then the patient needs to be transferred to an appropriate unit as a high priority. If this is a teenager who was in a motorcycle accident and thus if he/she was skeletally mature there might be less need for specialist paediatric services.

What are your treatment options for this limb injury?

The priority in this injury is to provide urgent stabilization of the fracture to facilitate management of the vascular injury and repair. There has been no mention of the neurological status of the limb but given the nature of the injury I would think it likely that there was an associated neurological injury. In this age group, flexible nails can be used to provide adequate stability with minimal intervention and rapid fixation: but for stability the nails might have to cross the physis. The alternative options include plate fixation or external fixation. There are pros and cons of each approach. Plate fixation in the presence of an open wound carries the risk of infection, as well as the potential need for subsequent removal of metalwork, which would involve soft tissue dissection around the site of the vascular repair. External fixation in this scenario has limited options for stabilization of the proximal fragment without risking damage to the growth plate: in this age group and with this injury severity, this might only be a relative contra-indication. Care must be taken not to cause further neurological injury.

What are your concerns for long term outcome?

The long term concerns centre around the risk of infection, growth arrest, deformity, and vascular sequelae of the axillary artery injury. These include cold intolerance and pain. Although no mention has been made of an associated neurological injury, if this was present, it could adversely affect the long term outcome.

British Orthopaedic Association and British Association of Plastic, Reconstructive and Aesthetic Surgeons, Standard for trauma—2009. https://www.boa.ac.uk/wp-content/uploads/2014/12/BOAST-4.pdf

Gustilo RB, Anderson JT. 'Prevention of infection in the treatment of one thousand and twenty-five open fractures of long bones: retrospective and prospective analyses'. *The Journal of Bone & Joint Surgery*, American volume, 1976 Jun; 58(4): 453–8.

Mark D, Miller MD, Stephen R. Thompson MBBS MEd FRCSC, Jennifer Hart MPAS PA-C ATC. *Review of Orthopaedics*, 6th Edition, 2012, an imprint of Elsevier, Philadelphia.

Whitehouse WM, Jr, Coran AG, Stanley JC, Kuhns LR, Weintraub WH, Fry WJ. 'Pediatric Vascular Trauma: Manifestations, Management, and Sequelae of Extremity Arterial Injury in Patients Undergoing Surgical Treatment'. *Archives of Surgery*, 1976; 111(11): 1269–75.

Viva 4   Questions

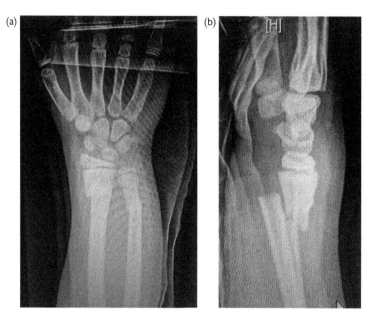

Fig. 3.4 X-rays

This 6-year-old boy fell off monkey bars onto his left wrist. What do you see on his X-rays (Fig. 3.4).

How would you manage this injury?

Tell me your tactics for reducing this fracture.

You mentioned a 'well-moulded plaster cast'. Could you explain what you mean?

Viva 4   Answers

This 6-year-old boy fell off monkey bars onto his left wrist. What do you see on his X-rays (Fig. 3.4)

These are Posterior-Anterior (PA) and lateral wrist radiographs of a skeletally-immature patient showing complete fractures through the distal third of the radius and ulna. The fractures run transversely through the metaphyseal-diaphyseal junction with overlap of the fracture ends. It is 100% dorsally translated and ~25% radially translated, but minimally angulated.

How would you manage this injury?

I would manage this injury by first employing ATLS protocols and ensuring that the child sustained no other injuries as he fell. I would then undertake a full history and examination of the child ensuring that they are consistent with the injury pattern (ie. rule out non-accidental injury). In the examination in particular, I would look for any open wounds, especially on the volar aspect of the wrist and examine the neurological status of the limb carefully looking for signs of median nerve injury.

I would manage this injury operatively with reduction (closed +/- open) and stabilization with K-wires, and I would do this on a planned trauma list at the earliest opportunity or urgently if there was any evidence of median nerve compromise.

Tell me your tactics for reducing this fracture

I would perform this procedure in theatre under GA (general anesthetic). I would ensure that the child is appropriately consented and marked and would supervise the WHO (World Health Organisation) theatre checks. I would position the child in the supine position with an arm board and image intensifier present. With this fracture pattern, I expect the dorsal periosteum to be intact which will impede reduction with simple traction alone. Hence, with my assistant providing counter-traction at the elbow, I would gently apply traction and exaggerate the deformity with my left hand (in this case angulate it more dorsally) and with my right hand, thumb the distal fragment into place. Once reduced, I could test for stability by dorsiflexing and palmarflexing the wrist under image intensifier. If it was stable I would apply a well-moulded plaster cast. I would have a low threshold for providing additional stabilization of the fracture with K-wires as the risk of redisplacement has been shown to approximate 30%. Also, there is a higher risk of redisplacement when both radius and ulna are fractured, as opposed to isolated distal radial fractures.

If the fracture cannot be satisfactorily reduced by closed means, I would make a small dorsal incision over the fracture site and lever the fracture into position using an instrument such as a McDonald dissector.

You mentioned a 'well-moulded plaster cast'. Could you explain what you mean?

The key factors for good plaster cast application are good moulding, thin and uniform padding, and adequate three-point fixation of the fracture (you should be able to demonstrate this if asked). Objectively, there are several indices that can be used including the cast index, padding index, and Canterbury index. The most commonly used and reproducible is the cast index, which is the ratio of the internal cast width in the sagittal to coronal plane. A cast index > 0.8 predicts a higher re-displacement rate.

[Padding index is the ratio of the thickness of the padding at the fracture site in the plane of deformity correction to the maximum interosseous diameter. Canterbury index is the combined score of the cast and padding index. A padding index > 0.3 and a Canterbury index > 1.1 is predictive of failure.]

The literature supports a good quality cast mould ahead of cast length in maintenance of fracture position. Several prospective, randomized trials have shown equal efficacy of short- (below elbow) and long-arm (above elbow) casts.

Bae DS, Howard AW. 'Distal radius fractures: what is the evidence'? *Journal Pediatric Orthopedics*, 2012; 32(Suppl 2): S128–30.

Bhatia M, Housden PH. 'Redisplacement of paediatric forearm fractures: role of plaster moulding and padding'. *Injury*, 2006; 37: 259–68.

McLauchlan GJ, Cowan B, Annan IH, Robb JE: 'Management of completely displaced metaphyseal fractures of the distal radius in children. A prospective, randomised controlled trial'. *The Bone & Joint Journal*, 2002 Apr; 84(3): 413–7.

Zamzam MM, Khoshhal KI: 'Displaced fracture of the distal radius in children: factors responsible for re-displacement after closed reduction'. *The Bone & Joint Journal*, 2005; 87: 841–3.

Viva 5   Questions

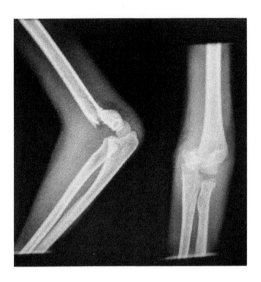

Fig. 3.5 X-rays

This 6-year-old boy falls off a trampoline onto his left outstretched arm.

What do you think about his X-rays shown in Fig. 3.5?

Are you aware of any classification system for this fracture?

How would you manage this fracture?

Would your management be different if the child had a pink hand but an absent radial pulse?

Viva 5   Answers

This 6-year-old boy falls off a trampoline onto his left outstretched arm. What do you think about his X-rays shown in Fig. 3.5?

This is an AP and lateral elbow radiograph of a skeletally-immature patient showing a displaced supracondylar fracture. The fracture has displaced posteromedially.

Are you aware of any classification system for this fracture?

Supracondylar elbow fractures can be classified as extension or flexion injuries. The most common is extension (98%), caused by a fall onto an outstretched hand which results in hyperextension of the elbow. Flexion injuries comprise only 2% and are usually the result of a direct blow to the posterior aspect of a flexed elbow.

The amount of displacement is then classified further according to Gartland:

> Gartland type I fractures are non-displaced or minimally displaced
> Gartland type II fractures are angulated with one cortex remaining intact
> Gartland type III fractures are completely displaced with no cortical contact*

Wilkins has modified the classification:

> IIA: non-rotated
> IIB: rotated
> IIIA: posteromedial displacement
> IIIB: posterolateral displacement (only 25% of Type III fractures but more commonly associated with neurovascular injuries)**

Leitch's group has also further modified the classification to add a Gartland type IV fracture which is multidirectionally unstable and can be displaced both into flexion and extension.

In this case, this is an extension, Gartland type IIB fracture.

How would you manage this fracture?

I would take a full history and examine the child and ensure that both are consistent with the injury, i.e. rule out non-acidental injury (NAI): supracondylar fractures are strong predictors of accidental trauma; however, transphyseal distal humeral fractures, which are frequently misdiagnosed as supracondylar fractures, are more common than supracondylar fractures in children younger than 2 years, and these may be associated with child abuse in up to 50% of cases.

I would then adhere to the BOAST/BSCOS standards for practice guidelines.

Firstly, a careful and thorough examination (and documentation) of the neurovascular status in particular is paramount; specifically noting the status of the radial pulse, digital capillary refill time and individual function of the radial, median and ulnar nerves. Neurologic injury is present in 10–15% of cases with the anterior interosseous nerve (AIN) most commonly affected. It is also

---

* Data from *Surgery, Gynaecology, Obstetrics*, 109, 1959, Gartland JJ, 'Management of supracondylar fractures of the humerus in children', pp. 145–154.
** Data from Wilkins KE. 'Fractures and Dislocations of the Elbow Region'. In: Rockwood CA, Wilkins KE, King R (eds), *Fractures in Children*. 1984. pp. 363–575

important to be vigilant for clinical signs of compartment syndrome. These injuries require early surgical treatment, ideally on the day of admission; however, night-time operating is not necessary unless there are indications for urgent surgery. Indications would include an absent radial pulse, clinical signs of impaired perfusion of the hand and digits, and evidence of threatened skin viability. If a child has an ischaemic limb, he needs urgent surgery and I would also discuss the case with the on-call vascular team.

Surgical stabilization would involve initial attempts at closed reduction; I would do this by applying continuous traction with the elbow in slight flexion for several minutes. I would consider and adjust the rotational alignment first, then the coronal plane (varus–valgus) deformity; then whilst maintaining traction, I would hyperflex the elbow whilst simultaneously thumbing the distal fragment anteriorly. Once the reduction is confirmed, I would stabilize it with two 2 mm K-wires, ensuring bi-cortical fixation. My personal preference would be to insert both wires laterally, ensuring that they are as far apart as possible, in a divergent fashion, and do not cross at the fracture site. I am aware that the crossed-wire configuration is biomechanically superior and an acceptable option. However, Skagg's retrospective study of nearly 350 supracondylar fractures treated with crossed or lateral entry only wires showed no difference in the maintenance of reduction but a 7.7% incidence of iatrogenic ulnar nerve injury with the crossed configuration.

I would also ensure that a cubitus varus deformity is avoided. Although mainly a problem of cosmesis (function is seldom impaired), O'Driscoll et al. identified posterolateral elbow instability with pain in adults presenting 20–30 years after varus malunion of supracondylar fractures sustained in childhood.

Would your management be different if the child had a pink hand but an absent radial pulse?

The BOAST/BSCOS standards for practice give guidance on this. The American Academy of Orthopaedic Surgeons also has similar recommendations in their clinical practice guideline. Urgent surgical treatment is required for children with an absent radial pulse, and this would include such a child with a pink, pulseless hand. I would still attempt a closed reduction and stabilization of the fracture with lateral entry pins. I would then observe the child after fracture reduction for ~ 15 min, ensuring the child (and in particular the arm) is kept warm and I would also consider using a Doppler probe to assess the radial pulse. The majority of vascular impairments resolve with anatomical fracture reduction and a perfused limb (even with an absent radial pulse) does not require brachial artery exploration. If the hand remains perfused, I would then cast the arm in 40–60° of flexion to avoid further vascular compromise. (Exploration of the brachial artery is only required if the limb remains ischaemic after closed or open fracture reduction, and I would ensure that this was done by a surgeon competent to explore/repair small vessels.) Post-reduction, I would be sure to monitor and document the child's neurovascular status closely and be vigilant for compartment syndrome which is more common in the presence of a pink but pulseless arm.

Despite specified standards for practice, I am aware that this topic continues to be controversial in the literature. A recent retrospective study by Weller et al. (2013) showed only 1 in 20 of their patients with a pink, pulseless hand (as assessed with a Doppler or capillary refilling time) after closed reduction and pinning required vascular repair (secondary to delayed ischaemia), whilst the other 19 all regained their pulse prior to discharge or at the first post-operative visit. However, a systematic review by White, Mehlman, and Crawford (2010) revealed that an absent pulse is an indicator of arterial injury in > 80% of cases with arterial spasm as a cause of pulselessness being only 9% in surgically-explored cases. The authors make a strong argument for more aggressive vascular evaluation, exploration, and repair in such cases.

Abzug JM, Herman MJ. 'Management of supracondylar humeral fractures in children: current concepts'. *The Journal of the American Academy of Orthopaedic Surgeons*, 2012; 20: 69–77. Review.

Leitch KK et al. 'Treatment of multidirectionally unstable supracondylar humeral fractures in children. A modified Gartland type-IV fracture'. *The Journal of Bone & Joint Surgery*, American volume, 2006; 88(5): 980–5.

Mahan ST, Osborn E, Bae DS, Waters PM, Kasser JR, Kocher MS, Snyder BD, Hresko MT. 'Changing practice patterns: the impact of a randomized clinical trial on surgeons preference for treatment of type 3 supracondylar humerus fracture's. *Journal of Pediatric Orthopedics*, 2012 Jun; 32(4): 340–5.

O'Driscoll SW et al. 'Tardy posterolateral rotatory instability of the elbow due to cubitus varus'. *The Journal of Bone & Joint Surgery*, American volume, 2001; 83(9): 1358–69.

Skaggs DL et al.: 'Operative treatment of supracondylar fractures of the humerus in children: the consequence of pin placement'. *The Journal of Bone & Joint Surgery*, American volume, 2001; 83(5): 735–40.

Weller A et al. 'Management of pediatric pulseless supracondylar humeral fracture: is vascular exploration necessary'? *The Journal of Bone & Joint Surgery*, American volume, 2013; 95(21): 1906–12.

White L, Mehlman CT, Crawford AH. 'Perfused, pulseless, and puzzling: a systematic review of vascular injuries in pediatric supracondylar humerus fractures and results of a POSNA questionnaire'. *Journal of Pediatric Orthopedics*, 2010; 30(4): 328–35.

Viva 6   Questions

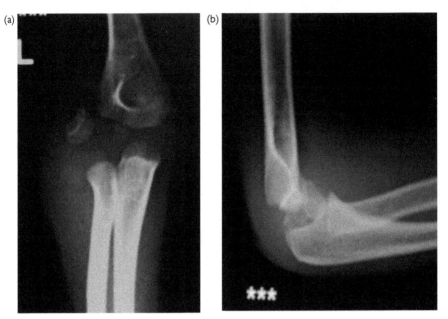

Fig. 3.6 X-ray

A 6-year-old boy fell from a trampoline onto his left elbow sustaining this injury. Tell me what you see in Fig. 3.6.

Are you aware of any classification systems for this fracture?

What are the principles of management of this injury?

What complications are you aware of with this injury?

Viva 6   Answers

A 6-year-old boy fell from a trampoline onto his left elbow sustaining this injury. Tell me what you see in Fig. 3.6

This is an AP and lateral elbow radiograph of a skeletally-immature patient that shows a widely displaced fracture of the lateral condyle. The fragment is also laterally rotated and there is substantial soft tissue swelling.

Are you aware of any classification systems for this fracture?

The most frequently used classification system is that described by Milch.

> **Milch type I** is a fracture that extends through the secondary ossification centre of the capitellum and enters the joint lateral to the trochlear groove

This has also been equated to a Salter–Harris IV fracture.

> **Milch type II** is a fracture that exits medial to the trochlear groove, thus the trochlea remains with the lateral fracture fragment. This makes the ulnohumeral joint unstable. Milch type II fractures have been equated more to a Salter-Harris II fracture (perhaps inaccurately as a Salter Harris II fracture, by definition, does not enter the articular surface)

Although used, the Milch classification provides little prognostic information regarding treatment and complications. An alternative is the Jakob classification system which is based on the presence of an intact articular hinge: in **type A,** the fracture is undisplaced with an intact articular surface; in **type B**, the fracture extends completely through the articular surface. Radiographically, this may be impossible to distinguish from the type A fracture; however, it is potentially unstable and at risk of late displacement. **Type C** is a grossly displaced (and may be significantly rotated) lateral condyle fragment.*

Finally, many surgeons classify the fracture based on the degree of displacement as this influences treatment: non-displaced (< 2 mm), minimally displaced (2–4 mm), or displaced (> 4 mm).

In this case, this is a Milch type I or Jakob type C, displaced fracture.

What are the principles of management of this injury?

I would firstly take a full history and then examine the child (to rule out NAI). In the examination, I would specifically look for gross soft tissue swelling, bruising and crepitus which are signs suggestive of an unstable fracture.

The management goal is to restore articular congruity and physeal alignment and achieve stable fixation.

In undisplaced cases, I would consider performing further X-rays to confirm the degree of displacement (the internal oblique view is the most useful) as the images can be deceptive, particularly in terms of fragment rotation, as most of the lateral condyle is cartilaginous.

In minimally displaced cases, one option would be to accept the position and apply an above-elbow cast or alternatively one could pin the fracture percutaneously: some might recommend using a

---

* Adapted from *The Journal of Trauma and Acute Care Surgery*, 4, 5, Milch H, 'Fractures and fracture dislocations of the humeral condyles', pp. 592–607. Copyright (1964) with permission from Wolters Kluwer Health, Inc.

single cannulated screw as a fixation method hoping that this would apply some compression and enhance fracture reduction. Again a cast should also be applied. Many surgeons advocate fixation for all minimally-displaced cases as there is a propensity for late displacement and non-union (Launay et al.). At the time of surgery an examination under anesthesia (EUA) and arthrogram can help define/confirm the degree of displacement and instability.

With this case, the child would require open anatomic reduction and fixation. I would utilize the anterolateral approach. The blood supply to the lateral condyle arises posteriorly, therefore I would be careful to minimize dissection of the posterior soft tissues. Dissection needs to be sufficient to visualize the articular surface as this is key to reduction, occasionally there is plastic deformation or comminution of the distal fragment, therefore judging reduction by the lateral metaphyseal fragment would not be adequate. Once anatomic reduction is achieved, the fracture can be stabilized with two 1.6 mm K-wires, ensuring they are separated as much as possible and that they do not cross at the fracture site. (Parallel pins are also acceptable, although they are biomechanically weaker.) The use of screws or bioabsorbable pins has also been described in the literature although the former requires secondary surgery to remove the metalwork.

I would test the stability of my fixation fluoroscopically, then place the child in an above elbow plaster with the elbow at 90° for 6 weeks.

What complications are you aware of with this injury?

The most common complications following lateral condyle fractures include delayed union and non-union with or without cubitus valgus and subsequent tardy ulnar nerve palsy. Growth arrest and fishtail deformity of the distal humerus can also occur. As the fracture heals, there may be formation of a lateral spur of new bone leading to the appearance of a (pseudo) cubitus varus. This has been reported to occur in upto 40% of patients, however it is generally mild and asymptomatic.

Delayed union and non-union is a frequent complication as the fracture is intra-articular and therefore constantly exposed to synovial fluid. It also has a poor blood supply and if not immobilized, there is constant motion at the fracture site from the pull of the wrist extensors on the distal fragment. The goal of management in such cases is to achieve union rather than attempt anatomic restoration of the articular surface. This is usually achieved with a screw to provide maximal metaphyseal contact.

The management of late-presenting fractures is controversial. Some have reported better results in patients treated with observation rather than delayed open reduction with the added risk of avascular necrosis (AVN) due to soft tissue stripping. Jakob et al. reported no difference in patients treated surgically after 3 weeks compared to no treatment. Others have reported good results with surgical treatment of late-presenting fractures (Roye et al.), with improved stability and reduced risk of cubitus valgus.

Jakob R et al.: 'Observations concerning fractures of the lateral humeral condyle in children'. *The Bone & Joint Journal*, 1975; 57(4): 430–6.

Launay F et al.: 'Lateral humeral condyle fractures in children: a comparison of two approaches to treatment'. *Journal of Pediatric Orthopedics*, 2004; 24(4): 385–91.

Roye DP, Bini SA: Infosino A. 'Late surgical treatment of lateral condylar fractures in children'. *Journal of Pediatric Orthopedics*, 1991; 11: 195–9.

Sullivan JA. 'Fractures of the lateral condyle of the humerus'. *The Journal of the American Academy of Orthopaedic Surgeons*, 2006; 14(1): 58–62.

Weiss JM et al.: 'A new classification system predictive of complications in surgically treated pediatric humeral lateral condyle fractures'. *Journal of Pediatric Orthopedics*, 2009; 29(6): 602–5.

Viva 7   Questions

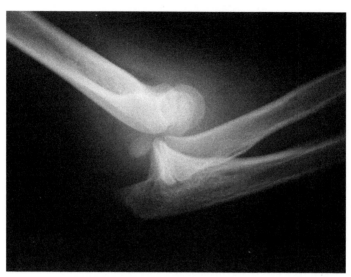

Fig. 3.7 X-ray

A 10-year-old national gymnast fell off the parallel bars and landed awkwardly onto her right outstretched arm. She has pain and swelling of her elbow. Please describe this X-ray (Fig. 3.7).

Are you aware of any classification systems for this injury?

How would you manage this injury?

Run through your technique for surgical management of this injury.

If the medial epicondyle was not incarcerated but simply displaced, say 8 mm, would you change your management?

Viva 7   Answers

A 10-year-old national gymnast fell off the parallel bars and landed awkwardly onto her right outstretched arm. She has pain and swelling of her elbow. Please describe this X-ray (Fig. 3.7)

This is a lateral radiograph of the elbow of a skeletally-immature patient which shows a joint dislocation. There is a well-rounded bone fragment within the joint: I would need to see an AP view to clarify whether or not this was a medial epicondyle. 50% of medial epicondyle fractures are reported to be associated with elbow dislocations.

Are you aware of any classification systems for this injury?

There are no widely accepted or validated classification systems. I am, however, aware of the Rang and the Watson Jones four-category systems which are very similar to each other:

Rang I/Watson Jones type I: minimally displaced/ < 5 mm displaced, no rotation
Rang II/Watson Jones type II: rotated/ > 5 mm displaced with rotation
Rang III/Watson Jones type III: trapped/incarcerated without dislocation
Rang IV/Watson Jones type IV: dislocated/incarcerated with dislocation

Treatment for type I injury is universally conservative, types III and IV require surgical intervention. The management of type II injuries is contentious.

In this case, this is a Rang or Watson Jones type IV injury.

How would you manage this injury?

I would take a full history and examination and ensure that they corroborate (i.e. rule out NAI which is highly unlikely in this age group and scenario). In particular, I would examine the ulnar nerve function as ulnar nerve dysfunction has been reported to occur in 10–16%.

The joint requires relocation and as the medial epicondyle may be or may become incarcerated, I would consent and mark the child's arm for closed or open reduction of the joint and internal fixation of the fracture.

Run through your technique for surgical management of this injury

I would place the child in a supine position with the arm abducted and externally rotated on an armboard. I would use an upper arm tourniquet. After ensuring the WHO checklist is complete, I would initially attempt to reduce the elbow joint. If the joint reduced but the fragment remained incarcerated it might prove possible to extract this using the Roberts manoeuvre which involves a valgus force to open the elbow joint followed by forearm supination and finger extension.

If the Roberts manoeuvre was successful in extricating the entrapped fragment, then I would proceed straight to reduction and fixation of the fragment. I would centre my incision over where the medial epicondyle should be and follow the haematoma down to the fracture site. By flexing the wrist and pronating the forearm, the flexor-pronator mass that attaches to the medial epicondyle is relaxed which would help reduction. I would reduce the fracture under direct vision and secure it with a partially-threaded compression screw with a washer. I would not deliberately explore the ulnar nerve.

If joint reduction and/or fragment extraction did not occur then I would need to open the joint.

If the medial epicondyle was not incarcerated but simply displaced, about 8 mm, would you change your management?

There is controversy about the definition as well as management of displaced fractures (type II injuries). A 3D computed tomography (CT) study by Edmonds (2010) suggests that plain X-rays are inaccurate in determining true displacement as fractures classified as undisplaced or minimally displaced on plain radiographs may have more than 1 cm of true displacement as measured on CT. There is also no consensus on what degree of displacement mandates operative fixation with recommendations ranging from as little as 2 mm to > 1 cm.

The management of displaced fractures is also controversial with evidence demonstrating good outcome following both operative and non-operative treatments. There is a current trend to manage competitive athletes more aggressively with surgical fixation. Proponents of surgical fixation believe that it would allow an earlier return to sports and more rapid return to pre-injury function. There are, however, no definitive studies supporting this and there are studies reporting full return to pre-injury level of sport for fractures treated non-operatively. A meta-analysis of conservative versus operative management of nearly 500 patients by Kamath et al. (2009) showed that radiographic union occurred in 92.5% of operatively-treated patients compared to 49.2% in non-operatively treated patients; however, pain at long-term follow-up was no different between the groups (15% operated versus 8.7% non-operated).

Edmonds EW. 'How displaced are 'nondisplaced' fractures of the medial humeral epicondyle in children? Results of a three-dimensional computed tomography analysis'. *The Journal of Bone & Joint Surgery*, American volume, 2010; 92(17): 2785–91.

Kamath AF et al. 'Operative versus non-operative management of pediatric medial epicondyle fractures; a systematic review'. *Journal of Child Orthopedics* 2009; 3: 345–57.

Lawrence JT et al. 'Return to competitive sports after medial epicondyle fractures in adolescent athletes: results of operative and non-operative treatment'. *American Journal of Sports Medicine* 2013; 41: 1152–7.

Mehlman CT, Howard AW. 'Medial epicondyle fractures in children: clinical decision making in the face of uncertainty'. *Journal of Pediatric Orthopedics,* 2012; 32: S135–42.

Pathy R, Dodwell ER. 'Medial epicondyle fractures in children'. *Current Opinion in Pediatrics,* 2015; 27: 58–66.

Viva 8   Questions

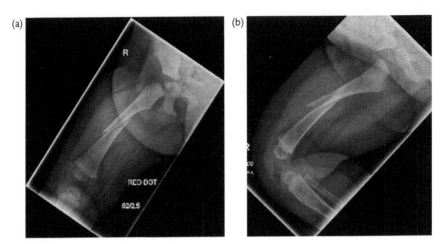

Fig. 3.8 X-rays

What does Fig. 3.8 show?

What is the initial management of this child if I tell you he is 6 months of age?

What are you worried about?

What are your management options and which would you choose and why?

Tell me briefly about traction.

Viva 8   Answers

What does Fig. 3.8 show?

This is an AP and lateral radiograph of a child . It shows a spiral fracture of the femoral diaphysis with no gross varus or valgus malalignment, there is an apex anterior (procurvatum) deformity, with shortening and some rotation. There is no significant translation.

What is the initial management of this child if I tell you he is 6 months of age?

I would perform a prompt, rapid, primary survey and manage the patient along ATLS guidelines. I would exclude other injuries, assess the vascular status of the limb and ensure this is a closed isolated injury. I would complete a full secondary survey and obtain the child's weight to guide my management.

After initial resuscitation I would ascertain a full, clear, consistent history from family and any other sources including collateral history from the paramedics. I would perform any other relevant clinical examination at this point including assessment for any bruises. If I had any concerns, I would contact the named doctor and named nurse for safeguarding in keeping with the guidance from the American Academy of Orthopedic Surgeons (AAOS). I would also refer to local hospital policies for pathway of management for paediatric femoral fractures.

What are you worried about?

A child of 6 months will not be mobile hence there is a high index of suspicion for non accidental injury (NAI). Spiral fractures are a common pattern for abuse-related femoral fractures although there is no clear association between specific fracture patterns in the femur and NAI. I will treat the fracture appropriately and follow the NAI pathway until I am certain this can be excluded.

What are your management options and which would you choose and why?

Firstly, I would admit the patient to the ward and continue following the NAI pathway until the possibility of NAI is excluded.

I would manage this fracture non-operatively. The most common options used to treat infants up to 1 year of age are the Pavlik harness or Gallows traction alone or followed by a period in a spica cast. For children with femoral shaft fractures up to 2 years of age, I would accept 30° of varus/ valgus deformity, 30° of anterior/posterior malalignment and up to 15–20 mm of shortening. I would accept only minimal rotational deformity as theoretically there is less remodelling potential. However, I recognize that the younger the child is, the more displacement (including rotational displacement) can be accepted due to the great remodelling potential in the infant. Theoretical complications of traction include compartment syndrome and Volkmann's ischaemic contracture. The skin must be examined daily.

Gallows traction can not be used in patients weighing more than 16–18 kg. If there is associated gross shortening, an initial period of traction can be applied with delayed spica cast application at the 2-week mark. There is a slightly higher risk of skin complications when managed with a spica cast however both the Pavlik harness and spica cast treatments result in good outcomes with minimal complications. In neonates and infants up to 3 months of age, the Pavlik harness is a useful device. The spica cast is usually reserved for slightly older infants.

Tell me briefly about traction

Traction is the application of a pulling force to a part of the body. It can be fixed, where the traction is applied to the limb against a fixed point of counter pressure, or sliding, which is used when all or part of the body, acting under the influence of gravity, is utilized to provide counter-traction. Traction can be either skeletal or skin, subdivided as to whether an adhesive or a non-adhesive bandage is used.

Are you aware of any evidence to support the management of femoral shaft fractures in children?

Yes, the AAOS published their guidance in 2009: it uses the child's age and weight to guide management.

Flynn JM, Skaggs DL, Sponseller PD, Ganley TJ, Kay RM, Leitch KK. 'The surgical management of pediatric fractures of the lower extremity'. *Instructional Course Lectures*, 2003; 52: 647–59.

Treatment of pediatric diaphyseal femur fractures guidelines and evidence report: Adopted by the AAOS Board of Directors June 19, 2009

Wang CN, Chen JJ, Zhou JF, Tang HB, Feng YB, Yi X. 'Femoral fractures in infants: a comparison of Bryant traction and modified Pavlik harness'. *Acta Orthopædica Belgica*, 2014 Mar; 80(1): 63–8.

Viva 9   Questions

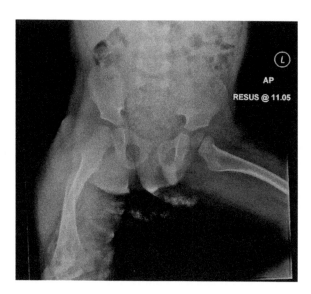

Fig. 3.9 X-ray

Describe Fig. 3.9.

The child is 3 years old, what is the most likely mechanism of injury?

What are your management options?

If you were to manage this in a spica, what would be the optimal position for a mid-shaft femoral fracture?

What are the disadvantages of using a spica cast?

What are the general complications you may expect following this injury?

Viva 9   Answers

Describe Fig. 3.9

This is an AP radiograph demonstrating a spiral, mid-shaft femoral fracture in a skeletally immature child. There is no gross shortening, however there is varus angulation with a rotational deformity as can be seen from the orientation of the femoral condyles in relation to the lesser trochanter. The radiograph has been performed in the resuscitation room indicating this may be part of a polytrauma, with other injuries to be considered.

The child is 3 years old, what is the most likely mechanism of injury?

An isolated femoral shaft fracture in an infant of walking age is more likely to be accidental than non-accidental. The likelihood of non-accidental injury (NAI) decreases with increasing age after the first year of life. NAI however should always be ruled out. Falls are the most common cause in toddlers, whereas high-energy trauma, motor-vehicle accidents, are responsible for the second peak in adolescence.

What are your management options?

My initial management would be in line with ATLS protocols and to exclude NAI. Shortening is the main factor, which dictates the type of treatment in this age group. If there is less than 2 cm of shortening, an early hip spica may be applied. If there is shortening of more than 2 cm I would consider intervention, as this is not an acceptable degree of shortening. Skin traction followed by a spica cast is an option as is traction as the sole method of treatment. If the injury is part of a polytrauma or the fracture is open, intervention is recommended. Flexible intramedullary nailing (and maybe even, external fixation and bridge plating) all have a place in this subgroup.

If you were to manage this in a spica, what would be the optimal position for a mid-shaft femoral fracture?

The affected thigh is placed in 20° of abduction with the opposite hip in moderate abduction to facilitate perineal hygiene. The hip is placed in 30° of flexion, 20° of abduction and neutral or slight external rotation. Excessive hip flexion may cause a femoral nerve palsy. There would need to be good molding of the cast to help maintain reduction.

What are the disadvantages of using a spica cast?

Skin care, hygiene and mobility issues. Most schools and nurseries in the UK will not allow a child to be in attendance with a hip spica cast on and access to education may be a factor to consider in the older child. More importantly, parents may not be able to work whilst the child is in the cast. Spica casts in toddlers can cause social isolation and behavioural changes (for example going back to nappy use after being toilet trained causes upset).

What are the general complications you may expect following this injury?

Femoral shaft fractures in children on the whole heal rapidly and well with minimal complications helped by the capacity for skeletal remodeling. A leg length discrepancy is the most common complication. Shortening may need follow up however but mostly it is of no clinical significance. Shortening is on average 1 cm in children between the age of 2 and 10 years with a range of 0.4 to 2.5 cm. Children with less than 2 cm of shortening rarely have long term sequelae. Overgrowth depends on many factors including fracture pattern and location. The amount of shortening and possibly the treatment method also influence outcome. There is an association, as suggested by Park et al., between the nail-canal diameter ratio and femoral overgrowth following flexible intramedullary nailing. Shortening of up to 2 cm is acceptable as there will be an anticipated overgrowth of 1–2 cm: the overgrowth is less if the femoral fracture is well reduced.

Non-union is uncommon, however, the risks are increased with load bearing devices such as external fixators and locking plates. The construct can be made too rigid to allow the fracture to unite. Re-fracture is mostly seen following removal of external fixators however it has also been reported after locking plate removal. Mal-union in the form of varus and flexion of the distal fragment is most common. Remodelling potential is higher in the plane of joint movement and rotational deformities rarely remodel.

Flynn JM, Garner MR, Jones KJ, D'Italia J, Davidson RS, Ganley TJ, Horn BD, Spiegel D, Wells L. 'The treatment of low-energy femoral shaft fractures: a prospective study comparing the 'walking spica' with the traditional spica cast'. *The Journal of Bone & Joint Surgery*, American volume, 2011 Dec 7; 93(23): 2196–202.

Flynn JM, Luedtke LM, Ganley TJ, Dawson J, Davidson RS, Dormans JP, Ecker ML, Gregg JR, Horn BD, Drummond DS. 'Comparison of titanium elastic nails with traction and a spica cast to treat femoral fractures in children'. *The Journal of Bone & Joint Surgery*, American volume, 2004 Apr; 86-A(4): 770–7.

Shemshaki HR, Mousavi H, Salehi G, Eshaghi MA. 'Titanium elastic nailing versus hip spica cast in treatment of femoral-shaft fractures in children'. *Journal of Orthopaedics and Traumatology*, 2011 Mar; 12(1): 45–8.

Viva 10 Questions

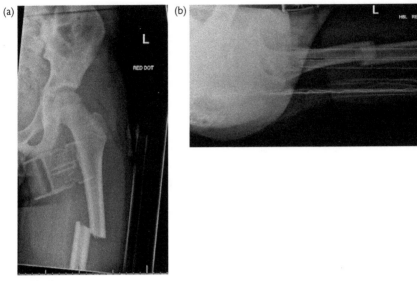

Fig. 3.10 X-rays

Describe Fig. 3.10—they are of a 10-year-old child.

How would you manage this?

What if I tell you he is a 14-year-old and weighs 55 Kg?

What are the risks with this chosen method?

What are the advantages and disadvantages of using external fixation?

Are you aware of any evidence for the management of femoral fractures in this age group?

Viva 10   Answers

Describe Fig. 3.10—they are of a 10-year-old child

These are AP and lateral radiographs demonstrating a transverse midshaft femoral fracture in a skeletally immature child. There is some varus angulation with translation of the fracture fragments and some minor shortening.

How would you manage this?

All trauma patients should be managed in accordance with the ATLS protocol hence the primary survey must be addressed first.

Assuming this was an isolated injury in a stable patient, I would manage this fracture operatively to allow rapid mobilization and to avoid the complications associated with traction and cast immobilization. This is a length stable fracture and in this age group, assuming the child was not overweight, I would consider flexible intramedullary nailing (FIN or ESIN) as my preferred treatment option.

Other surgical treatment options include internal fixation using a plating technique.

What if I tell you he is actually a 14-year-old and weighs 55 Kg?

In children who are approaching skeletal maturity, with the same fracture pattern i.e. a length stable fracture, I would consider adolescent / lateral entry femoral nailing or open reduction with plate fixation. My preferred method would be an antegrade adolescent lateral trochanteric entry point nail if available to avoid damage to the vascular supply to the femoral head.

What are the risks with this chosen method?

The main risk is osteonecrosis of the femoral head. There are reports of piriformis entry and even trochanteric entry nails causing osteonecrosis of the femoral head. The lateral ascending cervical branch penetrates the lateral capsule in the trochanteric fossa, close to the piriformis fossa and this can be damaged during nail insertion, causing osteonecrosis.

What are the advantages and disadvantages of using external fixation?

Advantages, in theory, include ease and speed of application and it is a robust method for restoring length and achieving satisfactory alignment. It avoids long incisions, without disturbing the fracture site and hence less blood loss. The technique also avoids the risk of physeal injuries and osteonecrosis. It also helps with the difficult problems which can be encountered with open fractures with severe soft tissue injuries. It is useful in the polytrauma setting especially with damage control surgery. In older children, the pins can be removed without the need for a general anaesthetic. Disadvantages include pin site irritation, infection and unsightly pin site scars. External fixators can be too rigid and this increased construct rigidity can cause delayed union and minimal callus formation. There is a documented increased re-fracture risk following removal of the fixator. This, once again, may be due to the fixator being too rigid and causing stress shielding of the fracture site, which ultimately prevents the development of satisfactory fracture callus.

Socially, some patients and their families have difficulty 'accepting' the fixator and return to school may be delayed until the fixator has been removed.

Are you aware of any evidence for the management of femoral fractures in this age group?

Flynn et al. performed a prospective trial comparing titanium elastic nails with traction and spica casting to treat femoral shaft fractures in children with a mean age of 10 and 9 years respectively. Recovery milestones, such as time to independent walking, were significantly earlier in the nailing group. Wright et al. performed a randomized trial comparing malunion rates after external fixation and after early application of a hip spica in the 4–10-year age group. They concluded there was a limited role for hip spica casting in this age group. Bar-On et al. found improved outcomes with flexible intramedullary nails compared with external fixation. The AAOS subsequently released guidelines for the management of femoral shaft fractures in children. These guidelines do not advocate routine use of external fixator in younger children. Depending on fracture type, age and weight of the child, flexible intramedullary nails are favoured. These guidelines have been adopted in the main in the UK but I believe we should develop our own guidelines.

Flynn JM, Luedtke LM, Ganley TJ, Dawson J, Davidson RS, Dormans JP, Ecker ML, Gregg JR, Horn BD, Drummond DS. 'Comparison of titanium elastic nails with traction and a spica cast to treat femoral fractures in children'. *The Journal of Bone & Joint Surgery*, American volume, 2004 Apr; 86-A(4): 770–7.

Kong H, Sabharwal S. 'External fixation for closed pediatric femoral shaft fractures: where are we now'? *Clinical Orthopaedics and Related Research* 2014 Dec; 472(12): 3814–22.

Miller DJ, Kelly DM, Spence DD, Beaty JH, Warner WC Jr, Sawyer JR. 'Locked intramedullary nailing in the treatment of femoral shaft fractures in children younger than 12 years of age: indications and preliminary report of outcomes'. *Journal of Pediatric Orthopedics*, 2012 Dec; 32(8): 777–80.

MacNeil JA, Francis A, El-Hawary R. 'A systematic review of rigid, locked, intramedullary nail insertion sites and avascular necrosis of the femoral head in the skeletally immature'. *Journal of Pediatric Orthopedics*, 2011 Jun; 31(4): 377–80.

Wright JG, Wang EE, Owen JL, Stephens D, Graham HK, Hanlon M, Nattrass GR, Reynolds RA, Coyte P. 'Treatments for paediatric femoral fractures: a randomised trial'. *Lancet*, 2005 Mar 26-Apr 1; 365(9465): 1153–8.

Viva 11   Questions

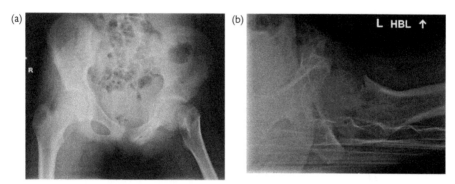

Fig. 3.11 X-ray

Describe Fig. 3.11.

How would you manage this child? He is 12 years old.

Tell me about your approach?

What is the blood supply of the femoral head in a child and how does it change with age?

Tell me about the ossification of the femur.

Viva 11 Answers

Describe Fig. 3.11

This AP radiograph shows a displaced intracapsular neck of femur fracture in an immature skeleton. It is a transcervical fracture (Delbet type 2).

How would you manage this child? He is 12 years old

A displaced transcervical fracture is an emergency: it requires anatomical open reduction and internal fixation. I would utilize the Watson-Jones approach to achieve direct visual reduction of the fracture before proceeding with my fixation, which will be with two or three partially threaded screws, depending on the size of the femoral neck. I would not penetrate the physis, however if I were in any doubt about the stability of the fixation, I would cross the physis to avoid complications associated with late displacement. I would also assess the child to see if they were safe and sensible enough for crutches and non-weight bearing with/without the use of a wheelchair. If there were significant behavioural difficulties, a spica cast might need to be considered. My postoperative plan would include a wound inspection at 2 weeks by the GP and a further review at 6 weeks with a repeat radiograph.

Tell me about your approach?

Under general anaesthetic and the patient supine I would mark out the anterior superior iliac spine (ASIS) and the greater trochanter. I would start the incision 2.5 cm distal and posterior to the ASIS and make a curved slightly anterior incision over the proximal femur anterior to the greater trochanter. There is no inter-nervous plane in the Watson-Jones approach as both the gluteus medius and tensor fascia lata are innervated by the superior gluteal nerve. The fascia lata is incised longitudinally and the approach deepened. The superior gluteal nerve must be protected as this is situated between 2–5 cm proximal to the greater trochanter. For deep dissection, the anterior most fibres of the gluteus medius may need to be detached. This will expose the capsule and a longitudinal casulotomy along the anterosuperior neck is made. This is an extensile approach.

What is the blood supply of the femoral head in a child and how does it change with age?

The femoral head blood supply changes according to growth plate maturity. There are three main sources including the lateral epiphyseal artery (LEA), which is the main vessel from the subsynovial ring anastamosis. The medial femoral circumflex artery (MCA); the main contributor to the synovial ring. The metaphyseal intraosseous vessels and the ligamentum teres (LT) are the other contributors.

The teaching is that from birth till 4 years of age, the metaphyseal vessels predominate and enter through where the physis will form. The LEA is also important. The ligamentum teres vessels are less important. They contribute very little up to the age of 8, and then only 20% as an adult.

The LEA consists of two branches; the posterosuperior and posterioinferior branches of the MCA. At the level of the intertrochanteric groove the MCA branches into these retinacular vessels which penetrate the capsule and traverse proximally.

As the physis becomes fully established it becomes impenetrable to the metaphyseal vessels.

From 4–7 years, the LEA predominates and is the sole blood supply at this stage.

From 7–13 years of age, the LEA contributes approximately 80% and the LT approximately 20%. Above 13 years of age, the adult pattern is adopted. As the physis fuses the metaphyseal vessels grow into the head. The LEA continues as well as the LT vessels.

Tell me about the ossification of the femur

It commences at the seventh foetal week. Early in childhood only a single proximal femoral physis exists. During the first year of life the medial portion of the physis grows faster than the lateral, causing the development of the femoral neck. The capital femoral epiphysis appears at approximately 4 months in girls and 6 months in boys. The trochanteric apophysis ossification centre appears at 4 years and is responsible for appositional growth of the greater trochanter. The proximal femoral physis is responsible for metaphyseal growth in the femoral neck.

Canale ST, Tolo VT. 'Fractures of the femur in children'. *Instructional Course Lectures*, 1995; 44: 255–73.

Maeda S, Kita A, Fujii G, Funayama K, Yamada N, Kokubun S. 'Avascular necrosis associated with fractures of the femoral neck in children: histological evaluation of core biopsies of the femoral head'. *Injury*, 2003 May; 34(4): 283–6.

Song KS. 'Displaced fracture of the femoral neck in children: open versus closed reduction'. *The Bone & Joint Journal*, 2010 Aug; 92(8): 1148–51.

Trueta J. The normal vascular anatomy of the human femoral head during growth. *The Bone & Joint Journal*, 1957 May; 39-B(2): 358–94.

Viva 12   Questions

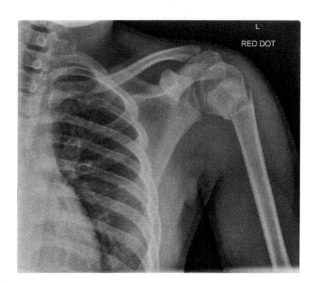

Fig. 3.12 X-ray

This 9-year-old boy fell heavily on his left arm whilst skateboarding. Can you comment on his X-ray (Fig. 3.12)?

Are you aware of any classification systems for this fracture?

How would you manage this injury?

If this injury occurred in an older child, for example a 15-year-old, would you manage it any differently?

If you were to manage this fracture surgically in this adolescent, run through the steps of your management.

Viva 12 Answers

This 9-year-old boy fell heavily on his left arm whilst skateboarding. Can you comment on his X-ray (Fig. 3.12)?

This is an AP radiograph of the left shoulder of a skeletally-immature patient showing a transverse fracture of the proximal humeral metaphysis. The fracture is angulated approximately 20° into varus. I would like to look at other views of a shoulder trauma series, specifically a scapular Y view and a (modified) axillary view to assess the degree of displacement further and to rule out a dislocation.

Are you aware of any classification systems for this fracture?

Paediatric fractures can be broadly classified into physeal or extra-physeal fractures. Physeal injuries can be further classified based on the Salter-Harris classification. For the proximal humerus, SH II fractures are the most common fracture type in the older child and SH I the most common in the neonate and younger child.

Alternatively, the Neer-Horowitz classification grades proximal humeral physeal fractures by the amount of displacement:

    Grade I: <5mm displacement
    Grade II: Displacement between 5 mm and 1/3 the width of the shaft
    Grade III: Displacement 1/3–2/3 the width of the shaft
    Grade IV: Displacement > 2/3 the width of the shaft*

How would you manage this injury?

I would manage this injury by first taking a full history and completing an examination of the child, in particular looking at the neurologic status of the limb (axillary nerve/brachial plexus). I would ask for plain X-rays (a full shoulder trauma series) and ensure that all features are consistent with the injury pattern (ie. rule out NAI).

The other pertinent points I would elicit are the presence of any open wounds, whether this is an isolated injury (or polytrauma) and the presence of a vascular injury. All of which would be indications for operative stabilization.

Other indications for surgical treatment are displaced SH III and IV fractures which are very rare and severe facture displacement in adolescent.

In this scenario, based on the age of the child and the minor degree of displacement, I would opt for conservative management with a collar and cuff sling with progression to mobilization as pain allows, usually within 3 weeks.

If this injury occurred in an older child, say a 15-year-old, would you manage it any differently?

In a 15-year-old child with this X-ray, I would still manage it conservatively with a sling. There is no controversy in the management of proximal humeral fractures in the younger child (< 10 years old), regardless of the degree of displacement, they do well with non-operative management as there

* Data from *Orthopedics* 41, 1965, Neer CS and Horowitz BS: 'Fractures of the proximal humeral epiphyseal plate', pp. 24–31

is tremendous remodeling potential (80% of longitudinal growth of the humerus takes place at the proximal physis) and a wide functional arc of motion of the shoulder.

However, I am aware of recent changes in thinking that suggests that the older child, particularly those with more displacement, may benefit from operative intervention. Previous studies advocating universal conservative management of paediatric proximal humeral fractures tended to include younger children with very few adolescents in the cohort. A recent systematic review of over 550 cases by Pahlavan et al. suggests that children over 13 years old may benefit from anatomic reduction and fixation due to poorer outcomes (shortening, varus malunion with restricted range of motion) with conservative management.

If you were to manage this fracture surgically in this adolescent, run through the steps of your management.

My treatment goal is to achieve an acceptable alignment, for which there is no absolute consensus in the literature, but I would aim for < 30° angulation and < 50% translation.

I would ensure the child is appropriately consented and marked. Ensure that the WHO theatre checks are made; then place the child in the supine position with a sandbag between the scapulae and using intra-operative fluoroscopy, attempt closed reduction with gentle traction, 90° of flexion, then 90° of abduction and external rotation.

If this fails, then I would proceed to open reduction via a delto-pectoral approach. Studies by Pandya et al and Bahrs et al showed that in the majority of cases, the periosteum or biceps tendon was a block to reduction. Other impediments to reduction include buttonholing of the diaphyseal fragment into the deltoid or the presence of comminution; and often, there is more than one structure blocking reduction.

Once the fracture is reduced adequately, I would stabilize it with percutaneous K-wires. I am aware of other techniques involving cannulated screws, plates and retrograde elastic nails. A recent study by Hitchinson, Bae and Waters (2011) comparing flexible intramedullary nails to percutaneous pinning showed both to be effective in stabilizing severely displaced fractures, with nails having fewer complications but requiring longer surgical time with higher blood loss. There was also a need for implant removal.

Bahrs C et al. 'Proximal humeral fractures in children and adolescents'. *Journal of Pediatric Orthopedics*, 2009; 29(3): 238–42.

Beaty JH, Kasser JR (ed). *Rockwood and Wilkins' Fractures in Children* 7th edition 2010. 'Proximal humerus, scapula and clavicle'.) Lippincott, Williams and Wilkins, Philadelphia, PA.

Hutchinson PH, Bae DS and Waters PM. 'Intramedullary nailing versus percutaneous pin fixation of pediatric proximal humerus fractures: a comparison of complications and early radiographic results'. *Journal of Pediatric Orthopedics*, 2011; 31(6): 617–22.

Pahlavan S et al. 'Proximal humerus fractures in the pediatric population: a systemic review'. *Journal of Child Orthopedics*, 2011; 5(3): 187–94.

Pandya NK, Behrends D and Hosalkar HS. 'Open reduction of proximal humerus fractures in the adolescent population'. *Journal of Child Orthopedics*, 2012; 6(2): 111–8.

Viva 13   Questions

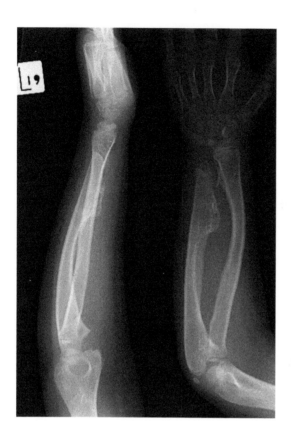

Fig. 3.13 X-ray

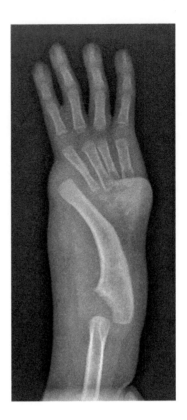

Fig. 3.14 X-ray

Describe what you see in this radiograph (Fig. 3.13).

Can you tell me anything about the genetic basis and/or inheritance pattern of this condition?

How would you assess this child who is age 4?

In this child's forearm, what would your indications for surgical treatment be?

Mother tells you she has looked online and there is a risk of cancer: how would you explain this to her?

Can you tell me a little about the X-ray in Fig. 3.14? It is a post-treatment radiograph.

Viva 13   Answers

Describe what you see in this radiograph (Fig. 3.13)

Fig. 3.13 shows an AP and a lateral view of the left forearm of a child. There are several exostoses visible and there is quite a considerable deformity present with a short ulna and a curved radius. On the AP view the prominent sessile exostosis appears to be growing towards the radius but on the lateral view it appears more prominent on the volar aspect.

The diagnosis is multiple exostoses. This is hereditary and termed HME

Can you tell me anything about the genetic basis and/or inheritance pattern of this condition?

It is an autosomal dominant inheritance pattern although the clinical phenotype can vary from generation to generation. The condition is due to a disorder in the EXT1, EXT2 or EXT3 (tumour suppressor) genes with some people suggesting that the clinical picture varies with which gene is involved. The gene defect is manifested as a growth disorder and may arise *de novo* and hence there may be no family history at the time that the index case presents.

How would you assess this child who is age 4?

A full history and complete examination are essential but at this young age, to my mind, some of the most important considerations are to discuss the family history of the condition and to gain insight as to how it has affected (or not affected) other members of the family. If they have had several surgical procedures and understand about the condition and its effects on function etc the clinician can adjust the consultation accordingly. If this is the first case in the family, more explanation and reassurance will be necessary.

It would be helpful to know at this young age, how many limbs are involved and to what extent. Hand dominance will be noted.

In this condition, involvement of the paired bones (such as in the forearm or in the lower leg) can lead to significant deformity and joint disruption so I would assess his/her lower limb alignment and upper limb function carefully.

I would have a low threshold for getting a baseline standing AP leg length/alignment radiograph to exclude any exostoses interfering with ankle growth for example.

I would want to define whether or not any symptoms were present: at this age, symptoms are rare but the lumps and bumps are becoming more noticeable with growth.

In this child's forearm, what would your indications for surgical treatment be?

The indications for treatment are open to interpretation and a holistic approach to the care of the child (and perhaps other siblings) must be undertaken.

In the forearm, my biggest concern would relate to the risk of progressive deformity leading to dislocation of the radial head. If I thought that the presence of any individual exostosis was, by direct pressure for example, interfering with growth and/or movement (such as pronation/supination) then I would consider simple excision. The distal ulna is one of the most frequently affected sites and an exostosis here may contribute to radial shaft deformity. The evidence that pronation/supination is improved after simple excision is limited.

If the deformity was progressive, then I would consider intervening to correct the radial deformity and perhaps to add length to the ulna. It is, however, impossible to restore a normal distal radioulnar joint and I would want to be careful not to make matters worse by lengthening the ulna. I would anticipate that if the radius remained straight and 'untethered' that the radial head would remain located during growth.

Lengthening for a short forearm could be considered but not at this age.

It is very rare for forearm exostoses to be associated with neurovascular compromise but if this did occur, appropriate treatment could be instigated.

Mother tells you she has looked online and there is a risk of cancer: how would you explain this to her?

I would explain that this is indeed a theoretical risk in patient with HME but it is extremely rare in growing children (according to the local bone tumour units in the UK, it essentially never happens). As the cartilage cap of the exostosis is the bit that is most active, and the defect is in the EXT (tumour suppressor) gene, malignant transformation to a chondrosarcoma can occur. The tumour is low grade in 90% of cases and does not usually present until the fifth decade or later. The proximal lesions are more susceptible to change and this is often associated with an increase or change in symptom level and a change in the shape or size of the lesion.

I would reassure her that there was no cause for concern at present or indeed in the forseeable future.

Can you tell me a little about the X-ray in Fig. 3.14? It is a post-treatment radiograph

This is an AP radiograph of the forearm and hand of a young child. There is only a single bone forearm and the bone resembles an ulna. There are only 4 digits and no thumb. The X-ray would be compatible with a diagnosis of a radial club hand where the radius is completely absent.

Treatment of this condition is complex and there are various principles that are involved. It is important to maintain function; for example, in many children elbow flexion is limited and the child can only get their hand to their mouth if the hand is allowed to radially deviate. In such circumstances, if the hand position is changed and/or stiffened, function is significantly worse.

Treatment also depends on the quality of the fingers and whether or not pollicization of an index finger is contemplated. Most surgeons would like to improve the wrist position: this often involves a release of the tight (deforming) soft tissue structures and repositioning the carpus in relation to the bone. Historically, centralization of the carpus on the distal ulna whilst preserving growth was the treatment of choice but now many surgeons perform a radialization of the distal ulna or a ulnarization of the carpus (both are in essence the same procedure but described from a different view point). Rebalancing of the soft tissues may be required in order to maintain position and movement.

In this radiograph it appears that this radialization/ulnarization procedure has been performed. The soft tissues around the digits appear 'featureless' and I would anticipate that all joints were quite stiff.

D'Ambrosi R, Barbato A, Caldarini C, Biancardi E, Facchini RM. 'Gradual ulnar lengthening in children with multiple exostoses and radial head dislocation: results at skeletal maturity'. *Journal of Child Orthopedics*, 2016 Apr; 10(2): 127–33.

Farr S, Kalish LA, Bae DS, Waters PM. 'Radiographic Criteria for Undergoing an Ulnar Shortening Osteotomy in Madelung Deformity: A Long-term Experience From a Single Institution'. *Journal of Pediatric Orthopedics*, 2016 Apr-May; 36(3): 310–5.

Kozin SH, Zlotolow DA. 'Madelung Deformity'. *Journal of Hand Surgery*, American Volume, 2015 Oct; 40(10): 2090–8.

Refsland S, Kozin SH, Zlotolow DA. 'Ulnar Distraction Osteogenesis in the Treatment of Forearm Deformities in Children With Multiple Hereditary Exostoses'. *Journal of Hand Surgery*, American Volume, 2016 Sep; 41(9): 888–95.

Waters PM. 'Forearm rebalancing in osteochondromatosis by radioulnar fusion'. *Techniques in Hand & Upper Extremity Surgery* 2007; 11(4): 236–40.

Viva 14   Questions

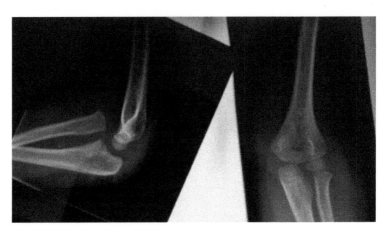

Fig. 3.15 X-ray

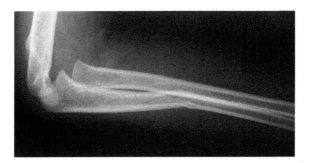

Fig. 3.16 X-ray

This 4-year-old child fell from a climbing frame onto her left arm. Tell me what you see on these X-rays (Fig. 3.15).

You obtain another X-ray (Fig. 3.16). What do you think now?

Can you classify this injury?

How would you manage this injury?

If, in a different case, the radial head remained dislocated despite reduction and stabilization of the ulna with a flexible nail; what would you do next?

Monteggia fractures are commonly missed. Are you aware of any literature on the management of such chronic or neglected injuries?

Viva 14   Answers

This 4-year-old child fell from a climbing frame onto her left arm. Tell me what you see on these X-rays (Fig. 3.15)

This is an AP and lateral X-ray of the elbow of a skeletally-immature patient. The AP film shows malalignment of the radiocapitellar joint and the lateral film confirms an anterior dislocation of the radial head. In the normal elbow, a line through the longitudinal axis of the radius passes through the centre of the capitellum. With a post traumatic dislocation of the radial head, I would be suspicious of a fracture of the ulna. I would therefore like further X-rays of the forearm to visualize the entire bone including the 'joint above and the joint below'.

You obtain another X-ray (Fig. 3.16). What do you think now?

This lateral X-ray of the forearm confirms a greenstick fracture of the ulna diaphysis which is angulated anteriorly. This is a Monteggia fracture-dislocation of the elbow.

Can you classify this injury?

Monteggia fractures can be classified by the Bado classification which is defined by the direction of the radial head dislocation. The radial head dislocation, in turn, is always in the direction of the apex of the ulnar deformity.

- In Bado type I fractures, which is the most common (70%), the radial head is dislocated anteriorly with an apex anterior fracture of the ulna.
- In Bado type II fractures, the radial head is dislocated posteriorly with an apex posterior fracture of the ulna. This fracture pattern is rare in children (3%).
- In Bado type III fractures, which is the second most common (23%), the radial head is dislocated laterally with a typical metaphyseal greenstick fracture of the ulna.
- In Bado type IV fractures (1%), both radius and ulna are fractured with anterior dislocation of the radial head.*

This case is therefore a Bado type I injury.

How would you manage this injury?

This child has fallen from a height, therefore in the first instance, I would employ ATLS protocols and ensure that she has no concurrent injuries. I would then take a full history and examine the limb and ensure that they corroborate. In the examination, I would look for open wounds and carefully examine and document the neurological status of the limb, especially that of the posterior interosseous nerve which is the most commonly injured nerve, complicating around 20% of cases.

This fracture would then need to be managed in theatre under a general anaesthetic. The principles of management are to reduce the ulna deformity and/or ensure that the bone is 'out to length' and typically the radial head will then reduce with direct pressure.

My treatment strategy would then depend on the ulna fracture pattern: for plastic deformation or greenstick fractures, such as in this case, manipulation and a well-moulded cast with the elbow in 90° flexion and supination would probably be sufficient.

* Data from *Clinical Orthopaedics and Related Research*, 50, 1967, Bado JL: 'The Monteggia lesion', pp. 71–86.

In a simple transverse or short oblique fracture pattern of the ulna (i.e. length stable), I would use an intramedullary flexible nail. In a comminuted or long oblique (i.e. axially unstable) fracture pattern, I would openly reduce the ulna and stabilize it with a short semi-tubular plate.

In all cases, the child would require close follow-up, weekly in the first instance as re-displacement of the radial head has been reported in up to 20% of cases.

This treatment algorithm has been corroborated by a recent multicentre study where treatment strategy based on ulna fracture pattern (or more rigorous treatment) yielded no failures.

If, in a different case, the radial head remained dislocated despite reduction and stabilization of the ulna with a flexible nail; what would you do next?

In this situation, I would re-evaluate the reduction of the ulna. It should be out to length with minimal angulation. If an anatomical reduction has not been obtained or maintained with the flexible nail, then I would proceed to open reduction of the fracture and stabilization with a semi-tubular plate. If the radial head was still dislocated following this, then I would explore the radio-capitellar joint, using the posterolateral approach to the elbow. Possible obstacles to reduction include the annular ligament or a cartilaginous or osteochondral fragment.

Monteggia fractures are commonly missed. Are you aware of any literature on the management of such chronic or neglected injuries?

Monteggia fractures are typically missed when there is only plastic deformation of the ulna; hence it is important to obtain adequate radiographs of the elbow and forearm and to analyse the radiocapitellar relationship (and the contour of the ulna) carefully.

A possible differential diagnosis to consider is congenital dislocation of the radial head. In such cases, the dislocation is typically posterior and often bilateral with hypoplasia of the capitellum, convexity of the radial head and shortening and bowing of the radius. It may be associated with syndromes such as Larsen's, Ehlers-Danlos or nail-patella syndrome.

The treatment of a child with chronic dislocation of the radial head represents a difficult dilemma. In the short term, several reports indicate that most children have minimal or no symptoms (Tachdjian). However, in the long term, pain, instability, restricted movement (prono-supination and flexion) and neuropathies may follow.

Reconstruction of ulna length and angulation can be performed acutely via a corrective osteotomy of the ulna or gradually using an external fixator with open reduction of the radial head if necessary and with/withour a formal annular ligament reconstruction. Such surgery is associated with problems such as residual radial head dislocation, ulnar nerve palsy, heterotopic ossification and fibrous synostosis.

Nakamura et al (2009) showed good long-term results after acute reconstruction for chronic missed Monteggia fractures in children under 12 or within 3 years of the initial injury.

Benson M, Fixsen J, Macnicol M, Parsch K (eds.). *Children's Orthopaedics and Fractures* 2010. 3rd edition: 'Fractures of the elbow and forearm'. Springer-Verlag, London, UK.

Exner GU. 'Missed chronic anterior Monteggia lesion. Closed reduction by gradual lengthening and angulation of the ulna'. *The Bone & Joint Journal* 2001; 83(4): 547–50.

Herring JA (ed.). *Tachdjian's Pediatric Orthopaedics* 5th edition 2014. 'Upper extremity injuries'. Elsevier Saunders, Philadelphia, PA.

Nakamura K et al. 'Long-term clinical and radiographic outcomes after open reduction for missed Monteggia fracture-dislocations in children'. *The Journal of Bone & Joint Surgery, American volume*, 2009; 91(6): 1394–404.

Ramski DE et al. 'Pediatric Monteggia fractures: a multicenter examination of treatment strategy and early clinical and radiographic results'. *Journal of Pediatric Orthopedics*, 2015; 35: 115–20.

Ring D, Jupiter JB, Waters PM. 'Monteggia fractures in children and adults'. *The Journal of the American Academy of Orthopaedic Surgeons*, 1998; 6(4): 215–24.

Viva 15 Questions

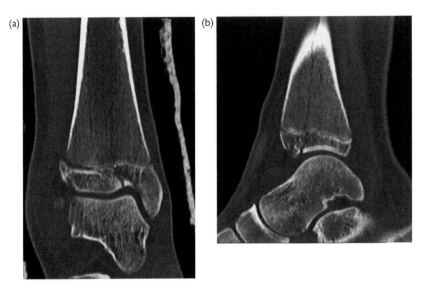

Fig. 3.17 CT images

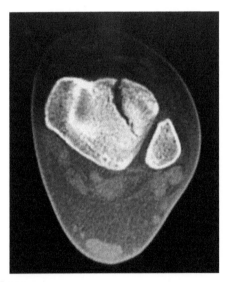

Fig. 3.18 Transverse CT scan

This 13-year-old boy twisted his ankle at football. He is not able to weightbear and his ankle is very swollen and bruised. What do you think of his images shown in Fig. 3.17?

Why do you think this fracture pattern (Fig. 3.18) has occurred?

Are you aware of any classification systems for triplane injuries?

How would you manage this injury?

Viva 15   Answers

This 13-year-old boy twisted his ankle at football training. He is unable to weightbear and his ankle is very swollen and bruised. What do you think of his images shown in Fig. 3.17?

These are an AP and lateral ankle CT images of a skeletally-immature patient. On the AP view, there is a Salter-Harris III fracture of the ankle; and on the lateral image, there is a Salter-Harris IV fracture. This is therefore a triplane ankle fracture—so called as there are different components in the sagittal, coronal and transverse planes.

Why do you think this fracture pattern (Fig. 3.18) has occurred?

Triplane and Tillaux fractures are unique to adolescents and are called transitional fractures due to the asymmetric closure of the distal tibial physis as a child progresses towards skeletal maturity. Over 18 months, the distal tibial physis closes sequentially: first centrally, then the anteromedial and posteromedial portions, and finally the lateral part. As such, Tillaux fractures tend to occur in older adolescents, typically in the last year of growth, whilst triplane fractures occur in a slightly younger age group.

Are you aware of any classification systems for triplane injuries?

Triplane fractures can be classified according to how medial or lateral the fracture exits the epiphysis as well as by the fact that the metaphyseal fracture occurs in the sagittal plane in medial triplane fractures and in the coronal plane in lateral triplane fractures. Lateral fractures are more common and they can be classified as 2-, 3-, or 4-part. The fibula can be fractured in conjunction with any of these patterns.

There are 2 fracture fragments in 2-part fractures—the medial fragment comprises the tibial shaft, medial malleolus and anteromedial aspect of the epiphysis, the lateral fragment includes the remainder of the epiphysis and the posterior metaphyseal spike.

In 3-part fractures, the coronal plane fracture line traverses the epiphysis and posterior metaphysis in their entirety. There are therefore 3 fracture fragments—the medial fragment remains the same and the lateral fragment is in 2 parts with a rectangular anterolateral quadrant of the epiphysis being a separate fragment (equivalent to a Tillaux fragment).

When the fracture extends more medially in the transverse plane, a 4-part fracture develops with the fourth fragment comprising the medial malleolus.

How would you manage this injury?

I would proceed with a full history and clinical examination of the child and ensure that they corroborate with the injury. This injury typically causes significant swelling, bruising and even blistering around the ankle. I would therefore ensure that the limb is well elevated and plan any operative intervention only when the swelling improves. I would also check the integrity of the skin, if there is tenting of the skin or signs of compromise, I would reduce the fracture urgently under conscious sedation in A&E and place the child in an above knee plaster with the foot in internal rotation; this reverses the deforming force that created the fracture.

The principle goal in the treatment of triplane fractures is to achieve anatomic reduction of the distal tibial articular surface. Rapariz et al. and Ertl et al. have shown that fractures with > 2 mm displacement developed degenerative changes and discomfort in the long term.

To define the fracture configuration further and help with surgical planning, as here, I would obtain a CT of the ankle. Studies have shown the inaccuracy of plain radiographs for articular surface displacement, especially those over 2 mm and Jones et al. have also demonstrated that surgeons changed their surgical planning for screw placement based on CT images.

If the CT showed that the fracture was < 2 mm displaced, I would attempt conservative treatment in an above knee plaster cast for 4 weeks, followed by a below knee cast for a further 2 weeks. I would monitor the child closely initially, and consider repeating the CT scan at 1 week if I am not confident about the reduction. If it is > 2 mm, I would treat this operatively with closed reduction (foot in plantarflexion with traction and internal rotation) and compression using a Weber bone reduction forceps and fixation with 4.0 mm cannulated screws. I would plan to place the screws orthogonal to the fracture line as analysed on CT and I would be careful to avoid damaging the physis any further, especially if the child has more than 2 years of growth remaining. If a closed reduction fails, perhaps due to interposition of a periosteal sleeve. I would have a low threshold for proceeding to open reduction (with direct visualization of the articular surface) and stabilization with a cannulated screw.

Are you aware of any complications of transitional fractures?

Residual articular incongruity with resultant degenerative change is the predominant concern with poor long-term outcomes (pain and swelling especially) noted in malreduced fractures > 2 mm.

Growth arrest is also a possible complication although less so considering transitional fractures (especially the Tillaux fracture) typically occur in adolescents with limited growth remaining. Rates of growth arrest following triplane fractures have been quoted from 0–21%. In theory, a growth arrest may result in a leg length discrepancy, fibular overgrowth with lateral impingement, and angular deformities.

I am also aware of a cadaveric biomechanical study that showed retained transepiphyseal screws (metallic or bioabsorbable) significantly increased peak intra-articular contact pressures over baseline (Charlton et al.), and thus I would recommend implant removal.

Charlton M, Costello R, Mooney JF III, Podeszwa DA. 'Ankle joint biomechanics following transepiphyseal screw fixation of the distal tibia'. Journal of Pediatric Orthopedics, 2005; 25(5): 635–40.

Ertl JP, Barrack RL, Alexander AH, VanBuecken K. 'Triplane fracture of the distal tibial epiphysis. Long-term follow-up'. The Journal of Bone & Joint Surgery, American volume, 1988; 70(7): 967–6.

Jones A et al. 'Triplane fractures of the distal tibia requiring open reduction and internal fixation: pre-operative planning using computer tomography'. Injury 2003; 34(4): 293–8.

Rapariz JM et al. 'Distal tibial triplane fractures: long-term follow-up'. Journal of Pediatric Orthopedics 1996; 16(1): 113–8.

Rosenbaum AJ, DiPreta JA, Uhl RL. 'Review of distal tibial epiphyseal transitional fractures'. Orthopedics, 2012; 35(12): 1046–9.

Wuerz TH, Gurd DP. 'Pediatric physeal ankle fracture'. The Journal of the American Academy of Orthopedic Surgeons, 2013; 21: 234–44. [Review]

Viva 16   Questions

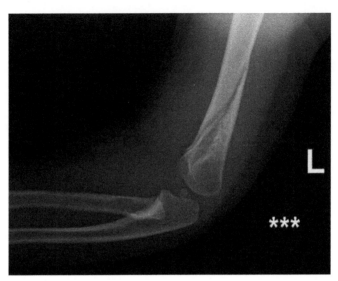

Fig. 3.19 X-ray

A 14-month-old girl was brought in by her father who is concerned that she is not using her left arm. Tell me about the X-ray (Fig. 3.19).

The child's father says that he found her crying in her cot after a nap. He thinks she probably caught her arm in the bars of the cot. He also becomes angry that you are asking so many questions, he just wants his daughter treated and to go home.

Tell me how you would manage this child.

What features on radiographs are suggestive of NAI?

What is your role in managing suspect NAI?

Viva 16 Answers

A 14-month-old girl was brought in by her father who is concerned that she is not using her left arm. Tell me about this X-ray (Fig. 3.19)

This is a lateral radiograph of a young child's humerus which shows an undisplaced spiral fracture of the distal humerus. A systematic review by Kemp A et al. (2008) and a large comparative review of NAI cases in a Level 1 paediatric trauma centre in the USA (Pandya et al., 2009) found that the prevalence of abuse was significantly greater in children under 18 months with a humeral fracture, whilst accidental injury was more likely in children > 18 months old. The most common type of humeral fracture resulting from abuse in children under 18 months of age was a spiral/oblique fracture. I would therefore be highly suspicious of NAI in this child.

The child's father says that he found her crying in her cot after a nap. He thinks she probably caught her arm in the bars of the cot. He also becomes angry that you are asking so many questions, he just wants his daughter treated and to go home

The story is vague, the mechanism seems improbable, the child has a spiral fracture which suggests a twisting injury to the humerus, and the father appears unnecessarily aggressive. I would remain concerned about the possibility of NAI. In this case, the child needs to remain in A&E or be admitted whilst further advice is sought from the child safe guarding team.

Tell me how you would manage this child

I would first take a thorough history from the parent and any other witnesses, examine the child after complete exposure. In my history the key points I would focus on are the age of the patient, mechanism of injury (looking for inconsistencies or improbability between the mechanism and injury pattern as well as any delay in presentation), antenatal and developmental history (as prematurity is a known risk factor for NAI), past medical history and family history (e.g. known osteogenesis imperfecta, osteopenia of prematurity, bone dysplasia or previous fractures; as well as any other previous attendances to hospital) and interaction between parent and the child (e.g. child fearful of parent, or parent evasive or aggressive).

I would be mindful of the risk factors of NAI: low socioeconomic class, parents with mental health or history of substance-misuse, exposure to domestic violence, vulnerable and unsupported parents, twins, developmental delay, preterm babies, and chronic illness.

I would ensure that I was meticulous with documentation in the child's medical notes. I would also gather collateral information, for example looking for any visual codes on the child's medical notes (depending on each hospital's policy) that indicate they are known to social services or are on the child protection register, or contact social services (day or night) directly to enquire whether the child is known to their services.

In my examination of the child, I would be certain to fully examine the child from head to toe as next to fractures, soft tissue injury like bruises and burns are the most common presentation of NAI (Baldwin and Scherl, 2013). In particular, I would be looking for signs of neglect, bruises with semblance to hand or fingerprints, or implements used to harm the child like a cigarette burn.

In addition to the above, the child's humeral fracture still requires appropriate management. In this case, I would immobilize the arm against the chest with a swathe or velpeau bandage.

Ultimately, if I have any concerns regarding the welfare of the child, I would inform my consultant and the named or designated nurse or doctor for safeguarding children depending upon local policies. My priority would be to ensure the child is in a safe environment. Out of hours it would be appropriate to admit the child to the ward for assessment. In cases where there is a high level of concern I would directly refer the child to children's social care, following Local Safeguarding Children Board (LSCB) procedures. In circumstances where there is risk of immediate serious harm, I would contact the police who can arrange emergency protection for the child.

Radiographic investigations should be performed in consultation with an appropriate radiologist. This would involve a skeletal survey, especially in children aged under 2, which includes plain films of the skull, chest, abdomen, spine, and limbs

Other investigations to exclude medical, skeletal, and biochemical abnormalities/differential diagnoses should also be considered.

What features on radiographs are suggestive of NAI?

There is no one fracture pattern or location that is specific for NAI. Fractures resulting from abuse have been described in virtually every bone in the body. More important is to consider the age and developmental stage of the child as there is a strong inverse relationship between age of the child and likelihood of a fracture from abuse (Kemp et al., 2008).

However, certain radiological findings should raise suspicions including presence of multiple fractures, rib fractures (particularly posteromedial, 71% probability of NAI), fractures of different ages, X-ray evidence of occult fractures (fractures identified on X-rays that were not clinically evident), metaphyseal corner (bucket handle) fractures of long bones, humeral fractures (1:2 chance of NAI), femoral fractures in children under 18 months old (1:3 chance), tibia/fibula fractures under 18 months old, and complex skull fractures.

What is your role in managing suspect NAI?

It is a legal responsibility of all clinicians to initiate child protection procedures if child abuse is suspected and we must all have a high index of suspicion for NAI. As orthopaedic surgeons, this is even more pertinent as most cases of maltreatment present with soft tissue injury or fractures, hence we are frequently the first doctor to see such children.

To ensure good medical practice, I am obliged to adhere to The General Medical Council's published guidance on cases of suspected abuse, 'Protecting children and young people: the responsibilities of all doctors'. NICE has also published guidelines on 'when to suspect child maltreatment'. It is also my responsibility to ensure that I have received the relevant training (minimum level 2 training) as a healthcare professional to recognize child maltreatment.

This is a difficult problem and must be managed sensitively as part of a multidisciplinary team, including paediatricians, orthopaedic surgeons, social workers, and allied health professionals. It is important to have a working knowledge of local procedures for protecting children and young people. In general, as an orthopaedic surgeon, my role is to consider the safety and welfare of my patient by being aware of risk factors and examining for signs of abuse or neglect. Each hospital will have a named nurse or doctor for child protection issues through which advice can be sought. The patient should not be allowed to leave the hospital if there are any concerns.

Baldwin KD, Scherl SA. 'Orthopaedic aspects of child abuse'. *Instructional Course Lectures*, 2013; 62: 399403.

General Medical Council (2012). 'Protecting children and young people: the responsibilities of all doctors' [http://www.gmc-uk.org/static/documents/content/Protecting_children_and_young_people_-_English_0414.pdf]

Kemp AM et al. 'Patterns of skeletal fractures in child abuse: systematic review'. *BMJ*, 2008; 337: a1518.

Jayakumar P, Barry M, Ramachandran M. 'Orthopaedic aspects of paediatric non-accidental injury'.
The Bone & Joint Journal, 2010; 92(2): 189–95.

National Institute for Health and Clinical Excellence (2009) 'When to suspect child maltreatment' [http://www.nice.org.uk/nicemedia/pdf/CG89FullGuideline.pdf]

Pandya NK et al. 'Child abuse and orthopaedic injury patterns: analysis at a level I pediatric trauma center'. *Journal of Pediatric Orthopedics* 2009; 29(6): 618–25.

Royal College of Paediatrics and Child Health (2014). 'Safeguarding children and young people: roles and competences for healthcare staff': intercollegiate document [http://www.rcpch.ac.uk/child-health/standards-care/child-protection/publications/child-protection-publications]

The Royal College of Radiologists/Royal College of Paediatrics and Child Health. 'Standards for radiological investigations of suspected non-accidental injury' (March 2008). [http://www.rcr.ac.uk/docs/radiology/pdf/RCPCH_RCR_final.pdf]

Viva 17   Questions

What do you know about the layers of the embryo that give rise to musculoskeletal tissues?

So when does a limb bud start to develop?

Do the upper and lower limbs develop at the same time?

Can you draw me a cross section of the embryo at that stage of development?

So how does the spine form?

Do they give rise to the entire vertebra? Is there a structure you have forgotten here?

What about the discs?

So what else do the somites give rise to?

So you mentioned the neural tube. What does that form?

And it also forms another part of the nervous system. Think about the arrangement of the peripheral nerves; the location of the anterior horn cells and dorsal root ganglia. How do you explain that?

So moving on to the limb, what germinal layer gives rise to bone?

So what controls the development of the limb bud?

Viva 17   Answers

What do you know about the layers of the embryo that give rise to musculoskeletal tissues?

In the early embryo, cells divide into 3 germ layers; ectoderm, endoderm and mesoderm. These layers all give rise to specific structures. Ectoderm gives rise to the nervous system, while mesoderm ultimately forms muscle, bone and connective tissue. Endoderm forms structures such as the gut.

So when does a limb bud start to develop?

Between the fourth and eighth foetal weeks.

Do the upper and lower limbs develop at the same time?

No—the upper limbs form first.

Can you draw me a cross section of the embryo at that stage of development?

This is a difficult and perhaps unexpected question to be asked. If this happens, collect your thoughts and remember to draw something that makes sense and allows you to convey some of the information you know. Outline the shape of the embryo, with limb buds on the outside, then start to add areas of ectoderm and mesoderm, describing them as you go (see Fig. 3.20). As always, if you don't know where to start, it is best to admit this, move on and score points on information you do know.

So how does the spine form?

The somites give rise to the vertebrae.

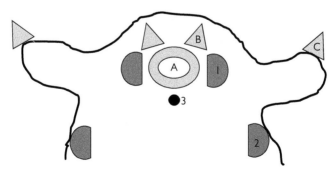

Fig. 3.20 This is the overall shape of the embryo in cross section (Fig. 3.20), with limb buds forming at the sides (C). Ectoderm gives rise to the neural tube (A) and neural crests (B). Mesoderm gives rise to the somites (1), which lie alongside the neural tube and the lateral plates (2)

Do they give rise to the entire vertebra? Is there a structure you have forgotten here?

In a difficult question, such as this, some prompting is expected and does not mean that you will fail the question.

Yes, the notochord. This is a structure that governs cell direction. It forms the anterior vertebral body, with the somites forming the remainder of the vertebra.

What about the discs?

The discs are also formed by the notochord and somites. The notochord forms the nucleus pulposus and the somites form the annulus fibrosus.

So what else do the somites give rise to?

Muscle and skin.

So you mentioned the neural tube. What does that form?

The neural tube forms the spinal cord.

And it also forms another part of the nervous system. Think about the arrangement of the peripheral nerves; the location of the anterior horn cells and dorsal root ganglia. How do you explain that?

Motor nerves arise from the neural tube and as a result the anterior horn cells are found within the spinal cord. In contrast, sensory nerves arise from the neural crest. Looking at my diagram, this explains why the dorsal root ganglion is located outside the spinal cord. The neural crest also forms the autonomic nervous system. This explains the location of the sympathetic chain and the distant parasympathetic plexi.

So moving on to the limb, what germinal layer gives rise to bone?

The mesoderm forms the lateral plates, which form bone for the limb bud.

So what controls the development of the limb bud?

Ectoderm gives rise to areas in the limb bud known as the Zone of Proliferating Activity (ZPA) and the Apical Ectodermal Ridge (both C).

Musculoskeletal System Development, https://embryology.med.unsw.edu.au/embryology/index.php/Musculoskeletal_System_Development

Moore KL, Persuad TVN:. *The Developing Human: clinically oriented embryology*, 8th edition. 2008. Philadelphia: Saunders.

Viva 18   Questions

Draw me a growth plate.

What about the blood supply?

Based on your picture, how do you explain growth plate injuries,?

Now, please illustrate on your diagram how the Salter-Harris Fracture types 1–5 injure the physis.

So apart from fractures, are you aware of any other conditions that affect the epiphysis and growth plate?

Is the growth plate the only part of the bone that contributes to growth?

Viva 18   Answers

Draw me a growth plate

When drawing in the exam it is essential that you follow these rules;

1) Fill the page
2) Talk as you draw—this type of question is used to test knowledge and understanding, not your ability as an artist
3) Simplify the drawing in a way that conveys your understanding of the topic, for example, when drawing a growth plate, 2 or 3 cells in each layer will suffice and save you time

The (discoid) physis at the end of a long bone links the epiphysis to the metaphysis. It consists of several zones defined by what the cells are doing in each zone or layer. In the *resting zone* of the physis, closest to the epiphysis, the cells are inactive and randomly dispersed within the matrix. Once stimulated, these cells start proliferating (*the proliferating zone, oxygen tension is high*) and they stack up in columns, the surrounding matrix is mainly collagen type II. In response to further stimuli, the cells then begin to hypertrophy (*the hypertrophic zone, oxygen tension is low*): as the cells grow, they take up more space leaving less room for the extracellular matrix which is now predominantly type X collagen. The micro-environment facilitates mineralization of the remaining matrix and chondrocyte apoptosis. The process of vascular ingrowth from the metaphysis brings osteoblasts to the scene and ossification takes place.

If the discoid physis is rolled up into a sphere, it then mimics the spherical physes seen in the small bones of the carpus and the tarsus. Such spherical physes are also seen as the secondary centres of ossification within the epiphyses of long bones. As they grow they take on the shape of the cartilage anlage that they are replacing. Abnormal pressures will lead to abnormal shapes.

The perichondrial ring of LaCroix and the fibrous groove of Ranvier lie at the periphery of the physis. They supply chondrocytes to the physis that allow appositional growth and by linking in to both the epiphysis and the metaphysis, these structures help to stabilize the physis and reduce the risk of physeal separation.

What about the blood supply?

The epiphyseal artery forms cascades within the epiphysis, with vessels that penetrate into the growth plate. These vessels bypass the resting zone and travel to the proliferative zone, which therefore has the highest oxygen tension. The nutrient artery of the diaphysis supplies the extensive network of capillary loops in the metaphyseal region, but these vessels do *not* supply the growth plate. As a result, as proliferating chondrocytes move away from the epiphyseal vessels, the conditions become increasingly hypoxic, which leads to hypertrophy, degeneration, calcification, and cell death. The metaphyseal vessels do supply the osteoblasts that lay down bone on the cartilage template: the initial woven bone is resorbed and replaced by lamellar bone.

Based on your picture, how do you explain growth plate injuries?

Fractures through the growth plate occur in the hypertrophic zone and specifically within the zone of provisional calcification where there is a division between the scanty and weak matrix and the mineralized and hence relatively strong matrix. This is the most hypoxic region.

Now, please illustrate on your diagram how the Salter-Harris Fracture types 1–5 injure the physis.

Type 1 injuries enter and exit through the hypertrophic zone. Type 2 injuries enter in the same place but exit through the metaphysis, taking with them a Thurston-Holland fragment. Type 3 injuries exit through the epiphysis and can therefore cause injury to the epiphyseal vessels and the proliferative zone. They disrupt the articular cartilage surface of the epiphysis. Type 4 injuries traverse both the epiphysis and the physis and continue in an essentially linear fashion into metaphysis: they also risk damage to the epiphyseal vessels and the articular surface. Type 5 injuries involve crushing of the growth plate, which can cause widespread damage.

There is an additional Type 6 injury which often involves a shearing mechanism to the periphery of the growth plate, injuring the perichondral ring and often leading to a growth arrest.

So apart from fractures, are you aware of any other conditions that affect the epiphysis and growth plate?

Yes, a wide range of conditions affect the growth plate. These include both congenital and acquired causes. Many congenital conditions such as the skeletal dysplasias can affect overall growth and congenital limb deficiencies are commonly associated with decreased growth rates (the affected limb is usually the shorter/smaller limb). Infections of both bone and joint can lead to damage to either the physis or the secondary ossification centres or both and metabolic bone disorders such as rickets or the much rarer mucopolysaccharidoses.

In some conditions the exact location of the growth disturbance has been identified, in others it has not.

Don't get too drawn on describing these: keep it simple and accurate!

But Table 3.1 may give you some additional extra pointers:

Table 3.1 Conditions that affect the epiphysis and growth plate

	Hypoplastic	Hyperplastic	Other
Epiphysis	MED, SED	Trevor's	
Resting zone	Pseudoachondroplasia, Diastrophic dysplasia		Gaucher's
Proliferative zone	Achondroplasia		
Hypertrophic zone	Kneist syndrome	Enchondroma	SUFE, rickets

Is the growth plate the only part of the bone that contributes to growth?

'No. Whilst the growth plate is responsible for longitudinal growth, bone width and shape is also achieved with appositional growth from the periosteum and, at the level of the physis, from the groove of Ranvier. Tension forces applied via muscular contractions to an apophysis also change the shape of the bone.'

Iannotti JP, Goldstein S, Kuhn J, Lipiello L, Kaplan FS, Zaleske DJ. 'The formation and growth of skeletal tissue'. In: Buckwalter JA, Einhorn TA, Simon SR, editors. *Orthopaedic Basic Science. Biology and Biomechanics of the Musculoskeletal System*: American Academy of Orthopaedic Surgeons; 2000.

P Rubin. 'On Organizing a Dynamic Classification of Bone Dysplasias'. *Arthritis and Rheumatism*, 1964 Dec; 7(6) 693–708.

Viva 19   Questions

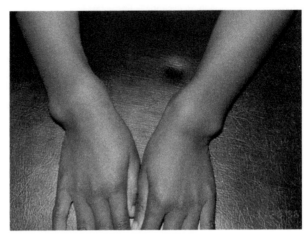

Fig. 3.21 Multiple joint pain
Courtesy of Tom D. Thacher, MD

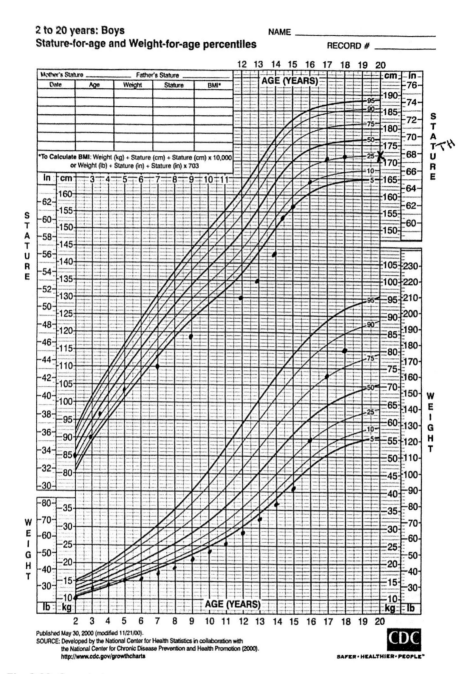

Fig. 3.22 Growth chart

Developed by the National Center for Health Statistics in collaboration with the National Center for Chronic Disease Prevention and Health Promotion (2000)

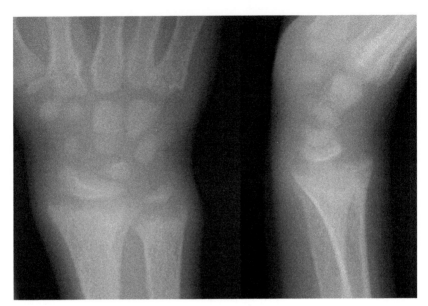

Fig. 3.23 Wrist X-ray

A North African woman brings her 3-year-old daughter into your clinic. The child is complaining of multiple joint pains, there is no history of trauma. What does the clinical photograph in Fig. 3.21 show? What other investigations might be useful?

We do not have the blood tests you have requested at the moment but Fig. 3.22 shows the growth chart for the child in Fig. 3.21—what does it demonstrate? What is happening at the arrow?

Fig. 3.23 is the wrist X-ray of the child. What does it show?

Viva 19   Answers

A North African woman brings her 3-year-old daughter into your clinic. The child is complaining of multiple joint pains, there is no history of trauma. What does the clinical photograph in Fig. 3.21 show? What other investigations might be useful?

This is a clinical photograph of a dark-skinned child (who appears older than 3 years of age) with wrist deformities. I would be thinking about a skeletal abnormality, a metabolic or inflammatory cause. I would like to have access to her clinical history and general examination findings in addition to basic information such as her charted weight and height measurements. I would request X-rays of her wrists (and other affected joints) and ask for appropriate blood tests. If I was suspecting a metabolic condition, I would want full blood count, electrolytes, vitamin D, parathyroid hormone, calcium, liver function tests with markers such as CRP and ESR if an inflammatory cause was more likely. In this case, I might also consider other markers of inflammatory arthropathies.

We do not have the blood tests you have requested at the moment but Fig. 3.22 shows the growth chart for a child similar to the one described above in Fig. 3.21– what does it demonstrate? What is happening at the arrow?

This growth chart for a boy in Fig. 3.22 demonstrates growth retardation; the child was on the 25th centile initially but then gradually fell off that centile. Both height and weight are affected in a similar way. This seems to show a chronic condition that has been present for some time. The arrow demonstrates an intervention/treatment and the gradual increase in weight and height lead to a crossing of the centiles towards (and past) the previous baseline.

The photograph and this chart would be in keeping with a diagnosis of Vitamin D deficiency rickets.

Fig. 3.23 is the wrist X-ray of the child. What does it show?

This is a plain radiograph of the wrist of a child. The physis is widened and there is significant cupping and flaring of the metaphysis. The metaphyseal trabeculae appear coarse, the cortices are a little thinned and indistinct. The 'swelling' due to the metaphyseal flaring is obvious. The diagnosis is consistent with rickets: vitamin D deficient or hypophosphataemic. A differential diagnosis would be a skeletal dysplasia affecting the metaphyses.

What are the associated clinical features of rickets in childhood?

Associated features of rickets in childhood are relative short stature (with respect to parental heights), chest wall deformities including a rachitic rosary and a pigeon chest. The ribs may become deformed and a Harrison's sulcus can be seen. The head may be enlarged. Swellings around the physes that are growing quickly may be apparent such as at the distal tibia and the wrist. The long bones may be bowed in both the coronal and sagittal plane leading to genu varum or genu valgum with anterior bowing.

What would you expect to see on blood tests in this child?

It depends on the underlying cause. In this scenario vitamin D-deficient rickets is likely: factors would include low vitamin D levels, high parathyroid hormone levels, normal or low calcium, normal or low phosphate levels. However we must consider the possibility of other causes of rickets such as X-linked or hypophosphataemic rickets; here one would expect normal vitamin D levels, high parathyroid hormone levels, normal or high calcium and low phosphate levels with high urinary phosphate levels.

How would you treat this condition?

Once again this depends on the underlying cause. Firstly I would refer to a paediatrician or metabolic bone physician. But the underlying principles in vitamin D deficiency are to provide vitamin D, remembering that there may be other aspects of malnutrition to address. In hypophosphataemic rickets treatment involves a combination of phosphate replacement and high 1,25-dihydroxy-vitamin D doses.

Herring JA. *Tachdijian's Pediatric Orthopaedics*, 5th edition. 2013, Elsevier.

Viva 20   Questions

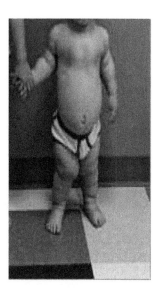

Fig. 3.24 Skeletal dysplasia

What do you understand by the phrase 'skeletal dysplasia' and which condition is shown in Fig. 3.24?

What are the features of achondroplasia? How might they present to an orthopaedic surgeon?

Do you know anything about the genetic pathology of Achondroplasia?

Viva 20 Answers

What do you understand by the phrase 'skeletal dysplasia' and which condition is shown in Fig. 3.24?

A skeletal dysplasia is a general disorder of bone growth: certain parts of the bone may be affected such as the epiphyses, metaphyses or spine; alone or in combination. The phrase is often used to describe disorders that feature disproportionate short stature (dwarfism) but actually a patient with a skeletal dysplasia may not be abnormally short.

This picture shows a child with short limbed (disproportionate) dwarfism as the hands only reach the iliac crest when they should normally reach mid thigh level. His head appears large. When looking at the limbs, the proximal arm segments seem particularly short in keeping with the rhizomelic nature of achondroplastic limbs: overall, I think the features are consistent with achondroplasia.

What are the features of achondroplasia? How might they present to an orthopaedic surgeon?

There are many features of achondroplasia. As described above the most obvious feature is a rhizomelic, disproportionate short stature (dwarfism) but there are other aspects. From head to toe they include: a prominent forehead with frontal bossing and a depressed nasal bridge. Some individuals might present with sleep apnoea or other symptoms suggestive of foramen magnum compression. Spinal aspects include a thoracolumbar kyphosis particularly during the first year of life and then an exaggerated lumbar lordosis which may be associated in adult life with the symptoms/signs of spinal stenosis. On the AP spine radiograph, there are the classical features of narrowing of the inter-pedicular distance in the lower lumbar spine. Lower limb claudication is a common symptom.

Classically, the upper limbs may demonstrate slight flexion deformities of the elbows and trident hands.

The lower limbs often demonstrate genu varum with overlong fibulae and patients may request deformity correction and/or limb lengthening.

Do you know anything about the genetic pathology of achondroplasia?

Achondroplasia is an autosomal dominant condition although most cases (approx 80%) present as a new mutation. The underlying problem is a mutation in the fibroblast growth factor receptor 3 gene (FGFR3). A single point mutation accounts for almost all cases with a glycine base being substituted by an arginine base. The gene is located on the short arm of chromosome 4.

The FGFR3 protein regulates the conversion of cartilage to bone by limiting ossification. The mutation leads to a 'gain-in-function' with increased limitation of endochondral (but not intra-membranous) ossification.

Wright MJ et al. 'Clinical management of achondroplasia'. *Archives of Disease in Childhood,* 2012; 97: 129–34.

Viva 21   Questions

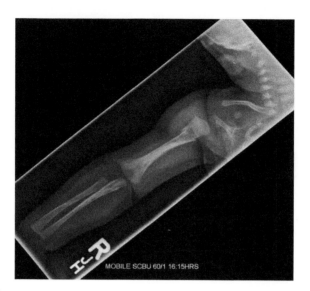

Fig. 3.25 X-ray

Fig. 3.25 shows an X-ray taken from a 1-month-old baby admitted to the hospital with pain and swelling in the upper limb. There is no specific history of trauma. Please describe the X-ray and your management.

How would you proceed the following day assuming that NAI was ruled out?

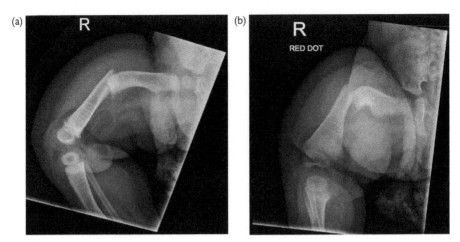

Fig. 3.26 X-ray taken 2 years later

This baby was diagnosed with OI type III due to a spontaneous mutation. Fig. 3.26 is an X-ray taken when she is 2 years old. What do you see?

How would you proceed?

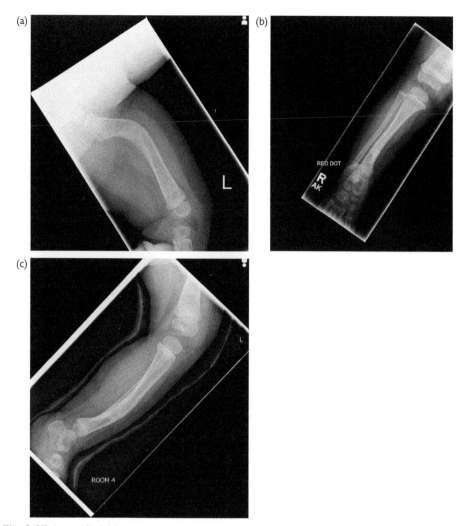

Fig. 3.27 Lower limb X-rays

Fig. 3.27 shows the other X-rays of the same girl. Assuming you have both AP and lateral films of both lower limbs how would you like to proceed?

Viva 21   Answers

Fig. 3.25 shows an X-ray taken from a 1-month-old baby admitted to the hospital with pain and swelling in the upper limb. There is no specific history of trauma. Please describe the X-ray and your management

This is an AP view of the right upper limb of a baby. There is a minimally displaced transverse fracture of the proximal humerus. I would take a complete history looking for the NAI 'red flags' with the aim of understanding the mechanism of injury. I would then proceed with a meticulous physical examination that would include body mapping and pictures of any positive findings. I would notify the safeguarding team and admit the child to the paediatric ward for further assessment. I would follow the local NAI guidelines and the hospital's management pathway until the possibility of NAI had been excluded. If this is an isolated injury I would provide analgesia and immobilize the arm in a vest close to the chest. I notice that the cortices are not well defined on the radius or the ulna which raises the suspicion of an underlying metabolic problem.

How would you proceed the following day assuming that NAI was ruled out?

I would proceed with assessment regarding a possible metabolic disorder or skeletal dysplasia. I would complete the physical examination focusing on colour of the sclerae, facial features, spinal alignment, skin quality and undertake blood tests to assess the bone profile including Vit D metabolism, a skeletal survey to assess the rest of the skeleton for signs of skeletal dysplasia and consider a referral to the geneticist.

This baby was diagnosed with Osteogenesis Imperfecta (OI) type III due to a spontaneous mutation. Fig. 3.26 is an X-ray taken when she is 2 years old. What do you see?

I see a mid-shaft transverse femur fracture in a previously bowed femur. I see growth arrest lines in keeping with bisphosphonate treatment for OI.

How would you proceed?

At this point I would need to make a decision regarding both short and longer term management of this fracture and limb alignment. This previous bowing could be a result of a previous fracture and this mal-alignment is potentially a risk factor for recurrent fractures.

I would need to decide whether I would simply treat the child symptomatically in traction and/or a spica cast to allow the fracture to heal and then assess the alignment following fracture healing/remodelling **or** whether I would advise early surgical intervention with fracture reduction and stabilization (with the use of additional osteotomies if necessary) to achieve normal bone shape and alignment. The use of a cast is associated with an increased risk of further fracture due to immobilization and/or the stress riser effect at the edges of the cast. I would also like to assess the alignment of the contralateral lower limb to plan any elective treatment for the other side.

Fig. 3.27 shows the other X-rays of the same girl. Assuming you have both AP and lateral films of both lower limbs how would you like to proceed?

These films highlight the involvement of both lower limbs with fractures at different stages of healing. Both femora and tibiae are bowed, risking repeated fractures.

Careful planning of corrective osteotomies around the CORA (centre of rotation angulation) and the use of an appropriate intramedullary device need to be considered. If the medullary canal is wide enough a telescopic intramedullary system (such as the Fassier–Duval rod or the Bailey-Dubow rod) is the treatment of choice. If not a Rush pin is also an option.

Anam EA, Rauch F, Glorieux FH, Fassier F, Hamdy R. 'Osteotomy Healing in Children With Osteogenesis Imperfecta Receiving Bisphosphonate Treatment'. *Journal of Bone and Mineral Research*, 2015 Aug; 30(8): 1362–8.

Harrington J, Sochett E, Howard A. 'Update on the evaluation and treatment of osteogenesis imperfecta'. *Pediatric Clinics of North America* 2014 Dec; 61(6): 1243–57.

Montpetit K, Palomo T, Glorieux FH, Fassier F, Rauch F. 'Multidisciplinary Treatment of Severe Osteogenesis Imperfecta: Functional Outcomes at Skeletal Maturity'. *Archives of Physical Medicine and Rehabilitation*, 2015 Oct; 96(10): 1834–9.

Viva 22   Questions

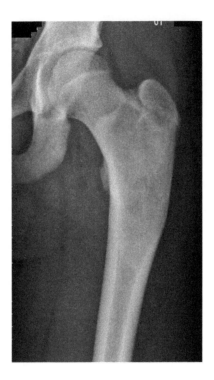

Fig. 3.28 X-ray

Fig. 3.28 is an X-ray of a 13-year-old boy who is complaining of 3 months of thigh pain. There is no history of previous fracture or injury. Could you talk about the radiograph and consider possible diagnoses?

The diagnosis is fibrous dysplasia. How would you investigate further?

If you remember the clinical presentation, a boy with a few months of pain, how would you manage this adolescent?

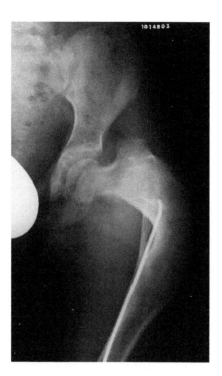

Fig. 3.29 X-ray

For some reason he has been lost to follow-up. He arrives in your clinic with a significant limp, and Fig. 3.29 shows his radiograph, what do you see? He has had treatment elsewhere a year ago. How would you manage the situation now?

Viva 22   Answers

Fig. 3.28 is an X-ray of a 13-year-old boy who is complaining of 3 months of thigh pain. There is no history of previous fracture or injury. Could you talk about the radiograph and consider possible diagnoses?

This AP X-ray shows a proximal femur in which there is an expansile lesion with thinning of the cortex laterally. The lesion itself has a narrow zone of transition with an eccentric margin. The lesion has a ground glass appearance lesion. There is also a varus deformity of the proximal femur (at the site of the lesion). These features are suggestive of a chronic process and there is no periosteal reaction that might indicate a malignant process.

I would suggest fibrous dysplasia is the most likely diagnosis. (*The lesion is so uniform in its appearance that there are no real obvious alternative diagnoses so resist the temptation to add other diagnoses to your list.*)

The diagnosis is fibrous dysplasia. How would you investigate further?

The focus of initial investigations is to establish whether the condition is polyostotic or monostotic and whether there are symptoms/signs suggestive of McCune Albright syndrome.

The first thing to do is a thorough clinical examination, looking specifically for signs of precocious puberty and irregular café-au-lait spots. These features would be consistent with McCune Albright syndrome. The clinical examination may also reveal other bony deformities, for example in the contralateral femur, tibiae, humeri, and the jaw. If such a deformity is seen, X-rays may reveal other lesions. However, multiple X-rays looking for possible lesions is not always a sensible approach and one could consider MRI of the relevant area instead. Occasionally, a radionuclide bone scan is indicated as it is better at detecting some lesions, especially in the ribs and skull.

If you remember the clinical presentation, a boy with a few months of pain, how would you manage this child?

The pain is likely to be coming from the cortical thinning and microfractures, so I would consider intramedullary fixation of the femur with fixation into the femoral neck to prevent further deformity.

If this was polyostotic fibrous dysplasia, I would discuss with the endocrinologists/metabolic bone disease specialists regarding a dexa scan for bone mineral density and treatment with systemic bisphosphonates.

For some reason the child has been lost to follow-up. He arrives in your clinic with a significant limp, and Fig. 3.29 shows his radiograph, what do you see? He has had treatment elsewhere a year ago. How would you manage the situation now?

This radiograph demonstrates that the lesion has progressed and the cortex has thinned further with an increase in the varus femoral neck alignment, creating a shepherd's crook deformity. There is a single flexible nail extending to the base of the neck.

With this degree of deformity, treatment should be aimed at realignment of the femur and the limb (a standing leg length/alignment film would be essential for pre-operative planning) by performing the appropriate number of osteotomies at thappropriate levels. These would then be stabilized with an intramedullary device which would include fixation into the femoral head/neck. It might be necessary to create a custom-made prosthesis and removal of the existing nail may prove challenging.

I would organize a 'cross-match' so that blood for transfusion would be available for the perioperative period. Fibrous dysplasia can be very vascular and major intraoperative bleeding can occur.

One of the aims of treatment is to improve bone density and advice from medical colleagues would be helpful.

Could you use plate fixation?

Historically, plate fixation has been shown to fail in shepherd's crook deformities either from osteogenesis imperfecta or fibrous dysplasia. However, some advocate a 2-stage procedure with a proximal plate initially to be replaced with a cephallomedullary device later on.

Kushare IV et al.: 'Fibrous dysplasia of the proximal femur: surgical management options and outcomes'. *Journal of Child Orthopedics*, 2014 Dec; 8(6): 505–11.

Livesley PJ et al.: 'The treatment of progressive coxa vara in children with bone softening disorders'. *International Orthopaedics*, 1994 Oct; 18(5): 310–2.

Viva 23   Questions

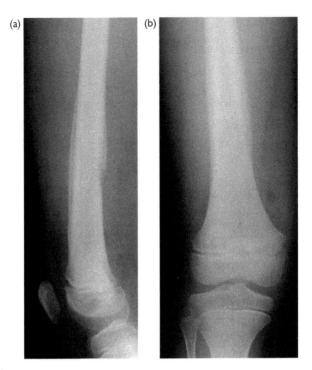

(a)   (b)

Fig. 3.30 X-rays

A 10-year-old boy presents with a 6-week history of thigh pain after a bad tackle and fall on the rugby field. What does Fig. 3.30 show?

What would be your top three differential diagnoses?

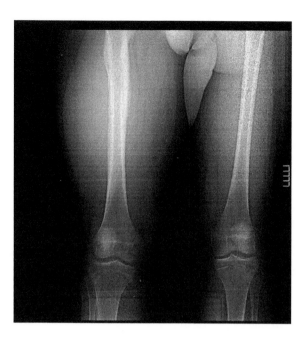

Fig. 3.31 X-ray

Fig. 3.31 shows a 15-year-old boy who presented in an identical way. How does this image differ? What would be your top two differentials here?

Yes, this was a Ewings sarcoma. Going back to the first case, what other investigations would you do?

Assuming that the investigations support a diagnosis of osteomyelitis, how would you treat this case?

When would you consider operative intervention?

Are you aware of any evidence regarding the duration of antibiotic treatment and IV antibiotic duration? What would you do in this case?

Viva 23   Answers

A 10-year-old boy presents with a 6-week history of thigh pain after a bad tackle and fall on the rugby field. What does Fig. 3.30 show?

AP and lateral radiographs of the knee and distal two thirds of a child's femur show diaphyseal changes involving the cortex and including a periosteal reaction with new bone formation. The cortex appears to be breached posteriorly.

What would be your top three differential diagnoses?

Without more history or investigations available, my top three differentials would be osteomyelitis, a healing undisplaced fracture and a primary bone tumour (Ewings or osteosarcoma) although there are no other typical features of malignancy.

Fig. 3.31 shows a 15-year-old boy who presented in an identical way. How does this image differ? What would be your top two differentials here?

This radiograph shows extensive soft tissue swelling with bony changes including new bone formation, periosteal reaction, cortical changes, and abnormal bony architecture. My concern here would be a neoplasm, possibly a Ewings sarcoma, or infection.

Yes, this was a Ewings sarcoma. Going back to the first case, what other investigations would you do?

I would do a full set of blood tests including inflammatory markers and blood cultures and I would request an MRI. If there was concern that other limbs were affected I would also consider a bone scan.

Assuming that the investigations support a diagnosis of osteomyelitis, how would you treat this case?

Provided that there was no collection seen on MRI, I would treat this case with IV antibiotics, converting to oral antibiotics when I was happy that we were using an appropriate antibiotic and that the patient was responding well to treatment clinically and with improvement in his inflammatory markers.

When would you consider operative intervention?

If there were signs of a significant subperiosteal collection or if there was a suggestion that this chronic osteomyelitis was associated with a sequestrum, I would have considered drainage or debridement.

Are you aware of any evidence regarding the duration of antibiotic treatment and IV antibiotic duration? What would you do in this case?

Yes, there is recent data from the UK and other countries suggesting that a short course of IV antibiotics e.g. 3–5 days followed by a further 3 weeks of oral antibiotics is sufficient for treating acute uncomplicated cases, however given the radiographic changes in this case it would suggest a slightly longer duration of infection and so I would prepare the patient/family for a longer IV duration depending on his response to antibiotics.

Dartnell J, Ramachandran M, Katchburian M. 'Haematogenous acute and subacute paediatric osteomyelitis: a systematic review of the literature'. *The Bone & Joint Journal*, 2012; 94(5): 584–95.

Jagodzinski NA, Kanwar R, Graham K, Bache CE. 'Prospective evaluation of a shortened regimen of treatment for acute osteomyelitis and septic arthritis in children'. *Journal of Pediatric Orthopedics*, 2009; 29(5): 518–25.

Peltola H, Paakkonen M. 'Acute osteomyelitis in children'. *The New England Journal of Medicine*, 2014; 370(4): 352–60.

Peltola H, Paakkonen M, Kallio P, Kallio MJ. 'Osteomyelitis-Septic Arthritis Study Short- versus long-term antimicrobial treatment for acute hematogenous osteomyelitis of childhood: prospective, randomized trial on 131 culture-positive cases'. *The Pediatric Infectious Disease Journal*, 2010; 29(12): 1123–8.

Viva 24 Questions

Anxious parents bring their 2-year-old child to A&E with a 24-hour history of a sore leg and unwillingness to weightbear, there is no history of trauma. What further information would you like from the parents and from examining the child?

There is not much to find in the knee or ankle, the child prefers to lie with their leg in external rotation and does not like you flexing it and despite all encouragement from his mother, he refuses to stand. Temperature is 38.2° C. What is your differential diagnosis?

What investigations would you like?

The radiographs are normal, the ultrasound scan confirms an effusion of the left hip (see Fig. 3.32) and the blood tests confirm a White Cell Count (WCC) of 20 and a C-Reactive Protein (CRP) of 37. Now what is your differential diagnosis?

How can you differentiate between septic arthritis and transient synovitis? Do you know any criteria that can help?

What options do you know for treating septic arthritis? Which would you choose in this case?

Describe your surgical approach to washing out this child's hip

How long would you give them antibiotics for? Would you keep them on IV antibiotics for the duration? Do you know of any recent evidence on the topic?

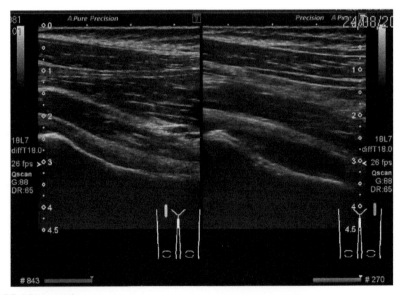

Fig. 3.32 Ultrasound

Viva 24   Answers

Anxious parents bring their 2-year-old child to A&E with a 24-hour history of a sore leg and unwillingness to weight bear, there is no history of trauma. What further information would you like from the parents and from examining the child?

I would like to know if there is any possibility of unwitnessed injury, any recent respiratory/ ENT viral infections or fever, and whether or not they are generally unwell with a loss of appetite. A history of previous similar episodes would be important. I would watch the child during the history taking to see how well (or not) they were moving. I would then examine the entire lower limb for swelling, erythema and pain on movement of the joints (hip/knee/ankle) and also document their vital signs: temperature, heart rate, respiratory rate and BP.

There is not much to find in the knee or ankle, the child prefers to lie with their leg in external rotation and does not like you flexing it and despite all encouragement from his mother, he refuses to stand. Temperature is 38.2° C. What is your differential diagnosis?

My differential would include infection of the bone or the joint (or the soft tissues, pyomyositis) an intra-abdominal abscess e.g. psoas, a femoral fracture, transient synovitis and inflammatory arthropathy. Personally I also have the rule: 'Think infection, think tumour' and would wish to exclude that possibility too.

What investigations would you like?

I would like plain radiographs of the pelvis and proximal femur, blood tests including, full blood count (FBC)/ CRP/ erythrocyte sedimentation rate (ESR), blood cultures and urea and electrolytes (U&E's) and an ultrasound scan.

The radiographs are normal, the ultrasound scan confirms an effusion of the left hip (see Fig. 3.32) and the blood tests confirm a WCC of 20 and a CRP of 37

I think it is septic arthritis.

How can you differentiate between septic arthritis and transient synovitis? Do you know any criteria that can help?

Kocher identified 4 factors to help distinguish between septic arthritis and transient synovitis: inability to weightbear, raised Erythrocyte Sedimentation Rate (ESR), raised temperature and raised WCC. Caird et al. introduced CRP as a further independent factor. The more factors that are raised, the higher the likelihood of septic arthritis. The two most important factors are CRP and weightbearing status.

What options do you know for treating septic arthritis? Which would you choose in this case?

The gold standard is surgical washout by way of arthrotomy. Given the known effusion and abnormal blood results in addition to the clinical picture I would proceed to wash out the hip and instigate IV antibiotics.

Describe your surgical approach to washing out this child's hip

I would do a small transverse incision 1 finger's breadth below the iliac crest and extending medially with a limited dissection between tensor fasciae latae (TFL) and sartorius, whilst protecting the lateral cutaneous nerve. I would then dissect down to and between gluteus medius and rectus femoris to identify the hip capsule. I would then perform a capsulotomy and excise a small corner of tissue. Samples would be taken for , microbiology and the hip would be irrigated well. I would leave the capsule open when closing the wound.

I would ask for an urgent Gram stain and microscopy and send the samples for culture in blood culture bottles.

How long would you give them antibiotics for? Would you keep them on IV antibiotics for the duration? Do you know of any recent evidence on the topic?

I would keep them on IV antibiotics until they had been apyrexial for 48 hours and were showing signs of starting to weightbear, then I would change to oral antibiotics if the inflammatory markers were improving too. Recent studies (Peltola et al.) have shown that in most cases of primary, uncomplicated joint sepsis only a few days of IV followed by a short course of oral antibiotics (e.g. 10 days total treatment time) are required.

Caird MS, Flynn JM, Leung YL, Millman JE, D'Italia JG, Dormans JP. 'Factors distinguishing septic arthritis from transient synovitis of the hip in children. A prospective study'. *The Journal of Bone & Joint Surgery*, American volume, 2006; 88(6): 1251–7.

Kocher MS, Mandiga R, Zurakowski D, Barnewolt C, Kasser JR. 'Validation of a clinical prediction rule for the differentiation between septic arthritis and transient synovitis of the hip in children'.
The Journal of Bone & Joint Surgery, American volume, 2004; 86-A(8): 1629–35.

Mignemi ME, Menge TJ, Cole HA, Mencio GA, Martus JE, Lovejoy S, et al. 'Epidemiology, diagnosis, and treatment of pericapsular pyomyositis of the hip in children'. *Journal of Pediatric Orthopedics*, 2014; 34(3): 316–25.

Peltola H, Paakkonen M, Kallio P, Kallio MJ. 'Osteomyelitis-Septic Arthritis Study G. Prospective, randomized trial of 10 days versus 30 days of antimicrobial treatment, including a short-term course of parenteral therapy, for childhood septic arthritis'. *Clinical Infectious Diseases*: an official publication of the *Infectious Diseases Society of America*, 2009; 48(9): 1201–10.

Singhal R, Perry DC, Khan FN, Cohen D, Stevenson HL, James LA, et al. 'The use of CRP within a clinical prediction algorithm for the differentiation of septic arthritis and transient synovitis in children'. *The Bone & Joint Journal*, 2011; 93(11): 1556–61.

Lyon RM, Evanich JD. 'Culture-negative septic arthritis in children'. *The Bone & Joint Journal*, 1999; 19(5): 655–9.

Viva 25   Questions

How would you define scoliosis?

How would you classify adolescent idiopathic scoliosis (AIS)?

What are the indications for a MRI scan?

What are the factors predictive of curve progression?

How does early onset scoliosis (EOS) differ from AIS and how will this affect your management?

How would you treat AIS?

Viva 25   Answers

How would you define scoliosis?

A deformity of the spine of more than 10° in the coronal plane with associated vertebral rotation.

How would you classify adolescent idiopathic scoliosis?

Scoliosis is classified by curve size and site: thoracic (apex T1–T12), thoracolumbar (apex T12–L1) or lumbar (apex below L1). Structural curves do not 'correct' on bending to less than 25°. Secondary or compensatory curves are usually non structural (and hence flexible).

True postural curves secondary to leg length discrepancy, muscle pain/spasm or nerve root irritation must be excluded.

What are the indications for a MRI scan?

The purpose of the MRI is to exclude intraspinal anomalies. The most common findings include syringomyelia and associated Chiari malformations, tethered cords, and tumours. Atypical curve patterns such as left thoracic curves, short angular curves, excessive kyphosis, neurological symptoms, excessive pain, and patients younger than 10 years with curves more than 20° are all indications for further investigation.

In some units, all patients undergoing surgery will have a pre-operative MR scan.

What are the factors predictive of curve progression?

In general terms, curve progression depends not only on age but also on skeletal maturity and of course curve severity. The more severe the curve, the greater the risk of curve progression. With curves between 5–20°, there is a 22% risk of curve progression. When curvatures increase from 20–30°, the risk again increases to 68%. From 30–60°, risk of progression increases to 90%. Remaining growth potential is also a major factor: Risser grades 0, 1, and 2, as well as an open triradiate cartilage are indicators of high risk for curve progression. Girls will grow for approximately 18 months following the date of menarche.

How does early onset scoliosis (EOS) differ from AIS, and how will this affect your management?

Early onset scoliosis is defined as a deformity that is present before the age of 10: it may be congenital, idiopathic, neuromuscular or syndromic in origin. Idiopathic scoliosis under the age of 10 is more common in boys and usually presents with a left thoracic curvature. The risk of curve progression is 10% however most resolve spontaneously. In young children, the main factor for risk progression is the apical rib-vertebral angle difference (RVAD). A difference of more than 20°, which is known as the Mehta angle, has a high risk for curve progression. The rib-vertebra relationship is also assessed and phase 2, which is overlap of the medial rib with the apical vertebral body, is also associated with curve progression. Neural-axis abnormalities need to be excluded, especially when RVAD is more than 20°. If the Cobb angle is < 30° and the RVAD < 20°, the child can be observed. Patients with a Cobb angle > 30 and a RVAD> 20 with a phase 2 rib-vertebrae relationship can be treated with serial plaster jackets to straighten the spine. Failed non-operative methods and curves greater than 50° should be considered for surgical intervention.

How would you treat AIS?

AIS are more common in females and usually presents with a right sided thoracic curvature. Curves less than 20° can be observed with regular reviews. Curves of 20–50° require bracing to prevent curve progression. If the curve is more than 50° spinal fusion remains the gold standard when patients are approaching skeletal maturity. In the younger, shorter patient you might consider a growing rod construct.

Helenius I. 'Anterior surgery for adolescent idiopathic scoliosis'. *Journal of Child Orthopedics*, 2013 Feb; 7(1): 63–8.

Mehta MH. 'Growth as a corrective force in the early treatment of progressive infantile scoliosis'. *The Bone & Joint Journal*, 2005 Sep; 87(9): 1237–47.

Weinstein SL, Dolan LA, Wright JG, Dobbs MB. 'Effects of bracing in adolescents with idiopathic scoliosis'. *New England Journal of Medicine*, 2013 Oct 17; 369(16): 1512–21.

Viva 26   Questions

How would you define congenital scoliosis and which age group does it affect?

What factors would you consider to be important during the clinical examination?

How would you investigate a child with congenital scoliosis?

How would you manage such a child?

What are the surgical options and when should each be considered?

What complications can you envisage?

Viva 26 Answers

How would you define congenital scoliosis and which age group does it affect?

Congenital scoliosis occurs secondary to a structural problem that produces a deformity. This problem is due to a failure of normal vertebral development during the fourth to sixth week of gestation and hence the deformity is present at birth although it may not be detectable at that stage. It usually presents clinically in the infant or toddler period. In some children (with more minor problems), it is not diagnosed until adolescence. In young children it can be difficult to detect the structural abnormalities on plain films due to the ossification patterns of the vertebrae and advanced imaging techniques might be necessary.

What factors would you consider to be important during the clinical examination?

From a spinal viewpoint, truncal imbalance can be a result of congenital spinal deformities. A head tilt, shoulder asymmetry, decompensation of the trunk, and pelvic obliquity must all be looked for and assessed.

A careful neurological examination is required to exclude spinal dysraphism, which can also manifest through cutaneous lesions such as skin tags, hairy patches, and skin dimples. The lower extremities should also be examined as vertical talus, TEV, calcaneovarus, and foot asymmetry have an association with congenital scoliosis and these findings alone may suggest a MRI of the spine and brain stem is indicated.

How would you investigate a child with congenital scoliosis?

In the older child, plain radiography is sufficient to confirm the diagnosis, and to classify the deformity. Radiographs are useful for measuring the curve magnitude and quantifying progression. In infants, radiographs are taken in the supine position; however, when the child is able to stand independently, PA and lateral weightbearing radiographs are taken. Apparent curve progression at this stage may simply be due to the change in orientation of the radiographs. In the infant, it can be difficult to identify the bony vertebral shapes. In the neonate, an ultrasound scan can confirm the presence of the posterior elements. The disc space sizes can give useful information regarding growth potential. Wide normal appearing discs have growth potential whereas poorly defined discs do not have growth potential. CT is best used for pre-operative planning, and 3D CT scanning defines anatomical anomalies better than radiographs. Any child who is being considered for surgery should have a MRI of the spine to assess for spinal dysraphism or other associated anomalies.

How would you manage such a child?

With the absence of documented progression a conservative approach can be adopted: this is most likely with a non-segmented (incarcerated) hemivertebrae and some partially segmented hemivertebrae (particularly if they are 'balanced' ie. facing each other). Bracing is generally much less successful in congenital scoliosis than in idiopathic scoliosis. Significant curve progression, a neurological deficit (or change in neurological status) and/or declining respiratory function demand consideration of surgical treatment. The aim of surgery is to achieve a balanced spine while maintaining flexibility and preserving as much spinal growth as possible. The main factors to be considered when surgical management is required are age, curve severity, and rate/liklihood of progression.

What are the surgical options and when should each be considered?

The aim of surgery is spinal stabilization rather than curve correction and thus 'early' in situ fusion techniques are often used. In children under the age of 10 with significant growth remaining, concerns of the crankshaft phenomenon can be a problem and this has led to the addition of an anterior arthrodesis to the in situ posterior fusion. Combined anterior and posterior fusions are commonly indicated in the management of curves with a poor prognosis.

Growth arrest procedures such as convex hemiepiphysiodesis are used for unilateral failure of formation. The convex lateral halves of the discs are removed adjacent to the hemivertebra as well as above and below. A posterior spinal fusion is then performed and the concave side is not disturbed. It is best reserved for children younger than 5 with short progressive curves.

Hemivertebra excision is associated with a high risk of neurological injury but is used when there is marked truncal imbalance as it allows for some correction of the deformity before the spine is fused. Combined anterior and posterior procedures are required. It is recommended in patients younger than 5 with progressive but flexible curves more than 40°. Correction and fusion with instrumentation are reserved for older children when partial curve correction is required. There needs to be flexibility in the segments below and above the deformity.

Deformities which are rigid require reconstructive osteotomies and instrumentation. Neurological compromise, truncal decompensation and pelvic obliquity are all indications for corrective osteotomies.

Growing rods maximize spinal growth however they are controversial in managing the curve progression.

What complications can you envisage?

The crankshaft phenomenon can occur when posterior spinal fusion alone is performed. Fusion of the spinal column can cause short stature. Surgical correction with shortening, over-distraction and overcorrection can lead to neurological injury. Early fusion can limit spinal and hence lung growth: it is important to keep the fusion as short as possible.

Chang DG, Suk SI, Kim JH, Ha KY, Na KH, Lee JH. 'Surgical outcomes by the age at the time of surgery in the treatment of congenital scoliosis in children under age 10 years'. *Spine Journal*, 2015; 15(8): 1783–95.

Murphy RF, Moisan A, Kelly DM, Warner WC Jr, Jones TL, Sawyer JR. 'Use of Vertical Expandable Prosthetic Titanium Rib (VEPTR) in the Treatment of Congenital Scoliosis Without Fused Ribs'. *Journal of Pediatric Orthopedics*, 2015; Apr 13.

Skaggs, DL et al. 'A Classification of Growth Friendly Spine Implants'. *Journal of Pediatric Orthopedics*, 2014; 34: 260–74.

Yazici M, Emans J. 'Fusionless instrumentation systems for congenital scoliosis: expandable spinal rods and vertical expandable prosthetic titanium rib in the management of congenital spine deformities in the growing child'. *Spine* (Phila Pa 1976), 2009 Aug 1; 34(17): 1800–7.

Viva 27 Questions

How do patients with kyphosis present?

Why do adults with kyphosis get pain?

What is the pathology in Scheuermann's kyphosis?

What are the radiographic findings of a patient with Scheuermann's kyphosis?

What would you see on the radiographs in postural kyphosis?

How would you manage a patient with kyphosis?

How would you manage a child with congenital kyphosis?

Viva 27   Answers

How do patients with kyphosis present?

Adolescents usually present because of the deformity and the attendant cosmetic concerns raised by family and/or friends. This differs from adults, where pain is usually the chief complaint.

Why do adults with kyphosis get pain?

The pain is usually felt distal to the thoracic kyphotic deformity. This is a result of compensatory hyperlordosis. Degenerative disc disease and facet arthropathy predispose adults to low back pain. Spondylolysis should also be considered if pain is primarily in the lumbar region.

What is the pathology in Scheuermann's kyphosis?

Halal et al. demonstrated an autosomal dominant mode of inheritance with high penetrance but variable expression. Anatomical findings include a thickened anterior longitudinal ligament, narrowed vertebral discs and wedged vertebral bodies. The cartilaginous end plates also have histological findings. The ratio of collagen to proteoglycan in the matrix of the endplate is below normal. This decrease in collagen results in abnormal end plate ossification and thus altered vertical growth of the vertebral body. There have been studies claiming Scheuermann's kyphosis is associated with osteoporosis, however this is still under debate. There may also be mechanical factors involved.

What are the radiographic findings of a patient with Scheuermann's kyphosis?

By definition, there will be anterior wedging across 3 consecutive vertebrae with a thoracic hyperkyphosis. There will be disc narrowing and endplate irregularities. Schmorl's nodes may be present. These occur where there is herniation of the disc into the vertebral endplate. Scoliosis and a compensatory hyperlordosis may also be present. Spondylolysis may be a secondary finding. A hyperextension lateral radiograph helps differentiate Scheuermann's from a postural kyphosis.

What would you see on the radiographs in postural kyphosis?

The thoracic kyphosis can be up to 60° but the radiographic findings of Scheuermann's kyphosis will be absent and the kyphotic angle should be fully correctable on the hyperextension lateral radiographs.

How would you manage a patient with kyphosis?

A thoracic kyphosis <50°, in an asymptomatic patient, can be observed with serial radiographs. A Risser assessment will establish how much further growth is expected. Closer monitoring around rapid growth periods is advised. Patients with curves between 50–70° may require bracing in an extension type orthosis. Bracing is continued for a minimum of 18 months and can be expected to provide up to 50% correction of the deformity. It is useful in adolescents with growth remaining. Bracing is ineffective in congenital kyphosis.

Indications for surgical intervention for Scheuermann's kyphosis include kyphosis exceeding 75°, deformity progression, neurological deficits including cord compression and severe pain in adults. Posterior spinal fusion with instrumentation is required. Advantages of a posterior only approach include decreased blood loss and reduced surgical time. Disadvantages of a posterior only approach include a higher rate of pseudarthrosis and less correction. Anterior release has been suggested when deformity does not correct to <50° on hyperextension lateral views. Good practice aims not to correct deformities > 50% of the original deformity to prevent junctional kyphosis. Newer thoracic pedicle-screw constructs may be sufficient to avoid the need for anterior procedures but an anterior release is required in the larger, more rigid, curves.

How would you manage a child with congenital kyphosis?

Surgery is indicated in most patients with type II and type III congenital kyphosis. In type II (failure of segmentation) patients who are younger than 5 and have curves < 55°, posterior fusion of the kyphotic deformity is recommended. Curves > 55° require vertebral resection, which has a high risk of causing neurological deficit.

Lowe TG, Line BG. 'Evidence based medicine: analysis of Scheuermann kyphosis'. *Spine* (Phila Pa 1976), 2007 Sep 1; 32(19 Suppl): S115–9.

Palazzo C, Sailhan F, Reve, I M. 'Scheuermann's disease: an update'. *Joint Bone Spine*, 2014 May; 81(3): 209–14.

Wood KB, Melikian R, Villamil F. 'Adult Scheuermann kyphosis: evaluation, management, and new developments'. *The Journal of the American Academy of Orthopaedic Surgeons*, 2012 Feb; 20(2): 113–21.

Viva 28   Questions

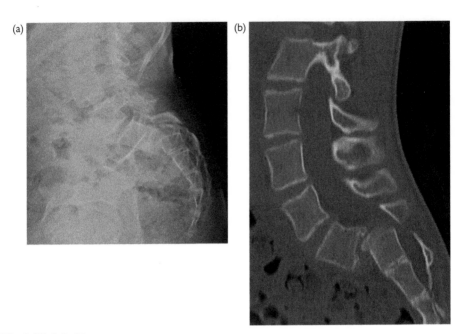

Fig. 3.33 Spinal images

How would you classify the pathology shown in Fig. 3.33?

Do all cases of spondylolisthesis develop a neurological deficit?

What other important radiographic findings do you know about and can you draw them on the X-ray provided?

How would you treat this condition?

Viva 28   Answers

How would you classify Fig. 3.33?

This is an isthmic type of spondylolisthesis, and according to the Wiltse–Newman classification, would be a type II. Type II has 3 subtypes:

A is where there is a fatigue stress fracture that does not heal normally. B is an elongated pars interarticularis as a result of healed micro-fractures. It is therefore intact and this can lead to diagnostic difficulties when distinguishing between this and type I (congenital/dysplastic). C is an acute pars fracture.

Meyerding also classified the spondylolisthesis according to the slip percentage. The width of the superior end plate of S1 is measured—A. The distance between the posterior edge of the inferior end plate of L5 and the posterior edge of the superior end plate of S1 is then measured—B. A/B x 100 will give the percentage slip.

- Grade I is a slip of 0% to 25%,
- Grade II is a slip of 26% to 50%,
- Grade III is a slip 51% to 75% and
- Grade IV is a slip of 76% to 99%.
- Grade V is named spondyloptosis, which is a 100% slip.

The CT image suggests a Grade II-III slip.

Do all cases of spondylolisthesis develop a neurological deficit?

No. Type I, dysplastic type, cases are more likely to develop neurological sequelae as the posterior elements are intact and the slip of L5 on S1 can cause radiculopathy as well as sacral nerve root compression. Even a slip of 25% can cause neurological deficit. Type II, isthmic type, cases rarely develop a neurological deficit. Hamstring spasm is the most common finding.

What other important radiographic findings do you know about and can you draw them on the X-ray provided?

The slip angle can be calculated which is the most sensitive indicator of potential instability and clinical symptoms. It is the angle between the superior endplate of L5 and a line perpendicular to the posterior border of the sacrum which passes through the cephalad point of S1. Slip angles of more than 50° are associated with greater risk of progression.

The pelvic incidence correlates with severity and has a direct correlation with the Meyerding-Newman grade. It is calculated by drawing a line from centre of the S1 superior vertebral end plate to the centre of the femoral head. A second line is then drawn along the superior end plate of the S1 vertebra and a perpendicular line is drawn from the centre point of the S1 end plate. The angle between these two lines is the pelvic incidence.

The pelvic tilt is calculated by drawing the same line from the centre of the S1 superior end plate to the centre of the femoral head. A vertical line is then drawn from the centre of the femoral head, which is parallel with the side margin of the radiograph.

The sacral slope is calculated by drawing a line parallel to the S1 end plate. A second line is drawn from the most anterior point of the S1 endplate horizontally, parallel with the inferior border of the radiograph.

How would you treat this condition?

Asymptomatic patients with low-grade (I–II) spondylolisthesis or spondylolysis require observation only with no activity modification. Symptomatic patients with low-grade slips and isthmic spondylolysis may require physical therapy including hamstring stretching, correction of their pelvic tilt and abdominal core strengthening.

Most patients with congenital spondylolisthesis with slip progression and symptoms require decompression and arthrodesis.

Indications for surgery include disabling pain unresponsive to conservative measures, neurological symptoms including cauda equina or radicular symptoms and Grade III or higher slips or progressive slips.

Goals of surgery include reduction in pain, prevention of further slips, stabilization of the spine, restoration of normal posture and gait and reversal and/or prevention of neurological deficit.

If neurological deficit is present, nerve root decompression is generally recommended. Posterolateral fusion with or without instrumentation may be performed. Pedicle screw constructs increase fusion rates and decrease postoperative slip rates. Fusion can be either in-situ or with reduction. Reduction for high-grade isthmic spondylolisthesis is controversial and there are no accepted guidelines.

Kasliwal MK, Smith JS, Kanter A, Chen CJ, Mummaneni PV, Hart RA, Shaffrey CI. 'Management of high-grade spondylolisthesis'. *Neurosurgery Clinics of North America*, 2013 Apr; 24(2): 275–91.

Liu X, Wang Y, Qiu G, Weng X, Yu B. 'A systematic review with meta-analysis of posterior interbody fusion versus posterolateral fusion in lumbar spondylolisthesis'. *European Spine Journal*, 2014 Jan; 23(1): 43–56.

Parker SL, Godil SS, Mendenhall SK, Zuckerman SL, Shau DN, McGirt MJ. 'Two-year comprehensive medical management of degenerative lumbar spine disease (lumbar spondylolisthesis, stenosis, or disc herniation): a value analysis of cost, pain, disability, and quality of life: clinical article'. *Journal of Neurosurgery Spine*, 2014 Aug; 21(2): 143–9.

Viva 29   Questions

What is spina bifida?

What are the risk factors?

How is it diagnosed?

How is it managed?

What about other orthopaedic manifestations?

Viva 29   Answers

What is spina bifida?

It is the name given to a group of neural tube defects caused by failure of closure of the neural crests. It is due to a failure of formation of the vertebral arch and posterior elements, which cover the spinal cord. There are different forms depending on where the neural elements are in relation to the spinal canal. The risk of neurological deficit is fairly low when the neural elements are located in the canal however with a myelomeningocele, the risk of neurological deficit is high.

What are the risk factors?

Folate deficiency has reduced over the years due to public awareness and cereal fortification with folic acid. Maternal hyperthermia and gestational diabetes are other factors. Exposure to valproic acid and other anti-epileptic medications has also been identified as a risk factor. There is a failure of function of the genes that control neural tube closure and up to 10% of foeti have a chromosomal abnormality such as trisomy 13 and 18.

How is it diagnosed?

Diagnosis can be made antenatally (by 18 weeks). Maternal serum and amniotic fluid levels of alpha fetoprotein levels are both important as are the appearances on the foetal ultrasound scan. Neurosegmental evaluation has prognostic implications, however the level may take several years to declare itself.

How is it managed?

A multidisciplinary approach to management is essential; those involved may change over time but will include a paediatrician, neurosurgeon, urologist, physiotherapist, orthotist, and a social worker as well as an orthopaedic surgeon.

With regards to the spine, infants with myelomeningoceles should be delivered by caesarean section to avoid any further neurological injury. Closure of the myelomeningocele is usually done within 48 hours and a shunt may be inserted for hydrocephalus. A tethered cord is a result of a fibrous band, which connects the conus medullaris to the bony sacrum, which prevents cranial migration of the conus with growth. It causes progressive scoliosis and spasticity and surgical release is indicated with neurological deterioration. Scoliosis is related to the level of the lesion and the higher the lesion the higher the incidence of scoliosis with > 90% being affected in high lumbar/thoracic lesions. Any developing deformity will require a MRI scan, as tethering and syringomyelia need to be excluded. A syringomyelia is a fluid filled cavity in the cord, which may in itself cause problems with neurological deterioration.

What about other orthopaedic manifestations?

Survival and neurological impairment depend on the level of spinal segment involved and this should be one of the key features to be identified. L4 is considered the key level differentiating who will walk and who will not, as L4 innervates the quadriceps. The level of spinal segment involved will dictate the aims of treatment. Orthopaedic management is to prevent deformity and to facilitate function. For example, in those who can walk, by the use of orthotics (KAFOs or AFOs knee-ankle-foot-orthotics) and/or surgery.

Hip flexion contractures are common and may require surgical release. Once again, the higher the lesion the more common the incidence of hip dislocation. Management of bilateral dislocations is controversial. Some groups say they should be left untreated, as there is a high failure rate following surgery with a significant complication risk including re-dislocation. If a child has a low lumbar lesion, and has a unilateral dislocation, there is an argument to consider treatment.

Knee flexion contractures are common and once again may require release. Flexion contractures can be treated with hamstring lengthening +/- guided growth techniques: extension osteotomies are less popular due to the high relapse rate. Extension contractures can be treated with serial casting and quadriceps lengthening. Knee valgus deformities are associated with external tibial torsion and femoral anteversion. Use of knee-ankle-foot orthoses can help this.

Foot and ankle deformities are very common. Several deformities including rigid clubfoot, planovalgus, cavus, and equinus contractures may be present and/or develop over time. The aim is to achieve a plantigrade braceable foot whilst avoiding pressure sores.

The variable sensation may lead to a delay in diagnosis of fractures and infections. Warmth, erythema and swelling should all point to a fracture until proven otherwise. Ulcers on the foot secondary to 'lack of care' or injury may be difficult to heal and can lead to amputation.

Chambers HG. 'Update on neuromuscular disorders in pediatric orthopaedics: Duchenne muscular dystrophy, myelomeningocele, and cerebral palsy'. *Journal of Pediatric Orthopedic*, 2014 Oct-Nov; 34 Suppl 1: S44–8.

Hopf CG, Eysel P. 'One-stage versus two-stage spinal fusion in neuromuscular scolioses'. *Journal of Pediatric Orthopedics*, 2000 Oct; 9(4): 234–43.

Swaroop VT, Dias L, 'Orthopedic management of spina bifida. Part I: hip, knee, and rotational deformities'. *Journal of Child Orthopedics*, 2009 Dec; 3(6): 441–9.

Viva 30   Questions

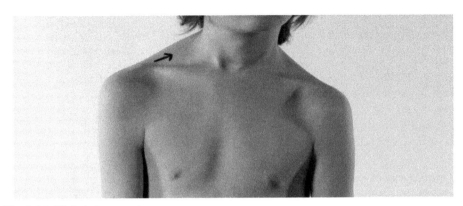

Fig. 3.34 Clinical photograph

Describe the clinical photograph in Fig. 3.34.

What are the causes of torticollis and what is the differential diagnosis?

What is atlantoaxial rotatory displacement (AARD)?

How would you investigate a child with torticollis?

How would you treat a child with torticollis?

Viva 30 Answers

Describe the clinical photograph in Fig. 3.34.

This clinical photograph demonstrates a child with torticollis, and this comes from the latin meaning 'twisted neck'.

What are the causes of torticollis and what is the differential diagnosis?

Torticollis depends on the age of the patient, the history and the examination. It can be present at birth, hence congenital, and may be the result of intrauterine 'compartment syndrome' of the sternocleidomastoid muscle. It may also be acquired. Whether the deformity is painful or not is also helpful for the diagnosis. Non-painful congenital causes include congenital muscular torticollis and other vertebral anomalies such as Klippel–Feil syndrome. Acquired painful causes include atlanto-axial rotatory displacement (traumatic) or juvenile rheumatoid arthritis (inflammatory). Neoplastic causes should also be in the differential. A correctible (flexible) torticollis may be secondary to a squint.

What is atlantoaxial rotatory displacement (AARD)?

It is a rotatory instability of the atlantoaxial (C1-C2) complex, ranging from mild displacement/ subluxation to a facet dislocation. It is held in a fixed position either due to muscle spasm or a mechanical block to reduction.

It is caused mainly by trauma, infection or inflammation. When AARD results from retropharyngeal irritation secondary to upper respiratory tract infections or a retropharyngeal abscess, it is named Grisel syndrome.

How would you investigate a child with torticollis?

I would start by taking a full history including prenatal, natal and post natal periods. I would then perform a physical examination, noting the range of movement possible and ensuring a neurological examination was performed.

It is reasonable to start with simple blood tests including full blood count, CRP and ESR. Although radiographs may not be diagnostic, they are useful to exclude fractures and congenital abnormalities. Other features such as basilar invagination should be excluded. McRae and McGregor lines are assessed on the radiographs. McRae's line is a line drawn from the basion to the opisthion. If the odontoid projects above this line, neurological sequelae will be encountered.

An open mouth view should help visualize the position of the odontoid peg relative to the lateral masses.

MRI may be useful to diagnose or exclude underlying tumour or infection.

How would you treat a child with torticollis?

Treatment of torticollis is dictated by the diagnosis, duration of symptoms and age of the child. Congenital torticollis is treated initially by non-operative methods. Excellent results, in up to 90% of patients, are achieved with massage and stretching. Whilst the untreated deformity is benign and the majority of cases develop adequate range of movement; permanent restriction of movement does affect facial growth and symmetry. The preferred surgical treatment is lengthening of the sternocleidomastoid, if indicated. This decision should be made when the child is of school age.

Klippel–Feil syndrome and other synostotic anomalies must take into consideration the deformity and potential neurological deficit. Halo fixation is used for deformity management involving head tilt and rotation. Surgical indications include progression of deformity and head tilt and rotation which are not correctable by positioning. Increasing rigidity is also an indication. Depending on the patients age, anterior and posterior fusion may be required to combat further growth of the spine.

Managing AARD aims to realign the neck into a reduced position and options include cervical collars, halter or skeletal traction, halo immobilization and surgery. The duration of symptoms dictates the treatment that will be offered. When a fracture or neurological compromise is not present, non-operative options should be tried first.

With an acute presentation, i.e. 2 weeks from onset of symptoms, a soft collar and anti-inflammatories should be trialled. If it resolves, we should monitor for recurrence. If it persists after 2 weeks, cervical halter traction and NSAIDS should be used. If it does not resolve after a further 2 weeks, C1-C2 fusion should be performed.

Chronic presentations, more than 2 weeks, require cervical halter traction, NSAIDS and benzodiazepines. The remaining algorithm remains the same.

Kahn ML, Davidson R, Drummond DS. 'Acquired torticollis in children'. *Orthopedic Review*, 1991 Aug; 20(8): 667–74.

Samartzis D, Shen FH, Herman J, Mardjetko SM. 'Atlantoaxial rotatory fixation in the setting of associated congenital malformations: a modified classification system'. *Spine (Phila Pa 1976)*, 2010 Feb 15; 35(4): E119–27.

Subach BR, McLaughlin MR, Albright AL, Pollack IF. 'Current management of pediatric atlantoaxial rotatory subluxation'. *Spine (Phila Pa 1976)*, 1998 Oct 15; 23(20): 2174–9.

Viva 31 Questions

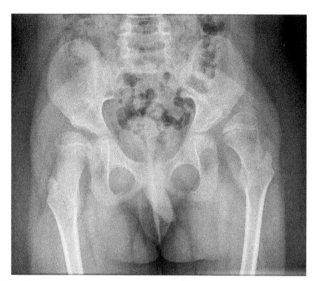

Fig. 3.35 AP pelvic X-ray

What do you see on Fig. 3.35 of an 8-year-old child?

What underlying condition do you think this patient may have?

How would you assess this patient?

The child is in pain and the hips are causing difficulty with washing and dressing. The parents would like to know what options are open to them.

What forms of surgical intervention are you aware of and what would be the appropriate surgical principles in this patient?

Are there any useful radiographic measures you could use for the right hip?

Would a Salter osteotomy be appropriate in this patient?

Do you know of any way in which this could have been picked up sooner?

Should we operate on this patient if they are asymptomatic?

Viva 31   Answers

What do you see on Fig. 3.35 of an 8-year-old child?

AP radiograph of a skeletally immature pelvis. The left hip is essentially dislocated (although by definition a dislocation implies no contact between the articular surfaces and this may not be completely true in this case) but does not appear degenerate. There is an increased acetabular index and an increased neck-shaft angle (although this may also represent increased neck anteversion). The right hip is subluxed: on both sides the migration percentage should be measured.

What underlying condition do you think this patient may have?

Most likely a neuromuscular condition and these images would be consistent with cerebral palsy.

How would you assess this patient?

I would take a history. In addition to the patient's perinatal and prior history I would like to know whether they have pain or problems with washing, dressing and seating. I would seek a history of other problems such as epilepsy and medications. If this patient is non-ambulant (*displaying knowledge that most of these patients are non-ambulant*) I would examine the patient seated, looking for spinal involvement or pelvic obliquity. I would then examine the patient on the couch noting (amongst other things) the position of their lower limbs and whether they are windswept, along with the range of abduction, rotation and flexion of both hips.

The child is in pain and the hips are causing difficulty with washing and dressing. The parents would like to know what options are open to them.

Non-surgical treatment includes analgesia, physiotherapy and wheelchair modifications. Sleep systems may also be helpful. Medications such as baclofen may improve spasticity and hence the pain. Botulinum toxin can be injected into the hip adductors to provide pain relief, although the effects are temporary and not without minor risk in GMFCS level IV and V patients (*respiratory complications have been reported*). Surgical treatment is an option for this patient.

It is important to remember that it can be difficult to identify the source of a child's pain and that reflux and constipation are common problems which can mimic hip discomfort.

What forms of surgical intervention are you aware of and what would be the appropriate surgical principles in this patient?

Soft tissue, bony and salvage surgery. Isolated soft tissue releases may be beneficial to arrest progression in a young child (*less than 6*) with an 'at risk' hip (*Reimer's migration index 15–40%*). Salvage surgery, such as a proximal femoral resection, is reserved for dislocated hips that are degenerate or cannot be successfully reconstructed. In this patient it would be appropriate to consider bilateral hip reconstructions: the soft tissue contractures are addressed by either direct releases or indirectly by shortening the femur. The femoral shape is improved via an intertrochanteric osteotomy to reduce the neck shaft angle to approx 110°, and to derotate such that the residual neck anteversion is normal. The dysplastic acetabulum would be addressed by a volume reducing acetabuloplasty.

If the femoral head is unlikely to relocate despite these measures, then an open reduction (prior to the osteotomies) would be indicated with a subsequent capsular repair.

Are there any useful radiographic measures you could use for the right hip?

Reimers migration index (RMI) describes the percentage of the femoral head lying lateral to Perkin's line. An increasing RMI has been linked to progressive subluxation and when it is greater than 40% this is strongly predictive for subsequent dislocation particularly in a child with GMFCS level 5 cerebral palsy.

Would a Salter osteotomy be appropriate in this patient?

The classic Salter osteotomy is a constrained redirectional osteotomy hinging on the pubic steymphysis and provides additional anterior cover at the expense of posterior cover. The acetabular deficiency is often predominantly posterior in cerebral palsy and therefore a Salter osteotomy would not be appropriate.

Do you know of any way in which this could have been picked up sooner?

Yes through hip surveillance programmes. The NICE guidance for spasticity suggests that all children with cerebral palsy other than hemiplegia should have an initial pelvic X-ray at 2 years of age. This should then take place annually in those who are GMFCS III to V. Ideally, as in the southern Swedish CPUP study (cerebral palsy follow-up programme) it would be combined with a record of the change in joint range of movement over time.

So should we operate on this patient if they are asymptomatic?

There is an argument for operating on hips that are likely to progress to dislocation. However, while we can predict to some extent which patients will progress, we cannot predict which of these patients will develop pain. There is evidence to suggest that less than 50% of asymptomatic dislocated hips develop pain in the long term. As such, observation of asymptomatic hips can be supported.

A body of respected opinion suggests that the gold standard of treatment is soft tissue or bony surgery for the migrating hip even in the absence of symptoms but equally many surgeons believe that the gold standard is a holistic, individualized treatment plan due to the complexity of the associated problems. 40–50% of the gross motor function classification system (GMFCS) V patients with severe associated difficulties have died by their mid 20s.

Knapp DR Jr, Cortes H. 'Untreated hip dislocation in cerebral palsy'. *Journal of Pediatric Orthopedics*, 2002; 22: 668.

Miller F, Bagg MR. 'Age and migration percentage as risk factors for progression in spastic hip disease'. *Developmental Medicine & Child Neurology*, 1995; 37: 449.

Naidu K, Smith K, Sheedy M, Adair B, Yu X, Graham HK. 'Systemic adverse events following botulinum toxin A therapy in children with cerebral palsy'. *Developmental Medicine & Child Neurology*, 2010; 52: 139.

Noonan KJ, Jones J, Pierson J, Honkamp NJ, Leverson G. 'Hip function in adults with severe cerebral palsy'. *The Journal of Bone and Joint Surgery*, American volume, 2004; 86: 2607.

Wheeler ME, Weinstein SL. 'Adductor tenotomy-obturator neurectomy'. *Journal of Pediatric Orthopedics*, 1984; 4: 48.

Viva 32   Questions

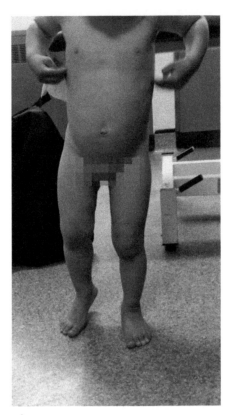

Fig. 3.36 Clinical photograph

What do you see in Fig. 3.36?

How will you assess her clinically?

If this girl was only 12 months old (and not the toddler in the photograph) and her radiograph confirms a dislocated right hip, how would you manage her?

What is the place of traction before closed reduction if the hip?

Viva 32   Answers

What do you see in Fig. 3.36?

I can see a toddler standing with pelvic obliquity and an equinus foot position on the right side which would suggest a leg length difference (or a neurological abnormality but I note the symmetrical upper limb posture). The right limb appears to be in slight ER.

How will you assess her clinically?

Following a full medical history including risk factors for developmental dysplasia of the hip (DDH), birth history and developmental milestone, I would proceed with a full clinical examination. As she is able to stand and walk, I would assess her standing posture and gait looking particularly for a Trendelenberg pattern (whilst also looking to exclude a neurological pattern). On the couch I would assess her leg length difference using the Galeazzi sign, assess hip range of motion particularly hip abduction in 90° of flexion.

If this girl was only 12 months old (and not the toddler in the photograph) and her radiograph confirms a dislocated right hip, how would you manage her?

I would counsel her family about the diagnosis and the management plan which would include in the first instance an attempt at a closed reduction.

I would admit her as soon as it was possible to do so. Under a general anaesthetic, I would perform a gentle EUA to determined whether or not the hip was reducible. An arthrogram would help my assessment. I would inject 2–4 ml of a dye (Omnipaque 300) into the hip either via a medial sub adductor longus approach or anterior approach under image intensifier control. In the at rest position, I would assess whether the hip was truly dislocated or subluxed. I would then reduce the hip with the Ortolani manoeuvre and look at the intra-articular structures such as the ligamentum teres and the labrum and assess the quality of the reduction by the width of the dye pool and the position of the maximal diameter of the femoral head relative to the labrum. If the safe zone (the range of available movement between maximal abduction and the point in the arc of abduction to adduction when the hip dislocates again) is small (< 30°) I would perform an adductor tenotomy. I am aware that some surgeons would also release the psoas tendon if the hip tended to sublux as the hip was extended below 90°.

If the safe zone was large and the medial dye pool small, no soft tissue release (tenotomy) would be indicated.

A hip spica cast (long leg or above knee) is used to immobilize the hip. Prior to discharge a plain radiograph or CT/MRI is required to confirm reduction. Further checks may be required during the period of immobilization. The duration in cast varies between surgeons: I favour 3 months in a cast and a further 6 weeks in a removeable abduction brace to allow time for the capsule to shrink and the acetabulum to remodel.

If the closed reduction failed, I would proceed to an open reduction: my preferred approach is the anterior approach.

What is the place of traction before closed reduction if the hip?

Pre-operative skin traction is rarely used in the UK currently although it remains popular in parts of Europe (France and The Netherlands for example). Skin traction was previously used routinely before closed reduction in an attempt to reduce the rates of AVN. A few studies including Salter et al. and Gage and Winter demonstrated a significant reduction in the rates of AVN when traction was used to bring the femoral head below the level of Hilgenreiner's line but other studies challenged those findings and reported low AVN rates with gentle reduction, holding the hip in the human position rather than the 'frog' position with extreme abduction.

Herring JA. *Tachdijian's Pediatric Orthopaedics*, 5th edition. 2013. Elsevier.

Graf R. 'Fundamentals of sonographic diagnosis of infant hip dysplasia'. *Journal of Paediatric Orthopedics*, 1984; 4: 735.

Gardner ROE, Bradley CS, Howard A, Narayanan UG, Wedge JH, Kelley SP. 'The incidence of avascular necrosis and the radiographic outcome following medial open reduction in children with developmental dysplasia of the hip'. *The Journal of Bone & Joint Surgery*, American volume, 2014; 96-B: 279–86.

Viva 33   Questions

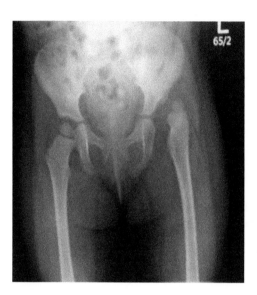

Fig. 3.37 X-ray

What do you see in Fig. 3.37?

She is 18 months old: what do you expect to find on her clinical examination?

What would your management plan be (assuming you have not treated her before) and how urgent is it?

What approach will you use for the open reduction and for the osteotomies if required?

What are the steps involved in an open reduction of the hip? Please describe the stages of the operation.

Viva 33   Answers

What do you see in Fig. 3.37?

This is an AP pelvis of a toddler with a dislocated left hip. Both ossific nuclei are present and the left acetabulum appears dysplastic.

She is 18 months old: what do you expect to find on her clinical examination?

If she is already walking I would expect to find asymmetry in her gait pattern and a leg length difference. She might walk with her left foot in equinus. On the couch, the leg would lie short and in external rotation. I would expect to find a positive Galeazzi test indicating a 'short' femur with limited hip abduction in flexion on the left. There might be asymmetry of the thigh/groin skin creases.

What would your management plan be (assuming you have not treated her before) and how urgent is it?

Assuming this girl had not had any previous failed treatment I would add her to the list for an EUA and arthrogram and an attempted closed reduction. I would aim to do this as soon as possible after having counselled and prepared the family for the postoperative period in a spica cast. I would advise the parents that the outcomes of surgery are good; their child will walk and run etc whilst admitting that earlier treatment might have been more effective in terms of long term outcome.

If successful with a closed reduction, I would hold the reduction in a spica cast for a 3-months period with an EUA and change of cast under GA at the 6 week mark to ensure that the hip stability was improving.

If the closed reduction attempt failed, I would proceed to an open reduction of the hip with or without a femoral or pelvic osteotomy as indicated: at this age some surgeons might prefer to proceed straight to an open reduction.

What approach will you use for the open reduction and for the osteotomies if required?

For a hip open reduction at this age with or without a pelvic osteotomy I would do an anterior approach via a bikini incision and the tensor fascia lata-sartorius interval. If a femoral osteotomy was indicated, I would use a separate lateral incision and routine approach to the proximal femur.

What are the steps of open reduction of the hip? Please describe the stages of the operation

I would want to consider and address the soft tissue blocks to obtaining a reduction: extracapsular—the adductor and psoas muscles; the capsule and the intracapsular structures—ligamentum teres, transverse acetabular ligament, pulvinar and finally consider the shape of the labrum.

Before commencing the open reduction and after an EUA, I would perform an open adductor longus tenotomy via a small transverse incision just distal to the skin crease (*or I would perform a percutaneous adductor tenotomy*). Via a bikini incision, I would identify the TFL-sartorius interval, protecting the lateral cutaneous nerve of the thigh (LCNT), and then identify the straight head of rectus femoris (RF). The next stage would involve splitting the apophysis of the ilium, retracting the gluteui and identifying the capsule. Detaching and tagging the straight head of rectus, identifying the reflected head and detaching it 'long'. Psoas tendon lengthening over the pelvic brim. Exposing all the capsule, inserting stay sutures and then peforming a T-shaped capsulotomy. Excision of ligamentum teres, division of the transverse acetabular ligament, and removal of the pulvinar (if necessary). I would look at the acetabular shape and size and protect the labrum. I would then attempt a reduction of the femoral head and test its stability to identify if the hip can be stable with open reduction alone or whether a concomitant osteotomy will be required. If the hip would not reduce, I would re-evaluate my soft tissue releases before considering the need for a femoral shortening osteotomy.

Then a capsulorrhaphy is performed and following closure in layers the hip is placed in a one and a half spica cast for 6–8 weeks.

An X-ray (or CT/ MR scan) to confirm reduction is done prior to discharge.

Following spica removal the hip is then followed up to monitor development over time. If the acetabulum does not develop as expected a pelvic or femoral osteotomy can be performed at a later stage.

Chiari K. 'Medial displacement osteotomy of the pelvis'. *Clinical Orthopaedics and Related Research*, 1974 Jan-Feb; 98: 55–71.

Ganz R, Leunig M. 'Osteotomy and the dysplastic hip: the bernes experience'. *Orthopaedics*, 2002; 25: 945.

Herring JA: *Tachdjian's Pediatric Orthopaedics*, 5th edition. 2013. Elsevier.

Pemberton A. 'Pericapsular osteotomy of the ilium for treatment of congenital subluxation and dislocation of the hip'. *The Journal of Bone & Joint Surgery*, American volume, 1965; 87: 65.

Salter R. 'Innominate osteotomy in the treatment of congenital dislocation of the hip'. *The Journal of Bone & Joint Surgery*, American volume, 1966: 48: 1413.

Viva 34   Questions

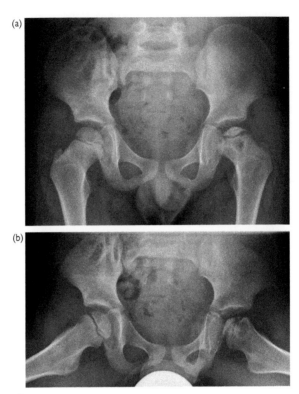

Fig. 3.38 Radiographs

Can you define what you understand by the term Perthes (Legg-Calve-Perthes) disease?

What do you see as the biggest challenges with this condition?

This child is 4-and-a-half years old, and this is his first consultation with you. The GP arranged these X-rays because of a short history of a limp. What can you tell me about his radiographs shown in Fig. 3.38? What features are you commenting on?

Have you enough information to know whether or not this child will do well or not?

This child's family are adamant that they will not consider any surgical management: is this a problem?

In what circumstances might you consider surgical intervention?

Is there a differential diagnosis for Perthes disease?

Viva 34   Answers

Can you define what you understand by the term Perthes (Legg-Calve-Perthes) disease?

In simplistic terms, this is a condition (not a disease) that affects the femoral head of children, particularly boys and particularly between the ages of 4 and 9. The blood supply to the epiphysis fails and as a consequence of this a chain of pathological events may ensue. The blood supply does return/recover but the end result of the process is linked to the extent of the avascular necrosis that occurs and the change in shape that results both in bone and in cartilage, if the avascular bone collapses before the blood supply has re-established itself.

What do you see as the biggest challenges with this condition?

There are many challenges; the first of which is accepting that we do not yet have a clear understanding of the pathoaetiology of the condition and although we can make generalizations about the condition, it is much more difficult to identify a specific child who would benefit from any specific management plan, be it surgical or conservative. If we could predict reliably which cases would result in a poor outcome in late adolescence or indeed in adult life, then we could consider treatments that would improve on this outcome.

We do know that the cartilaginous femoral head remains round, at least for some time, even after the bony epiphysis has become narrowed and sclerotic. Thus one challenge is to try and prevent the cartilaginous femoral head from deforming whilst its 'structural support' is undergoing necrosis, fragmentation, revscularization, and repair. The whole process takes quite some time and hence another obvious challenge is to find a way in which the process could be speeded up.

This child is 4-and-a-half years old, and this is his first consultation with you. The GP arranged these X-rays because of a short history of a limp. What can you tell me about his radiographs shown in Fig. 3.38?

Fig. 3.38 are AP and frog lateral radiographs of a child where the most obvious abnormality lies with the hip on the left side. The features are in keeping with Perthes disease.

What features are you commenting on?

On the AP view, there is a flattened, sclerotic epiphysis with perhaps some fragmentation laterally. On the lateral view, this area of fragmentation is confirmed. The whole head is involved and, if the pathology is in the fragmentation phase, I can apply the Herring Classification system. The lateral pillar is less than 50% of its normal height and thus this is a Herring C hip.

On both views there is evidence of a large metaphyseal cyst. There is a break in Shenton's line on the AP view but no major subluxation is seen. On the lateral view, the hip is obviously stiffer on the left than on the right as the obturator foramina are no longer symmetrical and the ischial spine is more obvious on the left than it is on the right so movement is not occurring in a normal fashion.

The prognosis depends on age but it is more related to bone age than chronological age.

Have you enough information to know whether or not this child will do well or not?

This child is young and should therefore do well but he has extensive disease. I would always want to match the radiographic features with the history and the findings from a clinical examination. One can also learn a lot about the functional range of movement by watching the child move around the consulting room and playing with toys. The formal examination may be more restricted due to anxiety, irritability and pain. I am also always influenced by how symptoms and signs are changing over time.

This child's family are adamant that they will not consider any surgical management: is this a problem?

This is not a concern at this, my first, consultation with the family and particularly given his age. I think it is entirely appropriate to offer the family an explanation of my understanding of the pathology, the natural history and the influence of treatment on this.

At this stage, I would suggest a conservative regime involving relative rest from activities that provoke the limp and/or pain, simple analgesic medication and physiotherapy exercises designed to obtain and then maintain a good range of movement in all planes of movement. Personally, I do not like the use of crutches in the first instance as I believe they encourage a flexed, adducted posture of the hip when I am particularly wanting to encourage maintenance of an abduction and extension range.

I would also explain to the family, that on occasion, 'early' surgery can help maintain a round femoral head and that this might be something I would consider at follow-up *if* the clinical and radiographic features suggested it might be indicated.

In what circumstances might you consider surgical intervention?

I think our understanding of when to intervene and how is evolving but I would become concerned with a child age 6–8 (or older) with a Herring B or B/C hip particularly if the hip is becoming stiff to clinical examination. At this stage, I would use some form of further imaging (my personal preference is an arthrogram as this allows me to look at the range of movement under anaesthetic too) to look at the shape of the cartilaginous femoral head. If this was shown to be spherical, I would like to 'protect' the vulnerable anterolateral portion of the femoral head by containing it or covering it. Thus I would advocate either a proximal femoral osteotomy to add slight varus to the hip or a pelvic osteotomy such as a Salter or Triple innominate. I would not wish to increase the pressure on the femoral head nor shorten the leg significantly. I might consider an opening wedge (rather than a closing wedge) femoral osteotomy.

Of course, I might also consider surgery to 'salvage' a poor mechanical situation towards the end of the Perthes process when revascularization has occurred and the epiphysis is essentially healed. At this stage residual deformity may well be causing impingement symptoms and signs and the acetabulum may be dysplastic.

Is there a differential diagnosis for Perthes disease?

Yes, there is a differential diagnosis and problems with sickle cell disease should always be considered as should hypothyroidism. There are a couple of other conditions that can mimic LCP especially if the changes are affecting both hips. If a child does have bilateral Perthes it is unusual for both hips to be at the same stage of the pathological process. If the changes are affecting both proximal femoral epiphyses and particularly if the child is short or shorter than expected for their parental heights, a skeletal dysplasia should be considered. In this circumstance, it might be reasonable to perform a standing leg length and alignment radiograph to look at the other epiphyses and consider a diagnosis of MED (multiple epiphyseal dysplasia) and perhaps to look at the spine to exclude a SED (spondyloepiphyseal dysplasia). Although patients with skeletal dysplasias are often shorter than average, these conditions do run in families and may be undiagnosed in which case the child is not abnormally short for his parental heights.

Herring JA, Kim HT, Browne R. 'Legg-Calve-Perthes disease. Part II: Prospective multicenter study of the effect of treatment on outcome'. *The Journal of Bone & Joint Surgery*, American volume, 2004 Oct; 86-A(10): 2121–34.

Herring JA, Kim HT, Browne R: Legg-Calve-Perthes disease. Part I: 'Classification of radiographs with use of the modified lateral pillar and Stulberg classifications'. *The Journal of Bone & Joint Surgery*, American volume, 2004 Oct; 86-A(10): 2103–20.

Huhnstock S, Svenningsen S, Pripp AH, Terjesen T, Wiig O, 'The acetabulum in Perthes' disease: a prospective study of 123 children'. *Journal of Child Orthopedics*, 2014 Dec; 8(6): 457–65.

Nguyen NA, Klein G, Dogbey G, McCourt JB, Mehlman CT. 'Operative versus nonoperative treatments for Legg-Calvé-Perthes disease: a meta-analysis'. *Journal of Pediatric Orthopedics*, 2012 Oct-Nov; 32(7): 697–705.

Perry DC, Skellorn PJ, Bruce CE. 'The lognormal age of onset distribution in Perthes' disease: an analysis from a large well-defined cohort'. *Bone Joint Journal*, 2016 May; 98-B(5): 710–4.

Rich MM, Schoenecker PL. 'Management of Legg-Calvé-Perthes disease using an A-frame orthosis and hip range of motion: a 25-year experience'. *Journal of Pediatric Orthopedic*, 2013 Mar; 33(2): 112–9.

Viva 35   Questions

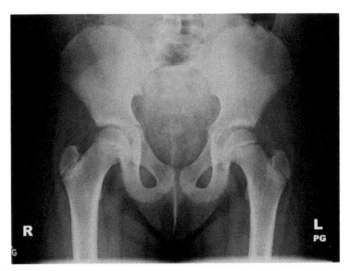

Fig. 3.39 X-ray

A 10-year-old girl presents with a 5-week history of atraumatic vague left thigh pain. She is otherwise well. What would your top three differential diagnosis be?

The GP has organized an X-ray (see Fig. 3.39). It was reported as normal by a consultant radiologist, what do you think, what further imaging would you request?

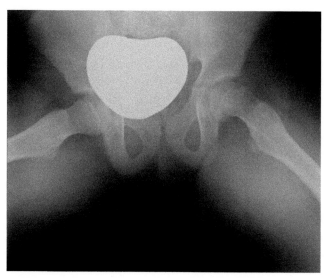

Fig. 3.40 X-ray

Does this X-ray (Fig. 3.40) help?

Does this fit with your interpretation of the AP view?

How could you grade/classify this condition?

Do these systems help?

How would you measure the severity of the slip?

How would you treat this patient?

Would you try to improve the angle of the hip from its current position by gentle manipulation?

Would you do anything to the contralateral asymptomatic hip?

What potential complications would you advise the parents about?

How would you minimize the risk of chondrolysis?

Given that she is only 10 years old would you have any other concerns?

Viva 35   Answers

A 10-year-old girl presents with a 5-week history of atraumatic vague left thigh pain. She is otherwise well. What would your top three differential diagnosis be?

Slipped capital femoral epiphysis, osteomyelitis, tumour.

Further down the list: Perthes (although she is a little old for a first presentation), hip dysplasia previously unrecognized (unlikely), septic arthritis (a little old and too well).

The GP has organized an X-ray (see Fig. 3.39). It was reported as normal by a consultant radiologist, what do you think, what further imaging would you request?

The physis of the left proximal femur looks different to that on the right: Klein's line does not intersect the left femoral epiphysis (Trethowan's sign). I would like a frog lateral view as well.

Does this X-ray (Fig. 3.40) help?

Yes the frog lateral shows a slipped capital femoral epiphysis.

Does this fit with your interpretation of the AP view?

Yes and it is now more apparent that Klein's line is abnormal and Trethowans' sign is present. On the AP view, the physis appears a little widened.

How could you grade/classify this condition?

There are different classifications related to severity, stability and chronicity. Mild/ moderate/ severe based on the Southwick angle which quantifies the amount of epiphyseal displacement relative to the metaphysis.

Loder's classification which defines the stability according to the patients ability to bear any weight on the affected side and the temporal classification based on whether the presentation is acute or chronic or acute-on-chronic: with a time point of 3 weeks defining acute from chronic.

Do these systems help?

They can aid decision-making regarding management, for example whether pinning in situ is possible, and whether there is a greater risk of complications such as avascular necrosis. However, the cut off between acute and chronic is somewhat arbitrary and although most surgeons would pin in situ a mild slip different practices exist for moderate and severe slips.

How would you measure the severity of the slip?

You can measure the slip angle (lateral epiphyseal shaft angle) and compare it to the asymptomatic side, subtracting the difference categorizes the severity; mild- less than 30°, moderate 30–50° and severe greater than 50° (Southwick classification), however there can be a contralateral mild slip present in 20–40% of cases which this method does not account for. The PSA (posterior sloping angle) method uses a very similar angle measurement but has a definitive cut off, recommending pinning in situ to be considered for any contralateral hips when the angle is greater than 14°.

How would you treat this patient?

I would need to measure the radiographs, but the slip appears to be mild and therefore I would pin it in situ (see Fig. 3.41).

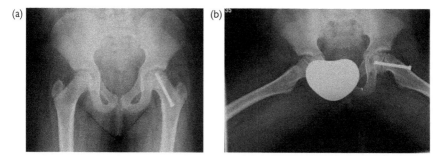

Fig. 3.41 X-rays

Would you try to improve the angle of the hip from its current position by gentle manipulation?

No this is a stable slip and it would not be mobile enough to reduce.

Would you do anything to the contralateral asymptomatic hip?

I would measure the PSA and if it was greater than 14° I would consider pinning it, however this would be in addition to discussion with the family about the potential pros and cons of doing so.

She is also young to have sustained a slip and this may heighten my awareness for an underlying metabolic condition and might increase my willingness to pin the contralateral side.

What potential complications would you advise the parents about?

The main complication of concern with this hip would be chondrolysis, avascular necrosis would also be a theoretical concern but it is a mild, stable slip and as long as I was careful with my screw insertion/positioning I think the risk of AVN is very small. I would also mention metalware failure and wound infection. There is also a risk of fracture. I would mention the risk of a future contralateral slip and discuss the pros and cons of prophylactic fixation.

How would you minimize the risk of chondrolysis?

The risk of chondrolysis is thought to be due to breaching the articular surface of the femoral head, I would therefore ensure that neither the guidewire nor the drill or screw tip went into the subchondral bone by regular imaging with the image intensifier during the procedure.

Given that she is only 10 years old would you have any other concerns?

I would be concerned about the possibility of a potential contralateral slip in the future and also an underlying metabolic disorder such as hypothyroidism.

Loder RT. 'What is the cause of avascular necrosis in unstable slipped capital femoral epiphysis and what can be done to lower the rate'? *Journal of Pediatric Orthopedics*, 2013; 33 Suppl 1: S88–91.

Loder RT, Skopelja EN. 'The epidemiology and demographics of slipped capital femoral epiphysis'. *International Scholarly Research Notices Orthopedics*, 2011; 2011: 486512.

MacLean JG, Reddy SK. 'The contralateral slip. An avoidable complication and indication for prophylactic pinning in slipped upper femoral epiphysis'. *The Bone & Joint Journal*, 2006; 88(11): 1497–501.

Novais EN, Millis MB. 'Slipped capital femoral epiphysis: prevalence, pathogenesis, and natural history'. *Clinical Orthopaedics and Related Research*, 2012; 470(12): 3432–8.

Sankar WN, McPartland TG, Millis MB, Kim YJ. 'The unstable slipped capital femoral epiphysis: risk factors for osteonecrosis'. *Journal of Pediatric Orthopedics*, 2010; 30(6): 544–8.

Viva 36 Questions

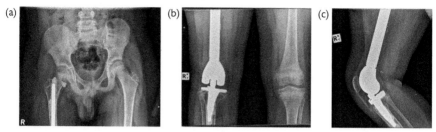

Fig. 3.42 X-rays

What do you see in Fig. 3.42?

Yes, this boy had excision of an osteosarcoma, with pre- and post-operative chemotherapy. He is now 12. How would you assess his leg lengths clinically?

What gait patterns might he have?

Carry on with your assessment.....

If the child has a stiff knee with a fixed flexion deformity of 10°, how can you then measure his leg lengths accurately in clinic?

This patient underwent a CT scanogram, with the right leg being 18 mm shorter. Without treatment, how much discrepancy will he have at maturity?

Viva 36   Answers

What do you see in Fig. 3.42?

An AP radiograph of the pelvis and AP and lateral radiographs of a child's right knee. There is an endoprosthetic replacement of the right distal femur and knee. On the contralateral left side, Harris growth lines are visible in the distal femur and proximal tibia: these are parallel to the physis and confirm that growth is taking place. The distance from the line to the physis should be greater in the distal femur than in the proximal tibia due to the differential growth rates.

Yes, this boy had excision of an osteosarcoma, with pre- and post-operative chemotherapy. He is now 12. How would you assess his leg lengths clinically?

I would ask whether he has noticed a difference in his leg lengths, whether he walks with a limp and if he has back or hip pain. I would observe him standing, looking at the level of his posterior inferior iliac spines (PSIS) and assessing for any obvious joint contractures (a flexed knee or an equinus foot). If there is a short side, I would use wooden blocks to build it up until the PSIS is level on both sides and he feels level. I would observe his gait.

What gait patterns might he have?

He might have a short leg gait. He might exhibit an abnormality on the short side, for example toe walking, or an abnormality on the long side, for example vaulting or circumduction or knee flexion.

Carry on with your assessment.....

I would examine his spine, looking for a scoliosis. I would then examine him lying on the couch, beginning by examining for hip, knee and ankle contractures, which can impede measurement of true leg lengths. I would then measure his true and apparent leg lengths, followed by a Galeazzi test to identify the limb segment that is short.

If the child has a stiff knee with a fixed flexion deformity of 10°, how can you then measure his leg lengths accurately in clinic?

I would place the other knee in the same position and then proceed with measurement. Alternatively, I could measure each segment separately between bony landmarks.

This patient underwent a CT scanogram, with the right leg being 18 mm shorter. Without treatment, how much discrepancy will he have at maturity?

Please could you remind me of his age?

Yes, he is 12 and had his tumour resected at age 11

Thank you. Assuming that boys reach skeletal maturity at 16, he has 4 years of growth remaining. His right distal femoral physis has been replaced and whilst the proximal tibial physis has been preserved at the time of surgery it does not appear to be growing well as judged by the lack of a Harris line on the right compared to the left. I am assuming that his remaining growth plates are unaffected by his chemotherapy regime. As per Menelaus' method, the distal femoral growth plate contributes 9 mm per year to growth and the proximal tibia contributes 6mm. As a result, he will lose 15 mm/year length and over 4 years, this will equate to 60 mm. So, his total discrepancy at maturity can be predicted as 78 mm. I am also aware that there are 'apps' that will do such calculations for me.

So, what treatment will you offer him and how will you council him and his family?

A discrepancy of 78 mm is not acceptable and although a shoe raise is possible, this is not well tolerated by most patients. Whilst in theory there are several surgical options that could be considered, one of the most important factors influencing our decision would be an appreciation of his original diagnosis and the treatment of this. Both these factors make leg lengthening on his affected side a less attractive option. I would, therefore, offer him surgical treatment in the form of an epiphysiodesis of the left distal femur and proximal tibia. I would explain that this will make him shorter on the left side by around 6 cm. (I am aware that usually the upper limit for an epiphysiodesis is 5cm) Although we would like to maintain height, it is more important to have leg lengths which are close to equal. He will still end up with the discrepancy that he has now and this operation is to prevent it from getting worse. A discrepancy of 18 mm is well tolerated but may require a shoe raise (approximately 1 cm would be enough).

How would you do the operation and when?

I would perform a percutaneous drill epiphysiodesis of the left distal femur and proximal tibia, using a 4.5 mm drill under image guidance, with subsequent curettage of the growth plate, taking care not to breach the cortex excessively or enter the joint. As there is more than 2 years' growth remaining, I would consider an open epiphysiodesis of the fibula (although recent evidence suggests this might be unnecessary). I would do this as soon as possible, as delay will risk a greater ultimate discrepancy.

Would you use uni- or bilateral-entry ports for the femur and tibia and are you aware of any evidence to support your choice?

I would use bilateral entry ports. Edmonds et al. described a lower complication rate with bilateral ports and, in particular, a lower rate of failed growth plate ablation.

Canale ST, Russell TA, Holcomb RL. 'Percutaneous epiphysiodesis: experimental study and preliminary clinical results'. *Journal of Pediatric Orthopaedics* 1986; 6: 150–6.

Edmonds E, Stasikelis P. 'Percutaneous epiphysiodesis of the lower extremity. A comparison of single versus double portal techniques'. *Journal of Pediatric Orthopaedics*, 2007; 27(6): 618–22.

Viva 37   Questions

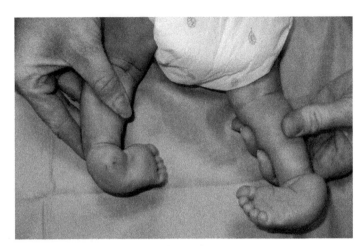

Fig. 3.43 Clinical photograph of a baby with foot deformities

What do you see in Fig. 3.43?

What is this deformity?

What elements make up the club foot deformity and are they all visible in Fig. 3.43?

Do you know of any classifications for clubfoot and what they are used for?

How would you treat this baby and when can the treatment begin?

Can you describe the Ponseti method of correction?

Does the Ponseti method confer any advantages to the patient compared with an open surgical approach?

When is surgical treatment required and what are the procedures you are familiar with.

Viva 37   Answers

What do you see in Fig. 3.43?

I see a baby lying prone with bilateral foot deformities suggestive of congenital talipes equinovarus (CTEV).

What is this deformity?

This is a congenital 3-dimensional deformity of the foot or feet: syndromic (non-idiopathic) feet have a higher tendency to be bilateral.

What elements make up the club foot deformity and are they all visible in Fig. 3.43?

The 4 elements are pronation of the first ray giving the appearance of forefoot cavus, forefoot adductus, heel varus and equinus. In this view it is difficult to see the hindfoot equinus. There are medial creases on the soles of both feet and both lateral borders are curved.

Do you know of any classifications for clubfoot and what they are used for?

Several classification systems have been described. The most popular is the Pirani classification. It is a descriptive classification with 6 components each graded 0, 0.5 or 1 depending on severity. The maximum score is 6 (3 points for the midfoot and 3 for the hindfoot) and this therefore represents the most severe deformity. The components include midfoot crease, lateral border, talonavicular reduction, posterior crease, empty heel and equinus. In this example the left foot has a deeper medial crease than the right but inspection of the foot from all angles and a clinical examination is required to apply the score effectively.

The Pirani score can predict the number of casts required for correction and the requirement for a tenotomy (increased with a Pirani score of 5 or above); but it has no long term prognosis.

(*The Dimeglio score is more complicated and less used in the UK, it introduces the concept of 'reducibility' of aspects of the deformity and highlights the problems associated with cases with known muscle imbalance. Again the higher the score, the more difficult the foot is to treat and the more likely that surgical intervention may be required.*)

How would you treat this baby and when can the treatment begin?

The treatment can start soon after birth (within 1 or 2 weeks) but there is no 'rush' as good outcomes are still easy to achieve if treatment starts later. In the UK, the standard of care is the Ponseti method.

(*The French functional method is also used in a few centres, it requires considerably more time and expertise with similar or inferior results.*)

Can you describe the Ponseti method of correction?

The Ponseti method corrects the deformity in stages with each episode of treatment involving manipulation of the foot to gain an improved position and then holding this in an above knee (flexed knee) cast for 7 days (the accelerated regime changes casts every 5 days). The acronym CAVE (for cavus, adductus varus and equinus) describes the order of deformity correction. The cavus (pronation of the first ray) is corrected first by supinating the forefoot so that it comes in line with the hindfoot: at this stage the foot deformity may look worse. The metatarsus adductus and hindfoot varus are corrected by abducting the foot with counterpressure on the lateral talar head. Abduction is achieved with the foot in equinus.

Once full (up to 70°) abduction has been achieved, the ankle can be dorsiflexed but if the ankle achieves less than 15° of dorsiflexion an Achilles tenotomy is required. This can be done under local anaesthetic in the clinic (or under general anesthetic in theatre) and this last cast is then left in place for 3 weeks.

Following removal of the last cast the feet are placed in a foot abduction brace that aims to maintain the external rotation under the talus. The brace is used 23 hours a day for the first 3 months and during naptime and nighttime thereafter for a minimum of 4 years. The total duration of treatment does vary from centre to centre.

Does the Ponseti method confer any advantages to the patient compared with an open surgical approach?

The short-term success rate of the Ponseti method is extremely high. Satisfactory correction is reported in 95% of idiopathic cases. The long-term success rates vary and depend on outcome definition. There are no prospective randomized trials comparing this method to extensive posteromedial release but stiffness with substantial loss of range of motion and pain are common complications reported following surgical release. About 35% of the patients corrected with the Ponseti method will require some form of surgery during the course of their childhood but this is usually limited to the soft tissues rather than involving major joint releases.

When is surgical treatment required and what are the procedures you are familiar with

Surgical treatment is normally reserved for the relapsed/ recurrent deformity or when the foot fails to correct. The required procedure will vary and will be dictated by the aetiology and the type/ degree of the deformity. In the idiopathic foot that relapses, (repeat) Achilles tendon lengthening for equinus, and a full tibialis anterior tendon transfer for dynamic supination are often indicated with occasionally, a more extensive soft tissue release (posterior or posteromedial) for a more severe deformity. The current 'a la carte' surgical approach was suggested by Bensahel and Dimeglio. It encourages the surgeon to consider what elements of the deformity remain and how much/how little surgery is required to correct them rather than to perform a standard peri-talar release as described by Simons, McKay, or Turco.

Recurrent deformity, particularly following surgery, requires careful analysis of all components of the deformity (which may by now be more planovalgus). By now, particularly in the older child or the child with non-idiopathic deformity, consideration should be given to addressing the bony components with either a shortening of the lateral column, a calcaneal osteotomy or supramalleolar osteotomy. The Ilizarov technique has also proved useful for recurrent deformity especially in the presence of severe scarring. It is important to maintain a holistic approach in the non-idiopathic cases and assess the joints above and overall function.

Dunkley M, Gelfer Y, Jackson D, Armstrong J, Rafter C and Eastwood D, 'Mid-term results of a physiotherapist-led Ponseti service for the management of non-idiopathic and idiopathic clubfoot'. Journal of Child Orthopedics, 2015; 9(3): 183–9.

Herring JA: Tachdijian's Pediatric Orthopaedics, 5th edition. 2013, Elsevier.

Ponseti IV: Clubfoot management. Journal of Pediatric Orthopedics 2000; 20: 699–700.

Viva 38   Questions

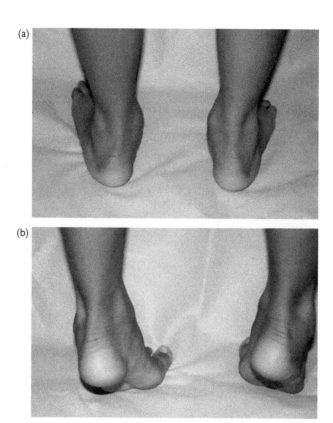

(a)

(b)

Fig. 3.44 Clinical photographs

Fig. 3.44 shows a 9-year-old boy who was asymptomatic until recently but who has developed foot and ankle pain over the last few weeks. Describe what you see.

What features are relevant in the history?

What would you look for when examining the child?

Fig. 3.45 shows the child's X-rays could you describe them please?

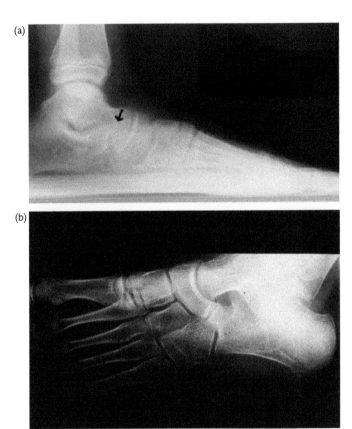

Fig. 3.45 X-rays

Would you investigate them further? What options do you have?

Do you think orthotics have a role here?

What types of coalition do you know of in the foot?

How would you manage this child?

What approaches do you know to a calcaneo-navicular coalition?

Viva 38   Answers

Fig. 3.44 shows a 9-year-old boy who was asymptomatic until recently but who has developed foot and ankle pain over the last few weeks. Describe what you see

The clinical photograph demonstrates a flat medial arch. The second photograph with the child on tip toes shows that the hindfoot valgus has corrected and the arch has returned.

What features are relevant in the history?

The most relevant feature is the age of the child and the complaint of pain in a previously painless but probably flat foot. The age of the child would be compatible with the presentation of an ossifying tarsal coalition and inflammation/infection/trauma should always be considered. I would be considering the following differential diagnosis:

1. A painful flexible flat foot
2. JIA
3. Tarsal coalition

What would you look for when examining the child?

In examining the child, I would make a brief overall assessment of the child to exclude obvious syndromic/neurological problems and watch him walking and standing. I would assess the overall limb alignment and length and foot posture.

In standing, focused assessment for flat foot would involvement examination of the longitudinal arches and mobility of the hindfoot in bilateral and single stance heel raise.

On the couch, I would look for signs of injury or inflammation and again assess joint mobility (ankle, subtalar, and midtarsal joints) and feel for areas of tenderness or pain.

Fig. 3.45 shows the child's X-rays could you describe them please?

Radiographs demonstrate an extended anterior process of the calcaneum: the anteater sign. The oblique view demonstrates the coalition more clearly.

Would you investigate them further? What options do you have?

This patient warrants further investigation. Some would argue that a MR scan would give the best chance of obtaining most useful information as to whether there is a coalition (or two), its exact location and its nature. Others feel that a MR image is often inconclusive and CT scans are better at delineating the anatomy of a bony or even fibrous coalition: in practice both are often required for operative planning.

Do you think orthotics have a role here?

Orthotics are designed to correct and support the arch in its corrected position: they are useful adjuncts for the treatment of the painful but flexible foot but they have a limited role as first line treatment for the painful, rigid foot that often occurs with a tarsal coalition: if the arch does not return on tip-toeing or a single leg heel raise, then an orthotic is unlikely to benefit the patient unless it is acting purely as a soft accommodative device.

What types of coalition do you know of in the foot?

Coalition in the foot classically presents as either a calcaneo-navicular coalition, which is the one most commonly identified, or a talo-calcaneal coalition (which may actually be the most common, but less frequently identified!).

How would you manage this child?

As the child is developing a painful flat foot, I would complete my examination looking for loss of mobility in the sub-talar joint or between the hind-foot and the mid-foot. If I identified a stiff STJ or if I suspected the subtalar movement was actually arising from the ankle joint, would investigate this child further, examining for a coalition (and excluding other causes) and counsel the child and the parents as to the likelihood that as the coalition ossifies, the flexibility of the foot will be reduced further and pain may continue to be an issue. In that scenario, excision of the coalition would be recommended.

What approaches do you know to a calcaneo-navicular coalition?

An Ollier's type skin incision can be used over the dorsolateral aspect of the foot. Dissection down to the anterolateral border of the calcaneum and onto the calcaneonavicular coalition via the sinus tarsi allows access for assessment and excision. Take care to protect an anterior branch of the sural nerve.

The examiner only asked for the approach but...

The procedure would involve excision of a trapezium shaped piece of bone and consideration should be given as to whether a 'spacer' must be placed in the gap: either EDB or fat or simply bone wax.

Churchill JA, Mazur JM. 'Ankle Pain in Children: Diagnostic Evaluation and Clinical Decision Making'. *The Journal of the American Academy of Orthopaedic Surgeons*, 1995 Jul; 3(4): 183–93.

Khoshbin A, Law PW, Caspi L, Wright JG. 'Long-term functional outcomes of resected tarsal coalitions'. *Foot & Ankle International*, 2013 Oct; 34(10): 1370–5.

Wenger DR, Mauldin D, Speck G, Morgan D, Lieber RL. 'Corrective shoes and inserts as treatment for flexible flatfoot in infants and children'. *The Journal of Bone & Joint Surgery, American volume*, 1989 Jul; 71(6): 800–10.

Viva 39   Questions

You are unlikely to spend the whole viva discussing a congenital vertical talus (CVT) but there could be a question at the end of a viva on the club foot.

What do you see in Fig. 3.46?

How would you treat this baby and when can the treatment begin?

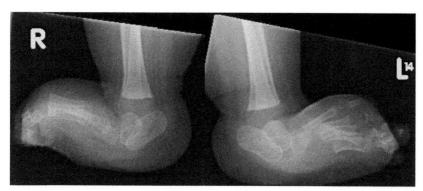

Fig. 3.46 X-ray

Viva 39   Answers

What do you see in Fig. 3.46?

This is a lateral radiograph of an infant's feet and the most striking abnormality is the hindfoot equinus and the position of the talar head in the sole of the foot. Although the navicular is not ossified in infancy, it appears that the forefoot/midfoot is not aligned with the talar head and thus there must be subluxation or frank dislocation of the talonavicular joint.

To confirm the diagnosis of a CVT I would want to examine the foot to see, amongst other things, whether or not the deformity was flexible and whether or not there were any other signs of a generalized neuromuscular or musculoskeletal condition. An X-ray with the forefoot in maximal plantarflexion would help me document the flexibility of the deformity and whether or not the talonavicular joint could be reduced.

How would you treat this baby and when can the treatment begin?

If this baby does have bilateral irreducible vertical tali, then treatment could begin within 1 or 2 weeks of birth using the 'reverse-Ponseti' technique which uses the principles defined by Ponseti for the stepwise correction of all facets of the club foot deformity but to a certain extent 'reverses' them to accommodate the opposite deformities seen in the foot with a vertical talus. These principles also take into consideration the fact that manipulation techniques that involve distraction of the soft tissues result in growth stimulation and can bring about a rapid change in shape of the cartilage anlages of the tarsal bones.

Before embarking on such treatment, it is always important to make a full assessment of the child and their co-morbidities as a holistic approach to the care of the child and their family is essential. For example, in children with a spina bifida lesion, surgical closure of this lesion will take priority. In arthrogryposis, associated knee deformities and/or hip dislocations may also need treatment and if all joints can not be treated simultaneously, an appropriate plan with an appropriate and realistic timescale will need to be determined on an individual basis.

Brand RA, Siegler S, Pirani S, Morrison WB, Udupa JK. 'Cartilage anlagen adapt in response to static deformation'. Medical Hypotheses, 2006; 66(3): 653–9.

Herring JA: Disorders of the foot. In Saunders, Tachdijian's Pediatric Orthopaedics, 5th edition 2013. Elsevier.

Miller M. Dobbs MB. 'Congenital Vertical Talus: Etiology and Management'. The Journal of the American Academy of Orthopaedic Surgeon, 2015 Oct; 23(10): 604–11.

Pirani S, Zeznik L, Hodges D. 'Magnetic resonance imaging study of the congenital clubfoot treated with the Ponseti method'. Journal of Pediatric Orthopedics, 2001 Nov-Dec; 21(6): 719–26.

Viva 40   Questions

(a)

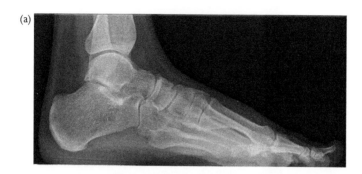

(b)

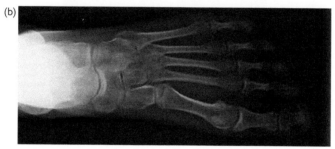

Fig. 3.47 X-rays

This 14-year-old girl presents with a 12 m history of multiple aches and pains in various joints and documented swollen knees. Her knees have no fluid in them today but her left foot is sore and she has a flat-ish foot with a stiff and uncomfortable subtalar joint. Her hind foot feels a little warm to the touch. Her X-rays are as shown in Fig. 3.47. Do need any further information or do you think you have a differential diagnosis in mind?

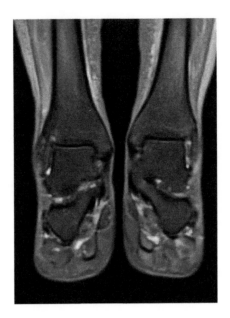

Fig. 3.48 MR image

Her FBC and CRP are normal, her ESR is 15. A representative MR image is shown in Fig. 3.48. Can you make any comments?

Which is your preferred method for evaluating a tarsal coalition: MRI or CT scan?

After review and discussion with the patient and her family you offer her a bar excision: what are the aims of the procedure and what risks would you counsel her about?

What are your comments about this X-ray (Fig. 3.49)?

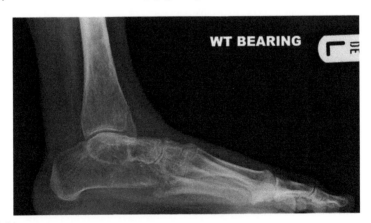

Fig. 3.49 X-ray

Can you tell me what the characteristic features of a fibula hemimelia are?

Viva 40 Answers

This 14-year-old girl presents with a 12 m history of multiple aches and pains in various joints and documented swollen knees. Her knees have no fluid in them today but her left foot is sore and she has a flat-ish foot with a stiff and uncomfortable subtalar joint. Her hind foot feels a little warm to the touch. Her X-rays are as shown in Fig. 3.47. Do need any further information or do you think you have a differential diagnosis in mind?

The AP and lateral radiographs of a skeletally mature foot show no obvious cause for her painful foot. There is no accessory navicular noted. The posterior facet of the subtalar joint appears reduced and there is some sclerosis around the angle of Gissane.

Her history of pains affecting other joints may need to be investigated more fully, particularly if her hindfoot is inflamed and stiff. I would want to take a full history and complete my examination and consider the diagnosis of a JIA (juvenile inflammatory arthritis).

Her FBC and CRP are normal, her ESR is 15. A representative MRI picture is shown in Fig. 3.48. Can you make any comments?

As far as a potential diagnosis of JIA is concerned these blood tests are reassuring. Also, her MRI shows no obvious joint effusion in either the ankle or the subtalar joint. It does however show a mature bony bar between the talus and the calcaneum at the level of the anterior facet of the subtalar joint. On this single image, there does not appear to be any significant bone oedema or soft tissue change suggestive of synovitis or an infective/inflammatory picture. Clinical judgement would help me decide whether this mature bar was responsible for some of her symtoms or whether it was a 'red herring'.

Which is your preferred method for evaluating a tarsal coalition: MRI or CT scan?

Opinion and the literature are divided on which imaging modality is most useful for evaluating a coalition. MRI avoids the radiation dose associated with a CT and is perhaps better at identifying fibrous and cartilaginous coalitions but the bony anatomy and the extent of the bar may be easier to evaluate on a CT scan. It can be difficult to know whether or not cartilaginous or fibrous bars are symptomatic but bone oedema or soft tissue change adjacent to the presumed coalition can be used to support the diagnosis, on the other hand, the dysplastic appearances of the sustentuculum tali may be better shown on a CT and allow better 3D appreciation of the site, extent and nature of the bar.

As with all investigations, the precise choice of investigations depends on the exact question being asked.

After review and discussion with the patient and her family you offer her a bar excision: what are the aims of the procedure and what risks would you counsel her about?

Excision of a talocalcaneal bar (or indeed a calcaneonavicular coalition) is an operation which is performed for pain relief rather than restoration of movement. It aims to relieve pain by reducing 'stress' on the abnormal area of bone and whilst it will restore some movement to the joint in question, this is not usually clinically significant and, to examination, the patient may well still have a flat foot and a stiff joint.

For a talocalcaneal coalition, the incision is medial at the level of the subtalar joint and the neurovascular bundle. Care must be taken not to damage these structures or the tendons of tibialis posterior, flexor hallucis and flexor digitorum longus. Dysaesthesia or numbness is a risk and wound healing can be slow.

My biggest concern would be the risk that this procedure would fail to alleviate her symptoms fully and that she would continue to have pain on activity and with attempted movement of the joint. There is no obvious hindfoot malalignment on her plain films or on the single MRI image that I have been shown, so there would be no indication for a concomitant osteotomy at the time of bar excision. Thus I would warn her that if pain persisted or recurred after the coalition had been excised, a subtalar joint fusion might need to be considered. Often, even when the coalition is limited to the anterior/middle facets of the subtalar joint, the posterior subtalar joint remains a a source of pain.

What are your comments about this X-ray (Fig. 3.49)?

This is a lateral radiograph of a skeletally mature patient. The hindfoot is abnormal and there is a complete coalition between the talus and the calcaneum. There is no fibula and I suspect that this may be a 4 ray foot (by counting the metatarsals). The diagnosis is a longitudinal deficiency of the lower limb: a fibula hemimelia.

Can you tell me what the characteristic features of a fibula hemimelia are?

Starting from distally and working proximally the following abnormalities may be identified:

1. Absent lateral rays
2. Tarsal coalition
3. Ball and socket ankle joint
4. Short/deformed/absent fibula
5. Short bowed tibia (apex antero medial)
6. Absent anterior cruciate ligament
7. Deficient lateral femoral condyle
8. Short, externally rotated femur and possibly
9. Features of a PFFD

Bouchard M and Mosca VS. 'Flatfoot deformity in children and adolescents: surgical indications and management'. *The Journal of the American Academy of Orthopaedic Surgeons*, 2014; 22(10): 623–32.

Mosca VS, et al. 'Talocalcaneal tarsal coalitions and the calcaneal lengthening osteotomy: the role of deformity correction'. *The Journal of Bone & Joint Surgery*, American volume, 2012 Sep 5; 94(17): 1584–94.

Murphy JS, Mubarak S. 'Talocalcaneal Coalitions'. *Foot and Ankle Clinics* 2015; 20(4): 681–91.

Viva 41   Questions

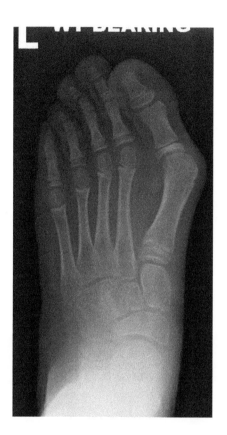

Fig. 3.50 X-ray

Describe the features on this X-ray (Fig. 3.50).

Would any other radiographs be helpful?

What features in the history and examination are you most interested in? She is a 13-year-old girl.

She has a history of ligamentous laxity and generalized aches and pains: her Beighton score is 8. Is this relevant?

She tells you she does not want to try any 'supports'; she simply wants an operation to fix it and she would like it done in the next summer holidays.

What operation will you offer her? Her IMA is 22°, her HVA 45°, and her DMAA nearly 50°. Her bunion is non tender.

As she is leaving, her mother asks you to look at the younger daughter's foot (age 7)—she appears to have a bunionette with a small fifth toe that overlaps the fourth toe. She asks you if there is a treatment for this?

We have talked about juvenile hallux valgus but is hallux varus a common problem too?

Describe the features on this X-ray (Fig. 3.51).

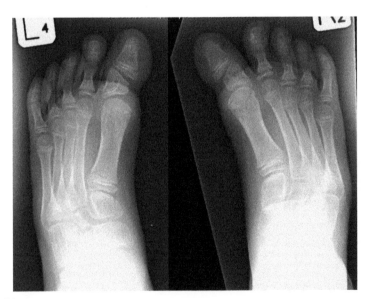

Fig. 3.51 X-rays

Viva 41 Answers

Please describe the features on this X-ray (Fig. 3.50)

This is an AP radiograph of the left foot of a skeletally immature patient. The most obvious features relate to a hallux valgus deformity with what appears to be a significant increase in the intermetatarsal angle and her hallux valgus angle. The lateral sesamoid is out of position. The writing at the top of the radiograph implies this is a weightbearing film.

Would any other radiographs be helpful?

It is my usual practice to ask for AP and lateral weightbearing radiographs to look at overall alignment and to help me judge the relationship of the hindfoot to the mid/forefoot. I would like to know whether she was significantly flat footed or not.

What features in the history and examination are you most interested in? She is a 13-year-old girl

Every patient deserves a full consultation which would include a complete medical history and examination but in this case my first 3 questions might relate to the following points: is there a family history, is the problem bilateral, and is she symptomatic? I would also want to know if she had any other medical conditions and whether or not she had tried any treatments prior to visiting this clinic.

She has a history of ligamentous laxity and generalized aches and pains: her Beighton score is 8. Is this relevant?

The Beighton score is out of 9 and I might assume that the point that is missing is that she is unable to place her palms on the ground with the legs straight and together: the other 8 points would represent symmetrical involvement of elbow and knee hyper-extension, hyper-extension of the fifth metacarpophalangeal (MCP) joint and an ability of the thumb to touch her forearm with a flexed wrist. It is consistent with generalized joint hypermobility but not necessarily the hypermobility syndrome. It has not been validated in children. Certainly a history of generalized aches and pains needs to be considered a little further: it could fit with a hypermobility syndrome, a Vitamin D deficiency/insufficiency or simply related to her growth but, as always, in the assessment of paediatric patients it is important to ensure that you distinguish the rare but worrying symptoms from the common, less worrying symptoms. It is important to listen carefully to what both the parents and the child are saying.

If she has uncomfortable flexible flat feet with pain related to her bunion, orthotic management of her foot deformity may well improve some of her generalized foot/lower limb symptoms. By altering foot posture, it could also relieve some of the pain related specifically to her bunion.

She tells you she does not want to try any 'supports'; she simply wants an operation to fix it and she would like it done in the next summer holidays. What operation will you offer her? Her IMA is 22°, her HVA 45°, and her DMAA nearly 50°. Her bunion is non tender.

Whilst I always respect the patient's opinion, the surgeon must also have an opinion which should also be respected. Based on the current literature, I would be reluctant to offer any teenager surgery for a hallux valgus deformity prior to skeletal maturity. Any offer of surgery would be designed primarily for relief of symptoms and I would want to ensure her symptoms were attributable to her bunion. Whilst the absence of tenderness at one clinic appointment, on its own, does not over-ride other features of the history and examination it is a point that I would note. I understand her reluctance to try 'supports' but I feel that if they were indicated, I would want her to try them first to see if we could manage her symptoms conservatively until later in adolescence. It is always important to keep the patient and their family 'on side' during these potentially difficult consultations.

Her deformity as described would be categorized as 'severe' and might therefore merit a double level osteotomy of the first metatarsal. However, her proximal physis is open which might make me consider an opening, medially based wedge osteotomy of the medial cuneiform but in this case there does not appear to be any significant problems with alignment at this level. The risk of disappointment with surgery and/or recurrence at this age and with this deformity would be high and, I feel, that I would prefer to wait until skeletal maturity to offer her any surgical procedure.

As she is leaving, her mother asks you to look at the younger daughter's foot (age 7)—she appears to have a bunionette with a small fifth toe that overlaps the fourth toe. She asks you if there is a treatment for this

An over-riding or overlapping fifth toe is a relatively common congenital deformity where the toe is small and poorly formed with soft tissue contractures that mean the toe rests in the dorsiflexed and adducted position (perhaps giving the appearance of a bunionette). The toe may rub on shoewear and cause problems in childhood or indeed in adulthood.

If surgery is indicated, the procedure usually involves essentially a circumferential soft tissue release at the level of the MTP joint via a racket handle incision. The toe is then placed in the corrected position and the soft tissues repaired. It is usually a very successful procedure.

We have talked about juvenile hallux valgus but is hallux varus a common problem too?

No, hallux varus is much more unusual and usually signifies an underlying pathology. The condition is often present at birth and may be associated with other local foot abnormalities such as a polydactyly, an abnormal first metatarsal and/or a bracket physis. Treatment is usually surgical and is often performed early so that any tethers of growth are released/removed.

Describe the features on this X-ray (Fig. 3.51)

AP radiographs of both feet of a child. The most obvious abnormality is a varus attitude of the great toes (particularly obvious on the right). The proximal phalanx of both left and right toes is an abnormal shape and on the left the appearance is of a delta phalanx or a bracket physis.

The treatment of a bracket physis involves the release of the physeal tether usually by excision of the longitudinal portion of the abnormal physis. The 'gap' can then be filled with an interposition material such as bone wax. Normal growth should then resume but may not match the contralateral foot. Further treatment may be required as the child grows.

Agrawal Y, Bajaj SK, Flowers MJ. 'Scarf-Akin osteotomy for hallux valgus in juvenile and adolescent patients'. *Journal of Pediatric Orthopedics, B*, 2015 Nov; 24(6): 535–40.

Barouk LS. 'The effect of gastrocnemius tightness on the pathogenesis of juvenile hallux valgus: a preliminary study'. *Foot and Ankle Clinics*, 2014 Dec; 19(4) :807–22.

Choo AD, Mubarak SJ. 'Longitudinal epiphyseal bracket'. *Journal of Child Orthopedics*, 2013 Dec; 7(6): 449–54. doi: 10.1007/s11832-013-0544-1. [Review]

Davids JR, Gibson TW, Pugh LI. 'Quantitative segmental analysis of weight-bearing radiographs of the foot and ankle for children: normal alignment'. *Journal of Pediatric Orthopedics*, 2005 Nov-Dec; 25(6): 769–76.

Viva 42   Questions

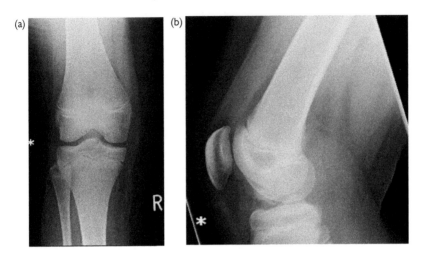

Fig. 3.52 X-ray

A 12-year-old girl fell whilst skiing. The following day, she attends A&E with a painful swollen knee and radiographs are taken. What do these radiographs in Fig. 3.52 show?

Can you describe the mechanism of the injury?

... and classify the fracture?

What would be the best way of attempting a closed reduction?

How do you think this injury would be best treated?

What surgical techniques do you know of? Do you know any pros and cons of either method?

How would you fix this case and what potential complications would you warn the parents about?

Viva 42   Answers

A 12-year-old girl fell whilst skiing. The following day, she attends A&E with a painful swollen knee and radiographs are taken. What do these radiographs in Fig. 3.52 show?

AP and lateral radiographs of a skeletally immature knee joint: the lateral view demonstrates a bony fragment within the joint and the AP view suggests a fracture of the tibial spine/eminence. There is a haemarthrosis.

Can you describe the mechanism of the injury?

Classically, it has been considered to be secondary to a hyperextension injury during which the ACL ligament avulses its attachment but often it occurs following a fall on the flexed knee.

... and classify the fracture?

The best known classification is that by Meyers and McKeever, grades 1–3: undisplaced, hinged and fully displaced, this one appears to be a grade 3.

What would be the best way of attempting a closed reduction?

Extending the knee can improve the position of the fracture fragment in a grade 2 injury but this closed reduction is rarely applicable to grade 3 injuries.

How do you think this injury would be best treated?

I think that closed reduction could be attempted in theatre but that it is unlikely to succeed and that surgical reduction and fixation will be required.

What surgical techniques do you know of? Do you know any pros and cons of either method?

Reduction and then fixation can either be achieved via an open procedure or performed arthroscopically. An open procedure is the more conventional and probably the easier method unless the surgeon is skilled at arthroscopy and arthroscopic surgery. The haemarthrosis may also hamper an arthroscopic approach. However, arthroscopic reduction and fixation is thought to shorten the patient's recovery time as there is less additional trauma to the soft tissues.

The method of fixation can be with either a cannulated screw or a suture anchor, particularly if the bone fragment is thin and/or comminuted. Screws enable the fracture fragment to be countersunk. This has been recommended as a way to 're-tension' the ACL as many surgeons feel that the ACL is stretched by the injury before its attachment to the bone fails and a fracture occurs. The screws should be angled appropriately so that they do not cross the physis. The screw often requires removal. A suture anchor or similar may avoid these issues but good fixation is still required.

How would you fix this case and what potential complications would you warn the parents about?

The fracture fragment appears to be in one large piece and therefore I would plan to fix it by open reduction and screw fixation (see Fig. 3.53). In addition to the usual risk factors such as non-union and infection I would discuss the proximity of the growth plate to the fixation and the likely need to remove the metal work once the fracture had healed. I would explain that the ACL may have stretched and that despite being intact, functional instability might be a problem. I would also explain that the post-operative rehabilitation requires around 8 weeks in a hinged knee brace and regular physiotherapy.

(a) (b)

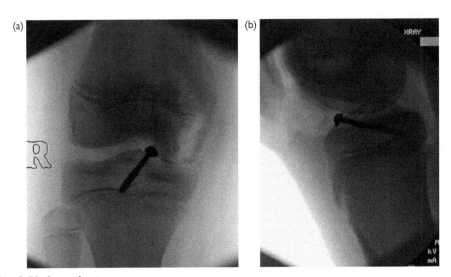

Fig. 3.53 Screw fixation

Chotel F HJ, Bérard J. 'ACL rupture in children'. In: Bonnin, ed, *The Knee Joint*: 2012. Springer-Verlag; pp. 291–323.

Leeberg V, Lekdorf J, Wong C, Sonne-Holm S. 'Tibial eminentia avulsion fracture in children—a systematic review of the current literature'. *Danish Medical Journal*, 2014; 61(3): A4792.

Merkel DL, Molony JT, Jr: Recognition and management of traumatic sports injuries in the skeletally immature athlete. *International Journal of Sports Physical Therapy*, 2012; 7(6): 691–704.

Mitchell JJ, Sjostrom R, Mansour AA, Irion B, Hotchkiss M, Terhune EB, et al.: Incidence of Meniscal Injury and Chondral Pathology in Anterior Tibial Spine Fractures of Children. *Journal of Pediatric Orthopedics* 2015; 35(2):130–5

Viva 43   Questions

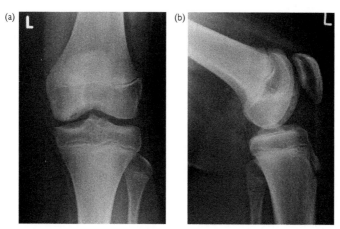

Fig. 3.54 X-rays

A 14-year-old girl presents to clinic referred by her GP with a 4-month history of swelling, discomfort and giving way of her knee. Pain is worse on exercise but there is no clear history of trauma. On examination there is a small effusion and joint line tenderness. Fig. 3.54 shows her radiographs. What do you think?

Is there another view you would consider obtaining?

Fig. 3.55 shows her MRI images, what can you see?

What treatment options would you discuss with the patient and family?

Do you know any way of broadly classifying osteochondritis dissecans (OCD) lesions in children?

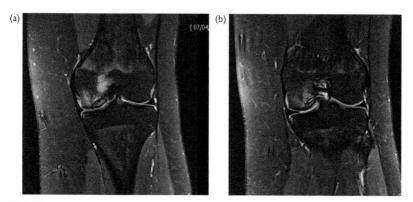

Fig. 3.55 MRI scans

Viva 43   Answers

A 14-year-old girl presents to clinic referred by her GP with a 4-month history of swelling, discomfort and giving way of her knee. Pain is worse on exercise but there is no clear history of trauma. On examination there is a small effusion and joint line tenderness. Fig. 3.54 shows her radiographs. What do you think?

These AP and lateral images show an osteochondral defect of the lateral aspect of the medial femoral condyle. Given the absence of trauma in the history the diagnosis is likely to be osteochondritis dissecans.

Is there another view you would consider obtaining?

A notch view can be helpful if there is a clinical history suggestive of OCD but no obvious abnormality on the AP and lateral images, however in this case I would request a MRI next.

Fig. 3.55 shows her MRI images, what can you see?

The images show a large osteochondral defect with a cleft between the fragment and condyle, which contains fluid. The fragment is not displaced but the cleft and fluid suggest that the fragment may be loose and unstable.

What treatment options would you discuss with the patient and family?

In the first instance I would recommend that the patient should be partially weightbearing using crutches and possibly use a range of movement brace. I would refer her for physiotherapy to prevent further quads wasting which has probably already started. I would discuss surgical options with the family including debridement, drilling and fixation with a bioabsorbable screw. Excising the lesion and debriding the base will result in a large residual cavity and risks ongoing pain and swelling. As the fragment is still partially attached I would recommend retaining it by doing a limited debridement and then reducing and stabilizing the fragment with a bioabsorbable screw.

Do you know any way of broadly classifying OCD lesions in children?

There is a classification by Guhl based on arthroscopic findings describing 4 stages:

I   Cartilage irregularity and softening, no fissures
II   Cartilaginous breach but non-displaceable lesion
III   Definable displaceable fragment but still attached
IV   Loose body and articular defect*

Can you think of any other classifications?

There is a classification based on MRI images that is similar to that of Guhl by Di Paola:

I   no articular breach
II   cartilage breach with low signal in the subchondral region

* Adapted from *Current Orthopaedic Practice*, 167, Guhl J.F, 'Arthroscopic treatment of osteochondritis dissecans. Clinical Orthopaedics and Related Research'. Copyright (1982) with permission from Wolters Kluwer Health, Inc.

III cartilage breach with high signal T2 changes suggestive of articular fluid escape

IV loose body and articular surface defect**

Edmonds EW, Polousky J: A review of knowledge in osteochondritis dissecans: 123 years of minimal evolution from Konig to the ROCK study group. *Clinical Orthopaedics and Related Research* 2013; 471(4):1118–26.

Dipaola JD, Nelson DW, Colville MR. 'Characterizing osteochondral lesions by magnetic resonance imaging'. *Arthroscopy*, 1991; 7(1): 101–4.

Guhl JF. 'Arthroscopic treatment of osteochondritis dissecans'. *Clinical Orthopaedics and Related Research*, 1982; 167: 65–74.

Pascual-Garrido C, Moran CJ, Green DW, Cole BJ. 'Osteochondritis dissecans of the knee in children and adolescents'. *Current Opinion in Pediatrics*, 2013; 25(1): 46–51.

** Reprinted from *Arthroscopy: The Journal of Arthroscopic & Related Surgery*, 7, 1,Dipaola JD, Nelson WD ,Colville MR, 'Characterizing osteochondral lesions by magnetic resonance imaging', pp, 101–104. Copyright (1991) , with permission from Elsevier.

Viva 44   Questions

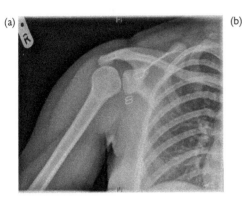
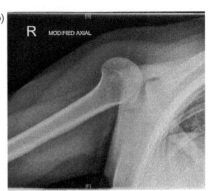

Fig. 3.56 X-rays

A 14-year-old girl presents to A&E with a recurrently 'clicking' shoulder that has now got stuck: she is in some discomfort and the shoulder movement is very restricted. What do these X-rays show (Fig. 3.56)?

On the same day, a 14-year-old boy is brought into A&E having fallen and injured his shoulder during a football tackle, his radiograph shows a classical anterior dislocation of the glenohumeral joint in a skeletally immature patient.

What do you know about shoulder dislocations in adolescence?

How would you classify shoulder dislocations in children?

How would you treat a first time dislocation?

If the patient were to represent with two further episodes of dislocation would this alter your management? Would an open physis change your management?

Do you know of any perceived differences between shoulder dislocation in the adolescent age group and in the younger child e.g. those less than 12 years?

Viva 44   Answers

A 14-year-old girl presents to A&E with a recurrently 'clicking' shoulder that has now got 'stuck': she is in some discomfort and the shoulder movement is very restricted. What does this X-ray show (Fig. 3.56)?

The AP view of the right shoulder of a skeletally mature patient suggests a posterior dislocation of the glenohumeral joint with a classical 'light bulb' appearance of the humeral head. The 'modified axial' view confirms that the humeral head is facing away from the glenoid and (without having directional markers on the X-ray) I assume the head is posterior.

For a teenage girl to have sustained a posterior dislocation of the shoulder without any obvious trauma or physiological event such as a tonic-clonic seizure is unusual. I am aware that multidirectional instability and/or teenage hypermobility/joint laxity can be associated with multidirectional instability and voluntary or involuntary dislocation.

The relative lack of pain suggests that this may be a manifestation of multidirectional instability: this is often inferior subluxation with a sulcus sign, but the humeral head can be unstable in all directions.

On the same day, a 14-year-old boy is brought into A&E having fallen and injured his shoulder during a football tackle, his radiograph shows a classical anterior dislocation of the glenohumeral joint in a skeletally immature patient.

What do you know about shoulder dislocations in adolescence?

They occur most frequently secondary to a sporting injury and are more common in boys. Anterior dislocation is the most frequent direction of dislocation and the risk of recurrence in this age group is high, even after 2 years of stability.

How would you classify shoulder dislocations in children?

There is no specific paediatric classification of shoulder instability. They can be classified according to direction, ie anterior, which is the commonest, or posterior or inferior; they can also be classified according to whether they are due to a traumatic injury or a traumatic in nature. The concept of multi-directional instability is relevant in some children as it is in some adults.

How would you treat a first time dislocation?

I would treat them with a brief period of immobilization, 1 week, followed by intense focused physiotherapy for the rotator cuff. Conservative management would be the treatment of choice.

If the patient were to represent with two further episodes of dislocation would this alter your management? Would an open physis change your management?

I would obtain an MRI scan and discuss the option of referral to a shoulder specialist for consideration of surgical stabilization; an open physis is not a contraindication to surgery although operative management in this age group may not have any benefit over continued conservative management. There is a lack of adequate data regarding the long term benefits of surgical intervention and recurrent dislocation can affect 30% of patients despite surgery in this adolescent age group.

Do you know of any perceived differences between shoulder dislocation in the adolescent age group and in the younger child e.g. those less than 12 years?

Traumatic dislocation of the shoulder in the preadolescent age group is rare and data is limited. It is therefore very important to consider the history carefully. Studies suggest that atraumatic and multidirectional instability may be more common than traumatic cases and that it may be more common in girls in this age range than boys.

Cordischi K, Li X, Busconi B. 'Intermediate outcomes after primary traumatic anterior shoulder dislocation in skeletally immature patients aged 10 to 13 years'. *Orthopedics*, 2009; 32(9).

Deitch J, Mehlman CT, Foad SL, Obbehat A, Mallory M. 'Traumatic anterior shoulder dislocation in adolescents'. *The American Journal of Sports Medicine*, 2003; 31(5): 758–63.

Khan A, Samba A, Pereira B, Canavese F: Anterior dislocation of the shoulder in skeletally immature patients: comparison between non-operative treatment versus open Latarjet's procedure'. *The Bone & Joint Journal*, 2014; 96-B(3): 354–9.

Lawton RL, Choudhury S, Mansat P, Cofield RH, Stans AA. 'Pediatric shoulder instability: presentation, findings, treatment, and outcomes'. *Journal of Pediatric Orthopedics*, 2002; 22(1): 52–61.

Li X, Ma R, Nielsen NM, Gulotta LV, Dines JS, Owens BD. 'Management of shoulder instability in the skeletally immature patient'. *The Journal of the American Academy of Orthopaedic Surgeons*, 2013; 21(9): 529–37.

Roberts SB, Beattie N, McNiven ND, Robinson CM. 'The natural history of primary anterior dislocation of the glenohumeral joint in adolescence'. *The Bone & Joint Journal*, 2015; 97-B(4): 520–6.

Viva 45   Questions

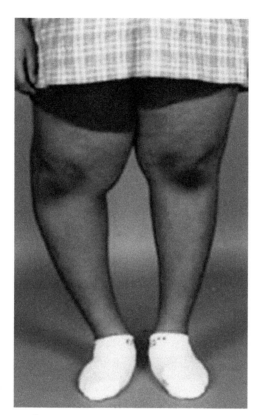

Fig. 3.57 Clinical photograph

This is a clinical picture of a 13-year-old boy who presents to your clinic with right knee pain. It seems that his knees had normal alignment up until 3 years ago. What does Fig. 3.57 show?

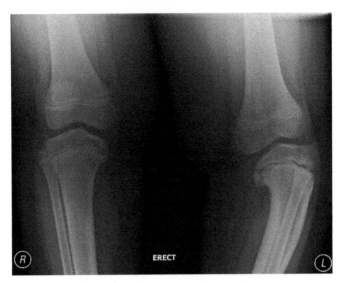

Fig. 3.58 AP X-ray

Fig. 3.58 shows an AP radiograph of both knees. What does it show and how would you classify and quantify the deformity?

How would you manage this patient?

Viva 45   Answers

This is a clinical picture of a 13-year-old boy who presents to your clinic with right knee pain. It seems that his knees had normal alignment up until 3 years ago. What does Fig. 3.57 show?

This is a clinical photograph of a large, heavy, dark-skinned child with a unilateral varus deformity of the right knee. There seems to be a strong tibial component to the deformity judging by the lateral border of the leg—but I would need long leg standing radiographs to confirm this and to confirm normal alignment on the opposite side.

Given his size and colour, the likely diagnosis is Blount's disease; both obesity and African or African-American origin are risk factors. In the late or adolescent form, this is usually a unilateral condition (in contrast to infantile Blounts which is more often bilateral).

Fig. 3.58 shows an AP radiograph of both knees. What does it show and how would you classify and quantify the deformity?

This X-ray radiograph confirms the diagnosis of Blount's disease affecting the right knee (with perhaps less obvious changes on the left knee too). On the right, there is tibia vara at the metaphyseal-diaphyseal junction with an irregular physeal line medially raising the possibility of a bony bridge. There is also beaking of the medial metaphysis and depression of the medial epiphysis and the articular surface. There also appears to be corresponding distal femoral valgus deformity but this may be positional as the child accommodates for the severe varus: a long leg film is essential to quantify the deformity. It appears as if there is a significant torsional element to the deformity.

The Langenskiöld classification of infantile Blount's is the most commonly used classification system. It has good prognostic value in infantile Blount's. It is less useful as a prognostic tool in late onset Blount's but it is still a useful tool to describe the radiographic appearance.

Given she is aged 12 years, this would be compatible with a Langenskiöld Stage VI.

How would you manage this patient?

In the first instance I would need more appropriate imaging including an AP limb alignment view and lateral views of the proximal tibia. The torsional component of the deformity must be acknowledged. Height and weight measurements would also be useful.

If his weight is an issue, the opportunity could be taken to discuss this and raise the awareness of obesity related problems in both childhood and adulthood. All treatment options would be easier in a slimmer child.

In terms of the tibia vara, the goals of treatment are to restore (and then maintain) the mechanical axis and achieve a well-aligned articular surface with equal leg lengths at/or around the age of skeletal maturity. At this stage of the disease a lateral epiphysodesis alone will not achieve correction as the medial physis is 'too sick' to correct with growth. Although a high tibial osteotomy, with either internal or external fixation, is a reasonable consideration this would not achieve good articular alignment. Personally, I would consider a hemi-plateau elevation held with a bone graft to improve articular congruity and a metaphyseal dome osteotomy below this to correct overall length; by using a circular frame, both alignment and length can be controlled. A lateral proximal tibial epiphysiodesis should be performed to prevent recurrent deformity. If the lengthening is planned to compensate for the absence of growth from the proximal tibial for the following 3 years, no further treatment should be required. Otherwise, a contralateral epiphysodesis should be considered at the appropriate time.

Whatever tibial intervention is considered, if the distal femoral alignment is truly in valgus (this would need to be checked carefully), the distal femur must also be corrected. Guided growth in the form of a medial eight plate or staple to the distal femur may be enough to achieve this.

Sabharwal S. 'Blount disease'. *The Journal of Bone & Joint Surgery*, American volume, Jul 2009; 91(7): 1758–76.

Salenius P et al. 'The development of the tibiofemoral angle in children.' *The Journal of Bone & Joint Surgery*, American volume, 1975; 57-A: 259–61.

Viva 46   Questions

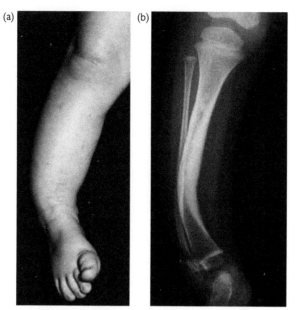

(a)   (b)

Fig. 3.59 Clinical and radiographic images

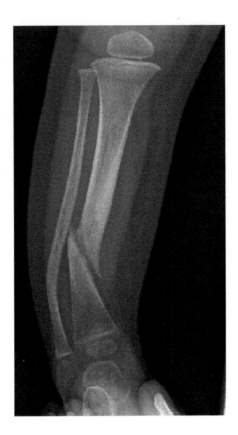

Fig. 3.60 X-ray

A 2-year-old child is brought to your clinic. The parents have noticed that whilst her toddler bow legs have improved on the left, on the right the deformity has worsened over the last 3 months. There is no history of trauma and no relevant family history. What do you see in Fig. 3.59? What do you think the underlying diagnosis could be?

What would your management of this patient be—at this moment?

6 months after your consultation the child reappears in your clinic. She fell in the orthosis and sustained a fracture which has not healed. She is not in pain and is still mobilizing. What can you see on Fig. 3.60? How would you manage this?

The pseudarthosis achieves union with your management and the limb is straight. However, as the child grows, a leg length discrepancy of 4 cm emerges. How would you manage this?

Viva 46   Answers

A 2-year-old child is brought to your clinic. The parents have noticed that whilst her toddler bow legs have improved on the left, on the right the deformity has worsened over the last 3 months. There is no history of trauma and no relevant family history. What do you see in Fig. 3.59? What do you think the underlying diagnosis could be?

The clinical picture shows a lateral bow to the tibia and fibula. All 5 digits are present and I can see no other noteworthy features (such as café-au-lait spots or neurofibromata). The accompanying radiograph confirms the lateral bow to the tibia and fibula with accompanying thickening of the cortex, particularly on the concave side. There is also disordered architecture of the bone in the tibial intramedullary canal. I would like to see a lateral radiograph but the most likely diagnosis is congenital pseudarthrosis of the tibia—although at the moment the tibia is in continuity.

The most likely underlying diagnosis is Type 1 neurofibromatosis. There are some cases of fibrous dysplasia giving rise to congenital pseudarthrosis of the tibia and very rarely a self-resolving benign form is encountered.

What would your management of this patient be—at this moment?

My management would be to establish the underlying cause and protect the child from impending fracture.

I would look for the features associated with a diagnosis of neurofibromatosis such as café-au-lait spots, axillary freckling, iris hamartomas and neurofibromata. I would also refer to a paediatrician/ geneticist so that the child and his/her parents can be counselled and managed as part of a Multi disciplinary team (MDT) if appropriate.

There is a real risk of impending fracture with subsequent non-union here, so I would protect the child in a clam-shell orthosis. This limits foot and ankle function but reassuringly stiffness is uncommon and we believe it reduces the risk of fracture. Children with pseudarthrosis of the tibia who fracture under the age of 4 years generally have a poorer prognosis than those who fracture later.

6 months after your consultation the child reappears in your clinic. She fell in the orthosis and sustained a fracture which has not healed. She is not in pain and is still mobilizing. What can you see on Fig. 3.60? How would you manage this?

This is an X-ray image showing an oblique fracture of the tibia with a bowed but intact fibula. The appearances are of a chronic 'injury'. There is alteration of bony architecture proximal to the fracture. The appearances are in keeping with a tibial pseudarthrosis.

The little girl is still only 2–3 years old and eventual treatment will involve resection of the whole pseudarthrosis site with intramedullary fixation with or without a frame, with or without a vascularized fibula graft or bone morphogenic protein (BMP). At this stage however, it is best to keep her in a protective orthosis while she continues to be comfortable and mobile. This will allow her bone to grow and will therefore make surgery easier later. If pain increased or mobility deteriorated, then surgery would be considered sooner.

Treatment of pseudarthrosis of the tibia is controversial. There is no consensus and outcomes are often poor. Although it is possible to achieve union initially, the refracture rates are high. Resultant limb length discrepancy and deformity are also common.

The basic principles are to maintain mechanical alignment of the limb and to perform a complete resection of all the hamartomatous tissue at the pseudarthrosis. This may include resection of the tibia and fibula at the pseudarthrosis site until normal medullary canal appears, the surrounding periosteum is also abnormal and should be excised. Given the frequency of recurrent fractures, I would use an intramedullary device to achieve alignment and stability. I would prefer to use some sort of growing rod that has male and female components that will elongate with longitudinal growth. Autologous bone graft can be used from the iliac crest if appropriate together with the rod. Some advocate the Masquelet technique (with intervening cement) but this has yet to be proven long-term. If this management failed or if I had a child of approximately 7 years or older, I would consider stabilization with a circular frame with either a vascularized fibula graft and/or BMP. An intramedullary device is still advocated by some even with a frame because of the risks of refracture and deformity progression.

At any stage of management, amputation can be considered. A Symes amputation with the pseudarthrosis incorporated into the prosthetic socket is the most frequently used in the younger child. In the older child, a below knee amputation is more functional.

The pseudarthosis achieves union with your management and the limb is straight. However, as the child grows, a leg length discrepancy of 4 cm emerges. How would you manage this?

My options are operative or non-operative but initially I would like to predict what the final discrepancy at maturity would be. The current discrepancy of 4 cm is too great a discrepancy to ignore; non-operative means would be a shoe-raise.

Operative options include a contra-lateral epiphysiodesis at the appropriate time (when there is only 4 cm of growth remaining, if this is the predicted final discrepancy). An alternative option would be to consider a circular frame and bone lengthening techniques, provided the metaphyseal lengthening site is well away from the pseudarthrosis site. It would be most appropriate to lengthen the affected tibia but there are risks so one should not ignore the possibility of doing a contralateral epiphysiodesis and a small femoral lengthening.

Dohin B et al. 'Masquelet's procedure and bone morphogenetic protein in congenital pseudarthrosis of the tibia in children: a case series and meta-analysis'. Journal of Child Orthopedics, 2012; 6(4): 297–306.

Nicolaou N et al. 'Congenital pseudarthrosis of the tibia: the results of an evolving protocol of management'. Journal of Child Orthopedics, 2013; 7(4): 269–76.

Pannier S. 'Pseudoarthrosis of the tibia' Orthopaedics & Traumatology: Surgery & Research, 2011; 97(7): 726–38.

Viva 47 Questions

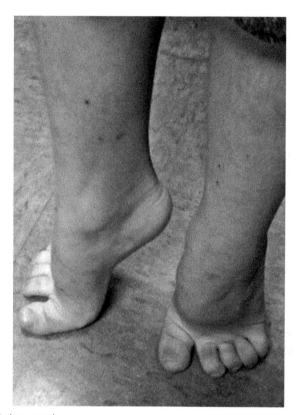

Fig. 3.61 Clinical photograph

Describe what you see in Fig. 3.61.

Assuming this is their normal walking pattern how do you know if the toe walking is habitual or not?

What abnormalities would you expect in the gait cycle?

What is the differential diagnosis of tip toe walking?

How would you treat a 2-year-old child with tip toe walking and concerned parents?

How do you treat resistant tip toe walkers over the age of 5?

Viva 47   Answers

Describe what you see in Fig. 3.61.

This is a toddler standing on their toes with the ankle in marked equinus. There is no obvious evidence of any other foot deformity

Assuming this is their normal walking pattern how do you know if the toe walking is habitual or not?

Firstly, I would take a history including a detailed account of the pregnancy, birth, and developmental milestones. I would want to know when the child started walking and whether or not they had toe-walked from the start. I would ask about a family history of toe walking and neurological conditions such as hereditary sensorimotor neuropathy (HSMN). A thorough clinical examination including a neurological examination needs to be performed. After this I would perform a focused lower limb examination including the Silfverskiold test to assess which of the calf muscles are limiting ankle dorsiflexion. Normally, the ankle should dorsiflex to 10° with the knee extended; with knee flexion and relaxation of the gastrocnemius, the ankle will dorsiflex slightly further to 20° in the typically developing child. However, with calf muscle contracture, ankle dorsiflexion will be limited to 10–20° short of neutral. The Silfverskiold test with the heel in neutral and the knee flexed and extended helps distinguish which muscles are most limiting ankle dorsiflexion.

What abnormalities would you expect in the gait cycle?

The normal heel strike i.e. first rocker is absent and most weightbearing occurs through the forefoot. During the second rocker, the ankle dorsiflexes and allows the tibia and body to move over the foot through eccentric contraction of the gastrocnemius-soleus complex. This does not occur if there is true tightness of the posterior muscle structures causing tip toeing. During the third rocker the ankle is in plantar flexion as the gastro-soleus complex contracts concentrically.

What is the differential diagnosis of tip toe walking?

Persistent toe walking beyond 2 years or unilateral toe walking at any age warrants further investigation. It may well be the first sign of an underlying neuromuscular condition or global developmental delay. Cerebral palsy, Duchenne muscular dystrophy, and autism all need to be excluded. Congenital contracture of the triceps surae muscle-tendon complex can also cause tiptoe walking. When neuromuscular aetiologies have been excluded this gait abnormality is defined as idiopathic toe walking. Idiopathic toe walking is the most common cause of toe walking.

How would you treat a 2-year-old child with tip toe walking and concerned parents?

As I mentioned earlier, I would take a full history and perform an appropriately detailed clinical examination. A gait history should include the age at which the child started to walk, onset of toe walking, the ability to stand with heels down and to walk with a heel-toe gait at any time, and the proportion of time spent toe walking now. If the child presents before the age of 2 and all pathological conditions have been considered and excluded, reassurance is given to the parents explaining that this pattern of walking is physiological and can be related to gait maturation.

How do you treat resistant tip toe walkers over the age of 5?

Surgery is reserved for resistant toe walking following failed non-operative measures, with fixed equinus and/or compensatory hyperextension of the knee. Children should be able to commit to a re-education program following the surgical correction. The parents should be aware of the success rates of these treatment methods.

The main objective is to lengthen the posterior calf muscles if they are tight. If there is limitation in dorsiflexion of the ankle, with combined tightness of the gastrocnemius and soleus, a percutaneous or open Achilles tendon lengthening procedure can be offered. Other procedures such as the Strayer and Baumann procedures aim to lengthen the triceps surae muscle-tendon complex at different anatomical levels. They are reserved for isolated gastrocnemius tightness. It requires a combined treatment of surgery and rehabilitation which can be prolonged and commitment from both patient and carer is essential.

Surgery can only allow the heel to contact the ground and it does allow the ankle a range of dorsiflexion. As the tendency to toe-walk originates centrally, once the contracture has been released, the child can stand with a plantigrade foot but may still 'choose' to toe walk: this tendency is difficult to overcome.

In persistent toe-walkers without significant contracture, the use of botulinum toxin injections may similarly allow a plantigrade position during stance. It may, due to the weakness caused, limit the ability to toe walk during gait but this effect will wear off and unless the patient has managed to 're-educate' their control of gait, the toewalking will return. Whilst such treatment is successful in children with a neuromuscular abnormality such as CP, in idiopathic toe-walking the results have been less impressive.

Engström P, Gutierrez-Farewik EM, Bartonek A, Tedroff K, Orefelt C, Haglund-Åkerlind Y. 'Does botulinum toxin A improve the walking pattern in children with idiopathic toe-walking'? *Journal of Child Orthopedics*, 2010 Aug; 4(4): 301–8.

van Bemmel AF, van de Graaf VA, van den Bekerom MP, Vergroesen DA: 'Outcome after conservative and operative treatment of children with idiopathic toe walking: a systematic review of literature'. *Musculoskeletal Surgery*, 2014 Aug; 98(2): 87–93.

van Kuijk AA, Kosters R, Vugts M, Geurts AC. 'Treatment for idiopathic toe walking: a systematic review of the literature'. *Journal of Rehabilitation Medicine*, 2014 Nov; 46(10): 945–57.

Viva 48   Questions

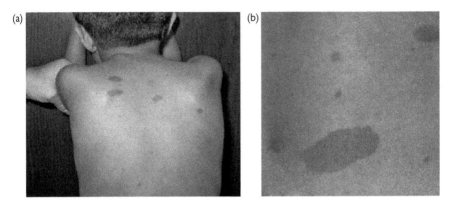

Fig. 3.62 Skin lesions

A 4-year-old boy attends your fracture clinic and during the course of your examination you notice these skin lesions (see Fig. 3.62). What do you think they are? What do you think the underlying condition could be?

How would you confirm the diagnosis?

What are the orthopaedic manifestations of this condition? How would you monitor them?

How would you manage tibial pseudarthrosis in a child with NF1?

Viva 48   Answers

A 4-year-old boy attends your fracture clinic and during the course of your examination you notice these skin lesions (see Fig. 3.62). What do you think they are? What do you think the underlying condition could be?

These are café-au-lait spots. They are on both sides of the body and have smooth edge indicative of an underlying diagnosis of neurofibromatosis type 1. The café-au-lait spots in McCune Albright syndrome have more jagged edges and tend to be unilateral.

How would you confirm the diagnosis?

I would look for the presence of 2 neurofibromatosis type 1 (NF1) associated features which include: axillary freckles, at least 6 café-au-lait spots, 2 or more neurofibromas, 1 plexiform neurofibroma, optic nerve glioma, 2 or more iris hamartomas (Lisch nodules), sphenoid dysplasia or tibial pseudoarthrosis and finally, as it is an autosomal dominant condition, I would ask about the presence of a first degree relative with NF1. However, genetic mutations can occur spontaneously and the condition has variable penetrance so the phenotype is variable.

Not all these clinical features are present from the beginning and they can emerge as the child grows so involvement of the paediatricians would be useful.

What are the orthopaedic manifestations of this condition? How would you monitor them?

The most common problem is scoliosis—particularly thoracic scoliosis. It is usually mild but children should be reviewed regularly for this, especially in adolescence when the bulk of spinal growth occurs. It is also important to consider pseudarthrosis of the tibia. This is usually a unilateral condition which is often preceded by a leg length discrepancy and some anterolateral bowing, however children can present even as old as 10 years of age which means some review is necessary. And lastly deformities of all limbs arising from deep plexiform neuromas are possible and can arise gradually, this means that regular detailed clinical examination is useful. For children with a more severe phenotype, management in a specialist centre may be preferred.

How would you manage tibial pseudarthrosis in a child with NF1?

The basic principles are, initially, to prevent fracture through the use of a clamshell orthosis. If a true pseudarthrosis is present then the key is to maintain mechanical alignment and achieve union. Union is difficult to achieve and even harder to maintain. I would consider intramedullary techniques with/without complete resection of the pseudarthrosis and accompanying hamartoma including periosteum. In young children, some surgeons would simply obtain alignment with out a major tissue resection at this first stage. I would use bone graft, initially iliac crest graft with BMP could be used or alternatively a vascularized fibula graft provided I had the relevant microvascular expertise available. Unfortunately all these techniques have a reported refracture rate which is the subject of current further study. All patients should be braced until skeletal maturity even if they are united. This inevitably leads to weakness and stiffness in the foot and ankle. For larger defects I would consider excision and bone transport using a circular frame. The results of this 'aggressive' plan are not very good in younger children. At all times I would have to be vigilant for leg length discrepancy and deformity and be ready to intervene for these if necessary.

Finally it would be important to counsel the family from the outset about a below-knee amputation or a through ankle Syme's amputation.

Herring JA. *Tachdijian's Pediatric Orthopaedics*. In Saunders, Elsevier, 5th edition. 2013.

Neurofibromatosis, Conference statement' National Institutes of Health Consensus Development Conference. *Archives of Neurology* May 1988; 45(5): 575–8.

Stevenson DA, et al. 'Approaches to treating NF1 tibial pseudarthrosis: consensus from the Children's Tumor Foundation NF1 Bone Abnormalities Consortium'. *Journal of Pediatric Orthopedics*, 2013 Apr-May; 33(3): 269–75.

Viva 49   Questions

A tall girl (aged 16, height 6 ft 1in, *or 1.84 m, and significantly taller than both parents*) with glasses comes into your clinic. She presents with multiple joint pains and an acute knee effusion after a twisting injury. She often has twisting episodes of her knees and ankles. What diagnosis are you considering?

What features of the history and examination would point you to a connective tissue disorder/dysplasia?

How would you quantify joint hypermobility?

Tell me about anterior cruciate ligaments (ACL) injuries in children. Are there any particular considerations in patients with Marfan or Ehlers-Danlos syndromes?

Viva 49   Answers

A tall girl (aged 16, height 6 ft 1 in, or 1.84m, and significantly taller than both parents) with glasses comes into your clinic. She presents with multiple joint pains and an acute knee effusion after a twisting injury. She often has twisting episodes of her knees and ankles. What diagnosis are you considering?

A girl so tall in comparison to her parents would be unusual so I would be thinking of a skeletal dysplasia such as Marfan syndrome. An acute knee effusion after a twisting injury could indicate any intra-articular injury; meniscal tear, ACL rupture, chondral injury, fracture for example.

What features of the history and examination would point you to a connective tissue disorder/dysplasia?

I would ask about a history of multiple joint pains, family history, cardiac symptoms/valve defects, ophthalmic history. I would be considering specifically a diagnosis of Marfan syndrome which is associated with increased height, mitral valve pathology, aortic regurgitation, and aortic dissection, lens dislocation and myopia, high palate and multiple joint pains. Ehlers-Danlos syndrome could be considered but is not specifically associated with increased height but multiple joint pains can be possible and there are subtypes associated with aortic dilatation and hyperextensible skin and widened scars. Marfan syndrome is autosomal dominant in most cases so a family history would be pertinent.

Features of Marfan syndrome on clinical examination include: high arched palate, long limbs, arachnodactyly, chest wall deformities (pectus carinatum, pectus excavatum), scoliosis, and joint hypermobility.

How would you quantify joint hypermobility?

I would use the Beighton score: The Beighton score is a score for hypermobility (maximal points 9); features include passive dorsiflexion of little finger beyond 90o with the forearm flat on a table, passive movement of the thumb to the volar aspect of the forearm, hyperextension of elbow, hyperextension of knee, touching palms to floor with legs straight. The score has not been validated for use in children.

Tell me about ACL injuries in children. Are there any particular considerations in patients with Marfan or Ehlers-Danlos syndromes?

ACL injuries are known to be a risk factor for further meniscal injuries and chondral injuries so there is a move towards ACL reconstruction. Both transphyseal and extraphyseal techniques such as all-epiphyseal ACL reconstruction are possible. No difference has been found between these techniques *if* transphyseal procedures utilize a more vertical tunnel placement in order to preserve the physis.

ACL injuries are more common in people with hyperlaxity disorders including Marfan syndrome and Ehlers-Danlos syndrome. Patients with hyperextension of the knees have been found to be over 5 times as likely to sustain ACL injury compared to normal controls. Patella tendon autografts may be better than hamstring grafts in patients with hypermobility from whichever underlying cause.

Christophersen C, et al. 'Ehlers-Danlos Syndrome' *Journal of Hand Surgery*, American volumes, 2014 Oct; 39(10): 207104.

Gebherd F et al. 'Multicenter study of operative treatment of intraligamentous tears of the anterior cruciate ligament in children and adolescents: comparison of 4 different techniques'. *Knee Surgery, Sports Traumatology, Arthroscopy* 2006; 14: 797–803.

Wolf JM, et al. 'Impact of Joint Laxity and Hypermobility on the Musculoskeletal System'. *The Journal of the American Academy of Orthopaedic Surgeons*, 2011; 19: 463–71.

Viva 50   Questions

(a)
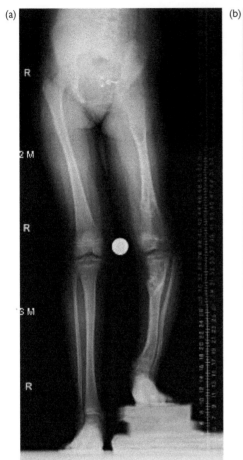
(b)
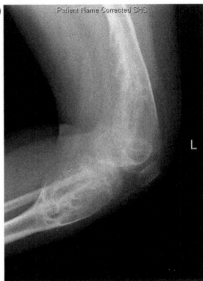

Fig. 3.63 X-rays

Describe the features on these radiographs: Fig. 3.63.

The child does have enchondromatosis: what are the main considerations for treatment?

What types of surgical procedures might you consider?

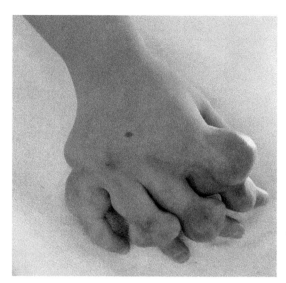

Fig. 3.64 Clinical photograph

Fig. 3.64 shows the non-dominant hand of a 14-year-old girl with multiple enchondromatosis, can you outline your management plan for this patient?

A 15-year-old boy was discovered to have a lesion in his left proximal femur as an incidental finding on an abdominal radiograph. The radiologists felt that the appearances were in keeping with an enchondroma: is biopsy to confirm this indicated?

Viva 50   Answers

Describe the features on this radiograph: Fig. 3.63

A standing long leg view of a skeletally immature patient shows extensive abnormalities throughout femur and the tibia of the left leg with a leg length discrepancy and malalignment leading to a significant pelvic obliquity. The right leg appears essentially normal. The condition is predominantly affecting the metaphyses and the lesions are radiolucent with cortical thinning but on the AP there is no major bone expansion. On the lateral view, however, there is obvious expansion. The features are in keeping with a polyostotic form of enchondromatosis (Ollier's disease). There is no speckled calcification within the lesion but this may not be apparent in the paediatric patient. The proximal femoral lesion may have a 'ground glass' appearance suggestive of fibrous dysplasia and this would be part of my differential diagnosis. I would ask for the radiographs to be reported by a radiologist with an interest in musculoskeletal pathology

The child does have enchondromatosis: what are the main considerations for treatment?

The main problems are the leg length discrepancy which is present in both the tibia and the femur and the deformity which, to naked eye assessment, appears to be affecting the tibia predominantly. The problems are likely to be progressive with growth. The deformity and cortical thinning may increase the risk of fracture.

I would make a full assessment of the patient clinically noting the deformities present and noting any torsional problems. Then I would analyse her radiographs to identify the site and severity of her deformity in both the tibia and the femur on the AP and lateral views.

I would develop a management plan, that would involve surgery and which would address these issues with the aim that at skeletal maturity, the patient would have well aligned limbs with no obvious leg length difference and good function. I would like to know what her height is now and what her parental heights are so that I could predict her final end height and perhaps the degree of discrepancy at skeletal maturity.

I would like to know if there was any obvious upper limb involvement that might, for example, restrict the patient's ability to use crutches.

What types of surgical procedures might you consider?

The options that are available to me to treat the angular deformity include:

1. The use of a hemiepiphysiodesis or guided growth technique to prevent increasing deformity and encourage gradual correction of deformity with further growth
2. An osteotomy (or osteotomies) with acute correction and internal fixation or gradual correction and external fixation
3. A combination of these techniques

For the leg length difference, my management might be influenced by her predicted final height at skeletal maturity. If this was a reasonable height, then I might counsel the family to undergo a distal femoral and/or proximal tibial epiphysiodesis on her longer (normal) right side. If both physes were closed surgically, the leg length difference would diminish by approx.1.5 cm per year (assuming that her growth continued at a reasonable rate on the left side).

If, the deformity correction method chosen for her left leg included an osteotomy and gradual correction with an external fixation device, then this technique could be adapted to include some lengthening (in addition to the length gained by correcting her deformity).

Again a combination of left and right sided surgery might be the most acceptable option.

Fig. 3.64 shows the non-dominant hand of a 14-year-old girl with multiple enchondromatosis, can you outline your management plan for this patient?

There is obvious significant deformity affecting all the digits and probably some of the metacarpals. The thumb is not well seen. Hands, like feet, need to be comfortable and functional and, if possible, cosmetically acceptable. It would be important to know whether her other (dominant) hand was similarly affected. I would want to know what problems she was complaining of and whether or not she had good function in this hand.

It would be feasible to address some of the lesions if they were causing a significant, specific problem: simple curettage can often improve the appearance and discomfort and may improve function.

A 15-year-old boy was discovered to have a lesion in his left proximal femur as an incidental finding on an abdominal radiograph. The radiologists felt that the appearances were in keeping with an enchondroma: is biopsy to confirm this indicated?

In general terms, it can be difficult to distinguish histologically between an active enchondroma (and in paediatric patients all enchondromas are active) and a low grade chondrosarcoma so if the clinical and radiographic appearances are both in keeping with the diagnosis, no pathological confirmation is required. The MRI appearances are typical on the T1 and T2 weighted images with a sharp margin and no surrounding oedema. Close follow-up may be indicated to judge the course of the lesion.

Most patients with a solitary enchondroma present with a pathological fracture or it is an incidental finding on a radiograph: they are often asymptomatic. 40% of enchondromas are found in the hands/feet but the distal femur and proximal humerus are the next most common sites: this site is therefore unusual.

Herring JA. *Tachdijian's Pediatric Orthopaedics*, 5th edition. 2013, Elsevier.

Krakow D and Rimoin DL. 'Review: Skeletal Dysplasias'. *Genetic Medicine*, 2010; 12(6): 327–41.

Viva 51   Questions

What do you understand by the term gait analysis?

Describe some of the features that *you* consider important when assessing a patients' gait pattern.

Do you recognize the gait graph in Fig. 3.65? Even if you cannot, can you describe the basic features.

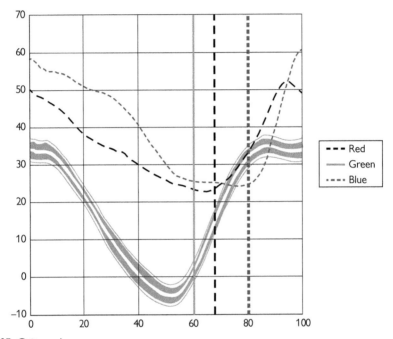

Fig. 3.65 Gait graph

Does this imply that there is a fixed deformity at hip level?

What do you understand by the term 'crouch gait'?

Viva 51   Answers

What do you understand by the term gait analysis?

In its simplest terms, gait analysis is the systematic study of human locomotion and it encompasses an assessment of movement/posture/behaviour by observation and/or by computerized analysis performed in at least two planes (from 'in front' and from 'the side'). Observational analysis can be helped by the use of video recordings reviewed in slow-motion to allow closer consideration of specific aspects of the gait cycle.

Computerized gait analysis also often includes the use of kinetics to look at the activity of muscle groups and the forces produced by this activity whilst surface electrodes can give information about the electrical activity of a specific muscle (for example tibialis anterior) and consider moments and lever arms.

Describe some of the features that *you* consider important when assessing a patients' gait pattern

(*This is a very open ended question and there are a myriad of features you could choose—so keep it simple and select something you are happy to talk about*).

Gait should be functional, comfortable and efficient with/without appropriate walking aids. Thus as part of a general assessment of the patient I look at the overall quality of their movement, their ability to co-ordinate and control their actions and the symmetry of the gait pattern. As they get up to walk, I note whether this action appears fluid or not and I note whether they can stop/start confidently or whether they need support to do so. I make particular note of their upper limb posture as they walk and look for any 'classical' gait patterns that I might recognize. My initial comments can be made with the child/adult still dressed and in their preferred footwear and/or splints but then it is essential to have the patient undressed sufficiently that all segments of the upper and lower limbs and the trunk are visible.

From the lateral side (assessing the sagittal plane), to start off with I simply look to see whether they are making forward progress with each step or whether one foot simply comes up to meet the other foot without overtaking it and whether the step length is adequate. I try to comment on whether or not there is a heel strike at initial contact, whether the knee extends during stance phase and whether there is good knee flexion in swing: in essence I am looking for the five parameters necessary for normal gait. (Stability in stance, foot clearance in swing, pre-positioning of the foot for initial contact, and an adequate step length with good energy conservation).

From the front (and/or behind ie the coronal and transverse planes) I look specifically for the foot progression angle and the position of the patellae in stance and swing. For example, if the foot progression angle is normal and yet the patellae face in, I might expect to find evidence of femoral neck anteversion and compensatory external tibial torsion on my clinical examination. I would also look to see whether there was any obvious scissoring of the legs or pelvic obliquity that might fit with a neuromuscular problem or a leg length difference.

In patients with an asymmetric gait I would be looking to see if the abnormality that I had noticed was the true problem or the compensation for the problem. For example, with a leg length difference I might notice a compensatory flexed knee posture on the long side but at other times or in another patient I might notice an equinus foot posture on their short leg. The 'hip hitch' and circumduction are other ways that patients may compensate for gait difficulties.

Do you recognize this gait graph in Fig. 3.65? Even if you do not, can you describe the basic features.

This gait graph represents hip movement in the sagittal plane (*if you are not sure, don't say but just describe what you see first...*).

The x axis represents the gait cycle and traditionally it starts with initial contact (IC). The green vertical line distinguishes the longer stance phase of gait (60%) and the shorter swing phase (40%)

The y axis usually represents movement in a particular plane (sagittal, coronal, or transverse) and the horizontal line represents the 'zero' line between, in this case, flexion and extension.

The green band represents the mean ±2SD values for the joint position at any stage of the gait cycle.

The blue and red lines represent the two limbs (in most gait laboratories—red is right). The gait cycles for both limbs are 'synchronized' rather than out of step as they are in normal walking. The single blue and red lines represents the mean 'line' for all the gait cycles tested and as such may not truly represent the actual gait *if* the gait pattern is highly variable.

On this graph, both the red and blue lines are well outside the normal values. There is asymmetry between the lines and hence between the right and left legs. The red and blue vertical lines confirm that there is a prolonged stance phase on both sides but more on the left (blue) side.

The graphs suggest that the normal movement for this joint is flexion at initial contact, but then as stance progresses the joint should extend fully before flexing again for swing phase: the range of movement is from some hyperextension to around 40° of flexion. This pattern of movement suggests this is a hip joint graph (*but all the preceding description can be given without knowing which joint you are looking at*).

The analysis suggests that the right and left sides (hips) are overly flexed throughout the gait cycle but that the actual range of movement is acceptable.

Does this imply that there is a fixed deformity at hip level?

Gait analysis can not tell you about fixed deformity, it tells you about the position of the joint during the gait cycle and the amount of movement that occurs at that joint. Clinical examination will tell you whether there is a fixed flexion deformity or whether, for example, the flexed hip posture is simply a compensation for a lumbar lordosis.

What do you understand by the term 'crouch gait'?

Crouch gait is a term usually applied to an ambulant child with cerebral palsy (CP) and it is characterized, in the sagittal plane, by hip and knee flexion and ankle dorsiflexion. It is possible that the heel might be off the ground at initial contact (particularly if there is a midfoot break posture with hindfoot valgus). The ground reaction force (GRF) remains behind the knee throughout the gait cycle. Muscles which act across two joints such as iliopsoas, the hamstrings and the gastrocnemius are considered important in the pathogenesis of this gait pattern but so is their functional lever arm and hence an assessment of torsional profiles (intoeing gait) and angular deformity (e.g. hindfoot valgus/everted foot) is also important. Reduced muscle excursion rather than a truly short muscle may the problem. Overlengthening of the gastrosoleus complex can lead to loss of the plantarflexion/knee-extension couple and in the past gave surgeons a bad name as it converted a child who could walk on tip toes to a child with flat feet but who could barely walk.

The flexion 'deformity' seen during gait may not be seen on formal examination confirming that it may be weakness as well as spasticity in the various muscle groups that is contributing to the problem.

Surgery may be indicated to correct fixed deformity, to improve lever arm function, to stabilize joints. Orthotics might help stabilize joint position and maximize muscle forces whilst the ability and motivation to comply with a physiotherapy regime designed to maintain range but also increase strength is essential.

A holistic assessment of the child and their family would be a pre-requisite before considering such a surgical intervention.

Herring JA. *Tachdijian's Pediatric Orthopaedics*, 5th edition. 2013. Elsevier.

Viva 52   Questions

(a) 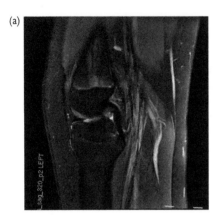   (b)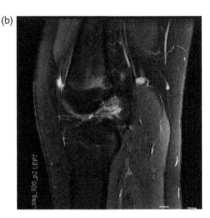

Fig. 3.66 MR Images

A 13-year-old sustains a knee injury as a result of a rugby tackle: he was carried off the field complaining of severe knee pain. You see him in fracture clinic 3 days later when a large haemarthrosis is still apparent. There is nothing abnormal to see on the radiographs. What would be your differential diagnosis and what would you do next?

What do these MRIs in Fig. 3.66 show and what would be your next step?

What do you know about ACL injuries in young people?

What other investigations may you consider?

If you were discussing surgery with the family what would you mention specifically?

What do you know about the controversies of ACL reconstruction in children/ adolescents?

If the family were keen to proceed with surgery would you undertake the procedure yourself?

Viva 52   Answers

A 13-year-old sustains a knee injury as a result of a rugby tackle: he was carried off the field complaining of severe knee pain. You see him in fracture clinic 3 days later when a large haemarthrosis is still apparent. There is nothing abnormal to see on the radiographs. What would be your differential diagnosis and what would you do next?

My differential diagnosis would include patella dislocation, anterior cruciate ligament (ACL) rupture, collateral ligament injury and meniscal injury. Depending on the exact examination findings, I would start mobilizing the child gently in a hinged range of movement knee brace as pain and swelling allowed and organize further imaging.

What do these MRIs in Fig. 3.66 show and what would be your next step?

The MRI scan shows an ACL rupture. There is no obvious joint effusion and I can not assess the menisci. I would continue to mobilize the patient in the hinged brace until they felt stable enough to mobilize without it, which may take a few weeks. I would arrange for physiotherapy to prevent further quadriceps wasting and to help provide knee stability. I would also discuss surgical options with the family.

What do you know about ACL injuries in young people?

They are relatively rare compared to the adult population but on the increase. They are more common in girls and tend to occur in the adolescent age group related to sporting activity. (*Prevention programmes have managed to reduce the incidence in some centres.*) They are often associated with concomitant meniscal tears.

What other investigations may you consider?

I would get a plain radiograph of the knee to assess the physes and if I was concerned about the bone age of the patient I would consider getting a radiograph of the non-dominant hand/wrist.

If you were discussing surgery with the family what would you mention specifically?

I would encourage physiotherapy from an early stage. If surgery was an option the family were keen to pursue, I would emphasize the importance of compliance with the post op knee brace and physiotherapy rehabilitation.

I would discuss the potential for physeal growth arrest and the pros and cons of operating now or waiting until the physes have closed. Also, the possibility of a meniscal tear and its repair if necessary.

Typically, a hamstring is used as the graft, I would discuss the fact that sometimes there is a requirement to harvest both left and right muscles if the hamstrings are thin (particularly in children and in girls). Other complications to mention include infection, increased laxity/stretching of the graft and early failure/ re-rupture which occurs in approximately 10% of children.

What do you know about the controversies of ACL reconstruction in children/adolescents?

The main issue I am aware of is drilling across the physis and the potential for physeal arrest. Animal studies have suggested that provided the hole is less than 7% of the surface area of the physis and provided that there is no metal fixation across the physis then there should not be any problem. There are reconstruction methods where the entire fixation is within the epiphysis and other methods that are extra anatomical. The concerns with these options are achieving good fixation and correct tensioning and also the non-anatomical aspect of the reconstruction may lead to early failure and ongoing instability. In younger patients some surgeons would advocate an intense physiotherapy programme to build up the quadriceps and help stabilize the knee and postpone surgery until the child is older.

If the family were keen to proceed with surgery would you undertake the procedure yourself?

No, I would not. I would refer this case to a colleague. It is an operation that should be performed by surgeons that have experience doing ACL reconstructions in adults and are comfortable with the technical demands of operating on children.

Al-Hadithy N, Dodds AL, Akhtar KS, Gupte CM. 'Current concepts of the management of anterior cruciate ligament injuries in children'. *The Bone & Joint Journal*, 2013; 95-B(11): 1562–9.

Dodwell ER, Lamont LE, Green DW, Pan TJ, Marx RG, Lyman S. '20 years of pediatric anterior cruciate ligament reconstruction in New York State'. *The American Journal of Sports Medicine*, 2014; 42(3): 675–80.

Fabricant PD, Jones KJ, Delos D, Cordasco FA, Marx RG, Pearle AD, et al. 'Reconstruction of the anterior cruciate ligament in the skeletally immature athlete: a review of current concepts: AAOS exhibit selection'. *The Journal of Bone & Joint Surgery*, American volume, 2013; 95(5): e28.

Ramski DE, Kanj WW, Franklin CC, Baldwin KD, Ganley TJ. 'Anterior cruciate ligament tears in children and adolescents: a meta-analysis of nonoperative versus operative treatment'. *The American Journal of Sports Medicine*, 2014; 42(11): 2769–76.

Renstrom P, Ljungqvist A, Arendt E, Beynnon B, Fukubayashi T, Garrett W, et al. 'Non-contact ACL injuries in female athletes: an International Olympic Committee current concepts statement'. *British Journal of Sports Medicine*, 2008; 42(6): 394–412.

Viva 53   Questions

This 3-year-old girl presented with a painless lump in her antecubital fossa that had been noticed 2 weeks previously whilst her mother was applying sunscreen to her. Can you describe the features of this radiograph please (Fig. 3.67)?

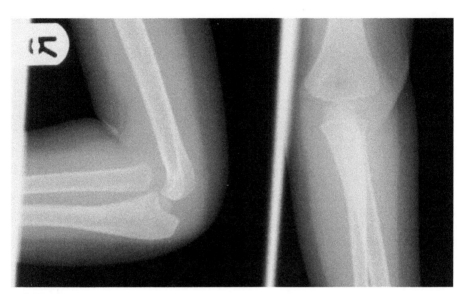

Fig. 3.67 X-rays

As there is no history of trauma do you have a differential diagnosis?

Would you consider any other form of imaging? Would an elbow arthrogram be useful?

This child subsequently underwent an open reduction of the radial head, annular ligament reconstruction and ulnar osteotomy: the latter took 6 m to heal. This is her 11-year follow-up radiograph (Fig. 3.68).

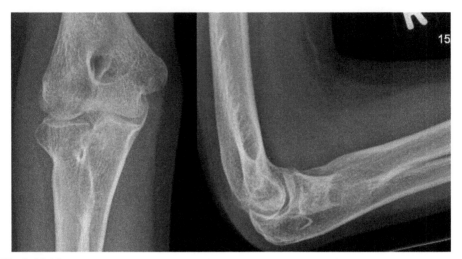

Fig. 3.68 X-rays

It is her non-dominant hand, she is in fixed supination of 10°, she has essentially full flexion and extension and no valgus/varus malalignment. She has no pain but she is concerned about the shape. She seems to be able to 'do' everything but she prefers to type using her dominant left hand only. Her left arm is normal. Does she have a problem that you can help her with?

Tell me about this X-ray: (Fig. 3.69).

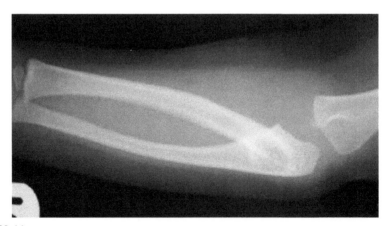

Fig. 3.69 X-ray

What is one of the more worrying complications of surgical treatment of this condition?

Viva 53   Answers

This 3-year-old girl presented with a painless lump in her antecubital fossa that had been noticed 2 weeks previously whilst her mother was applying sunscreen to her. Can you describe the features of this radiograph please (Fig. 3.67)?

The AP and lateral radiographs of a child's elbow show an anterior dislocation of the radial head. The longitudinal axis of the radius does not bisect the capitellum. There is no epiphysis visible in keeping with the girl's age. The radiographs do not show the whole forearm which would be essential to exclude a current fracture or given the history, evidence of a previous injury. I wonder whether the lateral might suggest a minor bow in the ulnar (apex anterior) which could be consistent with a late diagnosed Monteggia injury. Is there any history of trauma?

No, there is no history of trauma other than one episode 6 months previously when she stumbled whilst going down an escalator and was prevented from falling, by her father holding on to her hand. After this her arm hurt for 30 mins or so. Could this episode have been a pulled elbow? Is this X-ray compatible with that diagnosis?

The scenario described is classical for a 'pulled elbow'. The pain may be quite upsetting and the elbow will be held flexed and often the forearm is pronated. The child is reluctant to move the elbow and/or arm. The injury frequently resolves promptly and spontaneously but if formal reduction is required this can be done, with the child awake, by holding the child's hand (as if you were going to shake it) whilst holding her distal humerus with your other hand. A firm movement from pronation into full supination whilst the elbow is flexed to above a right angle usually results in a clicking sensation and the return of full movement.

The pathology behind this injury is a subluxation of the annular ligament from around the radial neck to around the broader radial head: the radial head does not dislocate. Radiographs are not usually necessary and this set of X-rays are *not* compatible with that diagnosis.

As there is no history of trauma do you have a differential diagnosis?

Children do frequently fall without their parents seeing the fall but if there had been unwitnessed trauma, I would still have expected a history of pain/reluctance to move or use the arm for a period of time. Trauma would still be my first consideration. Congenital dislocations of the radial head do occur and those that are not associated with more generalized problems can present at this age. The congenital radial head dislocations are generally posterior or posterolateral and they present with a posterolateral lump and restricted elbow extension. With an anterior congenital dislocation, the lump is palpable (as in this case) and there can be some restriction of flexion. The classic radiographic features include a hypoplastic capitellum and a dome shaped radial head with a longer neck than usual: whilst these features are described as classical, they can be difficult to identify in a young child where much of the elbow is still cartilaginous.

Would you consider any other form of imaging? Would an elbow arthrogram be useful?

Yes, I think further imaging would be helpful. Personally, I feel that a MRI would provide me with more useful information than an arthrogram. A MRI in a child of this age would probably require a general anaesthetic but it would outline the cartilaginous anatomy and detail the shape and size of the radial head and neck and perhaps help me determine whether the capitellum was hypoplastic.

An arthrogram would also require a general anaesthetic. It would give you the opportunity to perform an EUA which would probably simply confirm that the dislocation was irreducible. Technically, the arthrogram would be relatively simple to perform but, in my opinion, interpretation of the resulting images can be difficult. A CT scan would be an unnecessary amount of irradiation and unless the protocol was designed to look primarily at the softer (cartilaginous) tissues rather than the bone, I do not think it would give me any added information.

This child subsequently underwent an open reduction of the radial head, annular ligament reconstruction and ulnar osteotomy: the latter took 6 months to heal. This is her 11 year follow-up radiograph (Fig. 3.68)

These AP and lateral radiographs of a skeletally mature elbow confirm a located radial head but there appears to be a radio-ulnar synostosis. I would like to see radiographs of the whole forearm to show the wrist joint.

It is her non-dominant hand, she is in fixed supination of 10°, she has essentially full flexion and extension and no valgus/varus malalignment. She has no pain but she is concerned about the shape. She seems to be able to 'do' everything but she prefers to type using her dominant left hand only. Her left arm is normal. Does she have a problem that you can help her with?

Without taking a full history and completing a thorough examination it is difficult to answer this question well. If she was 3–4 years at the time of surgery and this is a 10 year follow-up with her growth completed she is now age 13–14 years. The actual shape of her elbow is likely to be within normal limits and therefore I am unsure why she is concerned about the shape. I note that she had a significant amount of surgery and a delayed union, thus there may be some prominence at the osteotomy site and there will be scars which she may be conscious of.

It is reassuring that she is able to 'do' everything with no pain. In order to type with both hands, she would need to pronate her right arm and as this can not happen at forearm level, she will have to abduct her shoulder in order to pronate her hand to type and use a keyboard. I wonder if it is this action which makes her feel that the shape is 'wrong'.

It is difficult to know what the precise best position for a hand is when there is no pronation/supination movement as it is dependent on many factors. These include, hand dominance, the movement in the contralateral limb, cultural factors and activity type/level. In theory, a position of 10° supination in a non-dominant arm is acceptable. I do not think that there is anything surgical I could or should offer at the moment but I would want to help her understand and cope with her function and an occupational therapy (OT) or physiotherapy assessment might help in this respect.

Tell me about this X-ray: (Fig. 3.69)

This is a lateral radiograph of a young child's forearm. The most obvious abnormality is a posterior dislocation of the radial head. The ulna appears to be bowed apex posteriorly. On this single view, I would be suspicious of a proximal radioulnar synostosis. If so, the forearm is likely to be fixed in pronation although the child might have developed compensatory hypermobility at the wrist level.

The condition may be bilateral. If the fixed position of this hand is compromising the child's function significantly then a derotation osteotomy might be considered: this simply exchanges one fixed forearm position for another one. The aim of surgery would be that the new position was more functional than the old position.

What is one of the more worrying complications of such a procedure?

The operation involves osteotomies of both bones and significant rotational change. The change in alignment can affect flow in the radial artery and/or result in a compartment syndrome. Other complications may also occur and whenever I consider vascular complications, I consider neurological complications too.

Jarrett DY, Walters MM, Kleinman PK. 'Prevalence of Capitellar Osteochondritis Dissecans in Children With Chronic Radial Head Subluxation and Dislocation'. *American Journal of Roentgenology*, 2016 Jun; 206(6): 1329–34.

Simcock X, Shah AS, Waters PM, Bae DS. 'Safety and Efficacy of Derotational Osteotomy for Congenital Radioulnar Synostosis'. *Journal of Pediatric Orthopedics*, 2015 Dec; 35(8): 838–43.

Viva 54 Questions

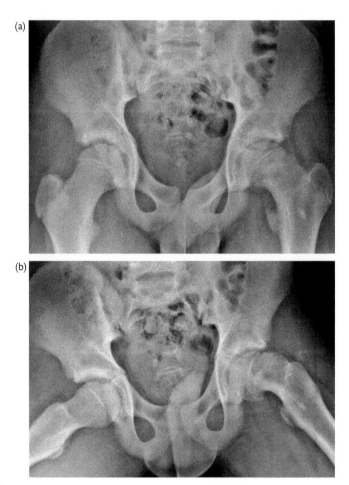

(a)

(b)

Fig. 3.70 X-rays

This 12-year-old presents to your outpatient clinic with an 18 month history of vague thigh pain. What do you think of these images (see Fig. 3.70)?

Do you think that this has happened recently?

How would you measure the severity of the slip? Can you measure it for me on this piece of paper?

How would you treat this case?

Why is there a risk of AVN?

Viva 54   Answers

This 12-year-old presents to your outpatient clinic with an 18 month history of vague thigh pain. What do you think of these images (see Fig. 3.70)?

The X-rays show a chronic slip of the left capital femoral epiphysis with metaphyseal remodelling and callus formation. The male patient is skeletally immature and the contralateral side appears normal.

Do you think that this has happened recently?

No, this has the history and appearance of a chronic slip that has occurred over time with remodelling and attempted healing occurring simultaneously.

How would you measure the severity of the slip? Can you measure it for me on this piece of paper?

I would measure the slip angle on the frog lateral view using the Southwick angle, these are the lines that I would draw.....

How would you treat this case?

I have measured this as a 60° slip on the left, so the true slip angle is 60–12 (of the contralateral side) = 48 i.e. moderate, I think that it would be best managed with a primary surgical dislocation of the hip and a subcapital realignment osteotomy such as described by Ganz, however this is a technically demanding operation with a moderately high risk of AVN and should be done by surgeons experienced in doing the procedure: I would refer this patient to a colleague with suitable expertise. Alternatively, the tried and tested treatment would be to pin the slip in situ. And treat the residual symptoms and deformity at a later date if necessary.

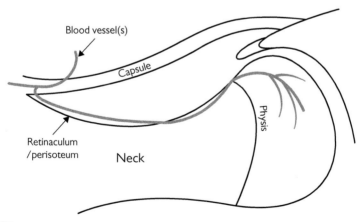

Fig. 3.71 Diagram

Why is there a risk of AVN?

When a Ganz or similar osteotomy is performed via a surgical dislocation approach, the femoral head is detached from the femoral neck within the capsule and the only continuity is that of the periosteum which contains the retinacular vessels supplying the femoral head. The amount of callus and remodelling will cause the capsule to be more adhesive and add further complexity to the case.

Can you draw the blood supply to the femoral neck at the level of the posterior femoral neck and capsule?

Southwick WO, 'Osteotomy through the lesser trochanter for slipped capital femoral epiphysis'. *The Journal of Bone & Joint Surgery*, American volume, 1967; 49(5): 807–35.

Uglow MG, Clarke NM. 'The management of slipped capital femoral epiphysis'. *The Bone & Joint Journal*, 2004; 86(5): 631–5.

Zenios Leunig M, Manner HM, Turchetto L, Ganz R. 'Femoral and acetabular re-alignment in slipped capital femoral epiphysis'. *Journal of Children's Orthopaedics*, 2017; 11: 131–7.

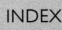

INDEX

Note: Questions, answers, tables, and figures are indicated by an italic *q, a, t,* and *f* following the page number.